Computers and Medicine

Helmuth F. Orthner, Series Editor

Springer

New York
Berlin
Heidelberg
Barcelona
Budapest
Hong Kong
London
Milan
Paris
Santa Clara
Singapore
Tokyo

Computers and Medicine

Marvin J. Miller, M.D.
Department of Psychiatry, Larue Carter Hospital, Indianapolis, IN, USA

Kenric W. Hammond, M.D.
Department of Psychiatry, Veterans Administration Medical Center, Tacoma, WA, USA

Matthew G. Hile, Ph.D.
Missouri Institute of Mental Health, University of Missouri-Columbia, St. Louis, MO, USA

Mental Health Computing

With 48 Illustrations

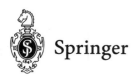 Springer

Marvin J. Miller
Department of Psychiatry
Indiana University School of Medicine
Larue Carter Hospital
Indianapolis, IN 46202, USA

Kenric W. Hammond
Department of Psychiatry
Veterans Administration
 Medical Center
Tacoma, WA 98493, USA

Matthew G. Hile
Missouri Institute of Mental Health
University of Missouri—Columbia
St. Louis, MO 63139, USA

Series Editor
Helmut F. Orthner
Professor of Computer Medicine
The George Washington University Medical Center
Washington, DC 20037, USA

Library of Congress Cataloging-in-Publication Data
Mental health computing/edited by Marvin J. Miller, Kenric W.
  Hammond, Mathew G. Hile.
      p.   cm. — (Computers and medicine)
    Includes bibliographical references and index.
    ISBN 0-387-94580-6 (hc: alk. paper)
      1. Psychiatry—Data processing.   2. Mental health services—Data
  processing.   I. Miller, Marvin J., 1946–   . II. Hammond, Kenric
  W.   III. Hile, Matthew G.   IV. Series: Computers and medicine (New
  York, N.Y.)
  RC455.2.D38M45   1996
  616.89′00285—dc20   95-37689

Printed on acid-free paper.

Production managed by Chernow Editorial Services, Inc., and supervised by Karen Phillips;
manufacturing supervised by Jeffrey Taub.
Typeset by Best-set Typesetter Ltd., Hong Kong.
Printed and bound by Braun Brumfield, Ann Arbor, MI.
Printed in the United States of America.

9 8 7 6 5 4 3 2 1

ISBN 0-387-94580-6 Springer-Verlag New York Berlin Heidelberg   SPIN 10508440

Dedicated to Dr. James L. Hedlund, a founder and leader in Mental Health Informatics. Jim, by his thorough scholarship and comprehensive understanding, provided the field with a common and comprehensive knowledge base. By his example, tutelage, and friendship, he encouraged and guided my activities in the field. He taught me to write (though he should not be blamed for the result), to think clearly, to deliver more than is required, and to behave with honor, humility, and courtesy.

Matthew G. Hile

Preface

We put this book together to help mental health clinicians use computers more effectively. With the help of my associate editors, Matthew G, Hile, Ph.D., and Kenric W. Hammond, M.D., we have assembled a variety of chapters that illustrate how computers can promote better care for our patients.

Computers generally enter the mental health facility through the business office, and sometimes do not venture beyond those walls. The main product of a mental health system, however, is not a balance sheet or a nicely printed bill, but mental health care. Administrators and clinicians will want to learn about up-to-date ways in which modern technology can help deliver better care and document ways that work the best. Computer programs do not offer an easy answer for the inadequately trained clinician or for the disorganized system. They can, however, be valuable tools for the skilled clinician and can force a thoughtful reexamination of procedures that were not carefully thought out in the past. The combination of human skills and computer tools can improve our delivery of mental health care.

Marvin J. Miller, M.D.

Series Preface

This monograph series intends to provide medical information scientists, health care administrators, physicians, nurses, other health care providers, and computer science professionals with successful examples and experiences of computer applications in health care settings. Through the exposition of these computer applications, we attempt to show what is effective and efficient and hope to provide some guidance on the acquisition or design of medical information systems so that costly mistakes can be avoided.

The health care industry is currently being pushed and pulled from all directions—from clinicians, to increase quality of care; from business, to lower cost and improve financial stability; from legal and regulatory agencies, to provide detailed documentation; and from academe, to provide data for research and improved opportunities for education. Medical information systems sit in the middle of all these demands. The generally accepted (popular) notion is that these systems can satisfy all demands and solve all the problems. Obviously, this notion is naive and is an overstatement of the capabilities of current information technology. Eventually, however, medical information systems will have sufficient functionality to satisfy most information needs of health care providers.

We realize that computer-based information systems can provide more timely and legible information than traditional paper-based systems. Most of us know that automated information systems provide, on average, more accurate information because data capture is more complete and automatic (e.g., directly from devices). Medical information systems can monitor the process of health care and improve quality of patient care by providing decision support for diagnosis or therapy, clinical reminders for follow-up care, warnings about adverse drug interactions, alerts to questionable treatment or deviations from clinical protocols, and more. Because medical information systems are functionally very rich, must respond quickly to user interactions and queries, and require a high level of security, these systems can be classified as very complex and, from a developer's perspective, also as "risky."

Information technology is advancing at an accelerated pace. Instead of waiting for 3 years for a new generation of computer hardware, we are now confronted with new computing hardware every 18 months. The forthcoming changes in the telecommunications industry will be revolutionary. Certainly before the end of this century new digital communications technologies, such as the Integrated Services Digital Network (ISDN) and very high-speed local area networks using efficient cell switching protocols (e.g., ATM) will not only change the architecture of our information systems but also the way we work and manage health care institutions.

The software industry constantly tries to provide tools and productive development environments for the design, implementation, and maintenance of information systems. Still, the development of information systems in medicine is, to a large extent, an art, and the tools we use are often self-made and crude. One area that needs desperate attention is the interaction of health care providers with the computer. Although the user interface needs improvement and the emerging graphical user interfaces may form the basis for such improvements, the most important criterion is to provide relevant and accurate information without drowning the physician in too much (irrelevant) data.

To develop an effective clinical system requires an understanding of what is to be done and how to do it and an understanding of how to integrate information systems into an operational health care environment. Such knowledge is rarely found in any one individual; all systems described in this monograph series are the work of teams. The size of these teams is usually small, and the composition is heterogeneous (i.e., health professionals, computer and communications scientists and engineers, biostatisticians, epidemiologists, etc). The team members are usually dedicated to working together over long periods of time, sometimes spanning decades. Clinical information systems are dynamic systems; their functionality constantly changes because of external pressures and administrative changes in health care institutions. Good clinical information systems will and should change the operational mode of patient care, which, in turn, should affect the functional requirements of the information systems. This interplay requires that medical information systems be based on architectures that allow them to be adapted rapidly and with minimal expense. It also requires a willingness by management of the health care institution to adjust its operational procedures and most of all, to provide end-user education in the use of information technology. Although medical information systems should be functionally integrated, these systems should be modular so that incremental upgrades, additions, and deletions of modules can be done to match the pattern of capital resources and investments available to an institution.

We are building medical information systems just as automobiles were built early in this century (1910s) (i.e., in an ad hoc manner that disregarded even existing standards). Although technical standards addressing computer and communications technologies are necessary, they are insufficient. We still need to develop conventions and agreements, and perhaps a few regulations, that address the principal use of medical information in computer and communication systems. Standardization allows the mass production of low-cost parts that can be used to build more complex structures. What are these parts exactly in medical information systems? We need to identify them, classify them, describe them, publish their specifications, and, most important, use them in real health care settings. We must be sure that these parts are useful and cost-effective even before we standardize them.

Clinical research, health services research, and medical education will benefit greatly when controlled vocabularies are used more widely in the practice of medicine. For practical reasons, the medical profession has developed numerous classifications, nomenclatures, dictionary codes, and thesauri (e.g., ICD, CPT, DSM-III, SNOWMED, COSTAR dictionary codes, BAIK thesaurus terms, and MESH terms). The collection of these terms represents a considerable amount of clinical activity, a large portion of the health care business, and access to our recorded knowledge. These terms and codes form the glue that links the practice of medicine with the business of medicine. They also link the practice of medicine with the literature of medicine, with further links to medical research and education. Because information systems are more efficient in retrieving information when controlled vocabularies are used in large databases, the attempt to unify and build bridges between these coding systems is a great example of unifying the field of medicine and health care by providing and using medical informatics tools. The Unified Medical Language System (UMLS) project of the National Library of Medicine, NIH, in Bethesda, Maryland, is an example of such effort.

The purpose of this series is to capture the experience of medical informatics teams that have successfully implemented and operated medical information systems. We hope the individual books in this series will contribute to the evolution of medical informatics as a recognized professional discipline. We are at the threshold where there is not just the need but already the momentum and interest in the health care and computer science communities to identify and recognize the new discipline called Medical Informatics.

Washington, DC   HELMUTH F. ORTHNER

Contents

Contributors

NORMAN E. ALESSI
Department of Psychiatry, University of Michigan Medical Center, Ann Arbor, MI 48109, USA

NEIL ALEX
Department of Psychiatry and Addiction Medicine, Kaiser Permanente, San Diego, CA 92110, USA

JOHN BENNETT
Taubman Center, Child/Adolescent Psychiatric Hospital, Ann Arbor, MI 48109, USA

YITZCHAK M. BINIK
Department of Psychology, McGill University, Montreal, Quebec H3A 1B1, Canada

PHILLIP W. CHRISTENSEN
Psychology Services, Veterans Administration Medical Center, Salt Lake City, UT 84108, USA

ALBERT D. FARRELL
Department of Psychology, Virginia Commonwealth University, Richmond, VA 23284, USA

ALLAN S. FINKELSTEIN
Psychology Services, Veterans Administration Medical Center, Albany, NY 12208, USA

DAVID R. GASTFRIEND
Department of Psychiatry, Massachusetts General Hospital, Harvard Medical School, Boston, MA 02114, USA

STUART GITLOW
Addiction Services, Massachusetts General Hospital, Cambridge, MA 02139, USA

ROGER L. GOULD
Interactive Health Systems, Santa Monica, CA 90401, USA

KENRIC W. HAMMOND
Veterans Administration Medical Center, Tacoma, WA 98493, USA

JAMES L. HEDLUND
Missouri Institute of Mental Health, University of Missouri—Columbia, St. Louis, MO 63139, USA

MATTHEW G. HILE
Missouri Institute of Mental Health, University of Missouri—Columbia, St. Louis, MO 63139, USA

MILTON P. HUANG
Adult/Child Psychiatric, University of Michigan Hospitals, Ann Arbor, MI 48109, USA

BRUCE W. JOHNSON
Johnson Consulting Services, Inc., Cincinatti, OH 45241, USA

JAVAD H. KASHANI
University of Missouri—Columbia, St. Louis, MO 63139, USA

ROBERT M. KOLODNER
Medical Information, Resources Management Office, Washington, DC 20420, USA

STEVEN LOCKE
Harvard Medical School, Beth Israel Hospital, Boston, MA 02215, USA

ROBERT MCCLAIN
Comprehensive Psychiatric Services, Missouri Department of Mental Health, Jefferson City, MO 65102, USA

LEIGH MCCULLOUGH–VAILLANT
943 High Street, Dedham, MA 02026, USA

MARTA MEANA
Department of Psychology, McGill University, Royal Victoria Hospital, Montreal, Quebec H3A 1B1, Canada

MARY P. METCALF
Department of Anthropology, University of Virginia, Charlottesville, VA 22906, USA

MARVIN J. MILLER
Department of Psychiatry, Indiana University School of Medicine, Larue Carter Hospital, Indianapolis, IN 46202, USA

MURRAY P. NADITCH
Strategic Advantage, Minneapolis, MN 55403, USA

SATISH S. NAIR
University of Missouri—Columbia, St. Louis, MO 63139, USA

JACK J. O'BRIEN
Research Services, Veterans Administration Medical Center, Tacoma, WA 98493, USA

ERIC P. OCHS
Department of Psychology, McGill University, Royal Victoria Hospital, Montreal, Quebec H3A 1B1, Canada

DORIS PICKERILL
Missouri Institute of Mental Health, University of Missouri—Columbia, St. Louis, MO 63139, USA

VIRGINIA S. PRICE
Department of Veterans Affairs, IRM Field Office, Tuscaloosa, AL 35401, USA

MARCIA E.H. REZZA
Harvard Medical School, Beth Israel Hospital, Boston, MA 02215, USA

JOHN C. REID
University of Missouri—Columbia, St. Louis, MO 63139, USA

JEFFERY E. SELLS
Psychology Services, Veterans Administration Medical Center, Salt Lake City, UT 84108, USA

CHRIS E. STOUT
Forest Hospital, Desplaines, IL 60016-4794, USA

T. BRADLEY TANNER
WPIC, University of Pittsburgh, Pittsburgh, PA 15213, USA

MORGAN THARP
Indiana Regional Cancer Center, 1500 North Ritter, Indianapolis, IN 46219, USA

BRUCE W. VIEWEG
Comprehensive Psychiatric Services, Missouri Department of Mental Health, Jefferson City, MO 65102, USA

RICHARD A. WEAVER
Psychology Services, Veterans Administration Medical Center, Salt Lake City, UT 84108, USA

EDWARD A. WORKMAN
Psychiatry Service, Veterans Administration Medical Center, Salem, VA 24153, USA

WILLIE KAI YEE
Psychiatric Applications Developer, PKC Corporation, Burlington, VT 05401-1530, USA

Part I
Clinical Evaluation and Treatment Software

1
MR-E The Mental Retardation-Expert: Performance Support for Clinicians
Matthew G. Hile

The Mental Retardation-Expert (MR-E)* is a performance support system (Gery, 1991) for clinicians treating individuals with mental retardation who engage in severe aggressive, self-injurious, or destructive behaviors. Performance support systems (PSS) are computer programs that provide information, technical assistance, and task training. The goal of these systems is to provide users with flexible and nonintrusive assistance, "where they need it, when they need it, in the forms most useful to them" (Carr, 1991, p. 46).

The definition of a performance support system emphasizes utility not form. A PSS is a collection of different tools and functions all geared to meet the various and specific job performance needs of its users. There are no systems that meet this definition in mental health or mental retardation, but there are programs that might serve as models for the components for such a system. Some important components include a user's library, documentation, training, and decision support or advising functions.

Library functions include collection, summarization, and organization of published materials; each of these functions is an important PSS component. For example, if the users need access to voluminous printed materials (e.g., regulations or diagnostic handbooks), a PSS might automate the text allowing the user to locate relevant sections by section number, index term, full text searching, conceptual maps, or by asking

*The Mental Retardation-Expert project was funded in part by the National Institute of Mental Health (Grant # 1 R29 MH43439). The opinions expressed in this paper are those of the author, and no official endorsement by any agency should be inferred. The author gratefully acknowledge the assistance of the Marshall Habilitation Center, Stephanie Patag, Linda Sage, and Danny Wedding. Correspondence should be sent to Matthew G. Hile, Missouri Institute of Mental Health, 5247 Fyler Avenue, St. Louis, MO 63139-1361. Internet: mimhmh@mizzou1.missouri.edu

the user a variety of questions that permit the system itself to define the desired information. The recent fourth edition of the Diagnostic and Statistical Manual of Mental Disorders on disk (DSM-IV; American Psychiatric Association, 1994) is an excellent example of this type of function for mental health practitioners.

Documentation functions, that help users complete diagnostic or treatment documentation could be beneficial. For example, a PSS might include functions to guide users in completing a problem-oriented medical record, as in the Computer Assisted Service Planning System (1994), or charting behaviors over time as in the Observer System (1993).

Training functions that provide users with new information, teach them new techniques, or review previously learned materials are a third potential component for a PSS. Training can involve a range of techniques including hypertext-based reading selections, programmed learning lessons, animation, experimental simulations, and video selections of treatment techniques in action or experts explaining a concept. Examples of training functions can be seen in the MediaMatrix (Ray, in press).

Advising functions, which provide expert assistance helping users deal with specific problems or questions, is a fourth useful PSS component. This function involves decision support systems (Michaelsen, Michie, & Baouanger, 1985) that capture human expertise in computer programs. They might help clinicians diagnosis problems and develop appropriate treatments, design functional assessment protocols, or suggest specific types of interactions with the client during therapy. Examples of these systems can be found in the areas of brief psychotherapy (Goodman, Gingerich, & de Shazer, 1989), psychiatric emergencies (Hedlund, Vieweg, & Cho, 1987), and sex therapy (Ochs, Meana, Pare, Mah, & Binik, 1994).

In a PSS for mental health and mental retardation professionals, these various components would be combined to provide the technical, scientific, and consultative services to support the individual's position. The specific features, and their functions, would be specific to the needs of the user. MR-E supports Master's level clinicians treating the undesirable behaviors of clients with mental retardation.

System Description

MR-E contains four major modules: a decision support system to provide expert assistance in the development of specific behavioral treatment plans, reviews and annotations to the scientific literature, a collection of sample behavioral treatment plans, and a comprehensive behavioral glossary. Each module focuses on a different aspect of clinical information, providing clinicians with an array of data.

Decision Support System

MR-E's decision support system was created by modeling a human expert's consultation approach (Hile, Campbell, Ghobary, & Desrochers, 1993). It takes a functional approach, helping clinicians identify the probable causes of the undesirable behavior. For example, a client could be aggressive because they wanted to avoid a difficult situation (e.g., attending a demanding vocational training program). Aggression in this case serves an avoidance function and is maintained by negative reinforcement. Another individual might act out when they want to obtain a desired item (e.g., attention from staff). Here aggression serves as an acquisition function and is maintained by positive reinforcement. MR-E helps the clinician examine the undesirable behavior in 21 different functional areas (see Table 1).

MR-E addresses each functional area by asking the clinician user a series of screening questions. In Figure 1, for example, the clinician is being asked if the behavior occurs because the client is in a nonstimulating, boring situation. Answering "Yes" would suggest that the behavior functions to get the client additional stimulation and cause MR-E to ask additional questions about this hypothesis. When the clinician responds "Yes" or "Maybe" to one of the 21 screening questions, MR-E asks further questions to clarify the functional hypothesis and to help identify appropriate treatments.

MR-E is built using production rules that take an IF–THEN format. These rules are clear to readers, easy to understand, and provide great flexibility. Production rules consists of one or more IF statements that, when supported, prove the THEN statement. For example:

IF   A is true and
IF   B is true and
IF   C is not true
THEN   X is true.

MR-E uses both uses backward and forward chaining in an opportunistic search strategy (Clancey, 1985). Backward chaining starts with the THEN portion of the rule and moves backward. Here the system takes each THEN statement and starts asking each of its associated IF questions. When it finds an IF statement that cannot be proved, it goes to the next THEN statement. In the above example, if A were not true, the system would not ask questions about either B or C. Backward chaining has the advantage of reducing the number of questions a user must answer. In contrast, forward chaining initially collects responses to all of the IF questions. The system then tries to find out which THEN statements are proved. Once all of the questions have been asked, this approach is both rapid and efficient.

Table 1. MR-E's 21 Functional Hypotheses

Anxiety/fear over specific event	The behavior reduces anxiety or fearfulness about specific events of conditions.
Aroused by future activity	An upcoming event is aversive or arousing. The behavior functions to reduce this state of arousal or to avoid the event or activity altogether.
Aroused by previous activity	A previous event is aversive or arousing. The behavior functions to reduce this state of arousal.
Aversive environment	Specific environmental stimuli are aversive. These stimuli may include excessive noises, crowding, temperature extremes, smoke, etc. Behavior is maintained (negatively reinforced by avoidance or escape) by the reduction or elimination of these aversive stimuli.
Aversive individuals	Specific individuals (peers, staff, parents, etc.) are aversive. The behavior allows the individual to avoid or escape those individuals.
Aversive physical condition	The behavior reduces or removes pain or other aversive physical condition.
Aversive physical deprivation	The behavior reduces or removes a state of physical deprivation.
Certain times are cues	A specific time (or times) of day serves as a cue for forthcoming aversive conditions or may coincide with excessive fatigue, hunger, or arousal associated with previous activities or experiences.
Consequences	The responses of others in the environment maintain the maladaptive behavior. This includes both positive and negative reinforcements.
Is hungry	The individual is hungry at this time of day. The inability to obtain food instigates this behavior.
Is tired	The individual is tired at this time of day. The inability to rest increases frustration and leads to this behavior.
Locations are aversive	Specific programs or locations contain aversive conditions that serve to instigate aggression or to disinhibit this individual's controls. The behavior decreases the aversiveness of these conditions.
Minimal stimulation	The individual is in a state of stimulus deprivation, boredom, or loneliness. The misbehavior is maintained by the resulting feedback. This feedback may be positive or negative.

Table 1. MR-E's 21 Functional Hypotheses

Models others' behaviors	The observation of others' maladaptive behaviors that serve as a cue for this behavior.
Part of chain	The behavior is the last link in a chain of behaviors that serve as discriminative events for this behavior.
Personal characteristics	The personality characteristics of the individual are the important factor in determining the problematic behavior and no other functional hypothesis seems appropriate.
Provoked by others	Being teased or taunted is aversive to this individual. The behavior is maintained by reducing or avoiding these provocations.
Related to aversive arousal	Aversive arousal serves as the setting event for this behavior. When aroused this individual is more likely to engage in the behavior.
Related to specific emotions	The behavior reduces or removes the conditions that produced the aversive emotional arousal. This reduction serves to maintain (negatively reinforce) the behavior.
Specific aversive requests	Specific requests or directives are aversive, or they interrupt specific positive events. The maladaptive behaviors are maintained (negatively reinforced) by the delay or avoidance of these requests or directives.
Specific aversive tasks	Specific tasks are aversive. The maladaptive behaviors are maintained (negatively reinforced) by escaping from these well-learned tasks.

MR-E's initial functional exploration uses backward chaining to direct its questioning. After completing this questioning, MR-E uses forward chaining to examine its "metarules" and to develop specific assessment and treatment suggestions.

Metarules are rules about rules. In MR-E, the system looks for patterns in the user's responses to discern the underlying function guiding the client's behaviors. In the psycho-educational model on which MR-E relies, three processes underlie all behaviors: positive reinforcement, negative reinforcement, and setting events. Reinforcement is well understood; however, the concept of setting events may be somewhat less clear. A setting event is anything that increases the probability of a behavior. For example, in children it is clear that fatigue makes it more likely that the child will become upset even in situations that would normally cause no

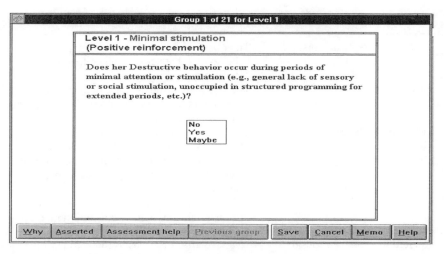

Figure 1. Sample question from decision support module.

difficulty. In this case, fatigue is a setting event. In its metarules, MR-E looks for the underlying mechanism that accounts for most of the client's undesirable behaviors. It then suggests interventions that rely on a similar mechanism. For example, if escape (i.e., negative reinforcement) is found most frequently, MR-E will recommend treatments that use escape to reinforce appropriate responding. When MR-E is unable to select a single underlying mechanism, it recommends specific functional assessments to differentiate between the likely alternatives.

Regardless of the results from the metaanalysis, MR-E creates a consultation report summarizing its findings and recommending specific types of treatments for all of the specific functional hypotheses identified by the clinician. Figure 2 is an example of a portion of such a report. The report highlights the various functional hypotheses found during the consultation and the treatment methods that would be appropriate for those hypotheses. Note that MR-E does not write a behavioral treatment protocol. Rather it is designed to provide the clinician with the support they need to create a treatment plan. In this way MR-E supports clinicians but does not replace them.

Scientific Literature

Often clinicians turn to the scientific literature for answers to specific questions and for help in treating individual clients. However, the literature is vast and ever growing and it may be difficult or impossible for practicing clinicians to get materials directly related to their needs. To facilitate the transfer of information from the scientific literature to clinicians, MR-E includes literature reviews and annotations of specific articles.

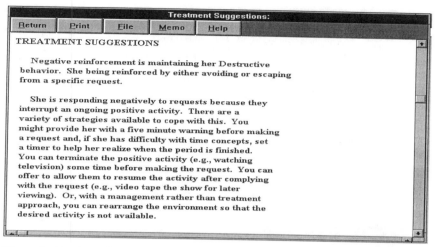

Figure 2. Portion of a consultation report.

Literature reviews are organized in terms of the intrusiveness of the particular intervention. This was done because clinicians frequently want to start treatments with the least intrusive alternative that has some chance of success. Within the reviews each article is briefly discussed and overall recommendations are made. However, these brief discussions do not contain sufficient information for clinicians to model the specific treatment paradigms. To minimize the need for finding the source document, MR-E includes stylized annotations of each of the articles in its reviews. These annotations are designed to fill the information needs of the clinician.

Each annotation contains three parts (see Fig. 3). The first part provides a scientific discussion of the articles, similar to journal abstracts. The second part describes the behavioral effects of the treatment and the specific procedures used. The third part is most critical to the goals of MR-E. In this section the specific methodology is described in such a way to allow the clinician to replicate the most effective treatment discussed in the article. This minimizes the clinician's need to locate the source document and maximizes the impact of the individual annotation. Additionally, although not displayed in this figure, the full citation is provided in case the clinician wishes to obtain the source document.

Notice in Figure 3 the underlined and highlighted word "DRI." This is one of MR-E's hypertext links. If the clinician is unfamiliar with this word they can select it to read the glossary entry for the procedure, that is, "differential reinforcement of incompatible behavior." In this way clinicians, who may be unfamiliar with some of the specific procedures, can expand their knowledge of available treatment options.

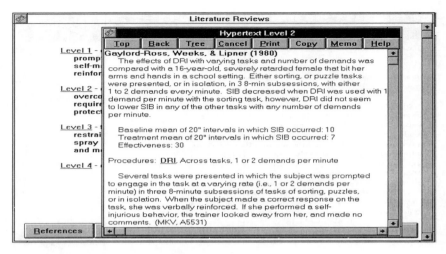

Figure 3. Three parts of a MR-E annotation.

Sample Treatment Plans

A third useful source of information for clinicians is treatment plans developed by others. From these plans clinicians can learn how to structure and implement interventions. They can use them as models for their own plans or take ideas from them to incorporate into their treatments. To find relevant plans clinicians conduct a search of the available treatments in a manner similar to conducting a literature search. They specify the target behaviors, level of severity of those behaviors, the client's diagnosis, and whether or not the client has a mobility difficulty. Multiple levels of each of these criteria can be selected to provide progressively more inclusive searches.

The results of a search are shown in Figure 4. In this search five treatment plans matched the relevant criteria. The clinician has selected two for further examination (mild restraint and token economy) and MR-E displays part of that additional information. In MR-E this module currently contains little information and is in place to allow for future expansion.

Behavioral Glossary

The behavioral glossary contains more than 350 terms used in MR-E. These include behavioral interventions, undesirable behaviors, medical conditions, functional hypotheses, and other words and concepts relevant to the clinician's task.

The glossary is accessible in two ways. The first, shown in Figure 5, provides a dictionarylike interface that allows the user to look up unfamiliar

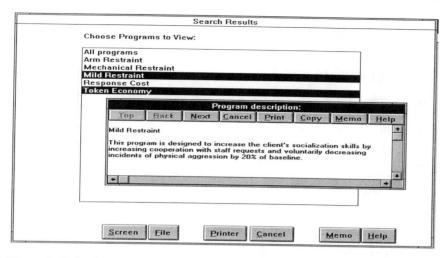

Figure 4. Behavioral treatment plan module.

terms. More frequently, however, the glossary will be used within the context of one of MR-E's other modules. MR-E uses hypertext to give clinicians information within the context of their current activity. For example, terms available in the glossary are highlighted in all of the modules. While the descriptions could have been included in each section, the use of hypertext allows the clinicians to get the information they need and only the information they need. Using this feature, clinicians are free

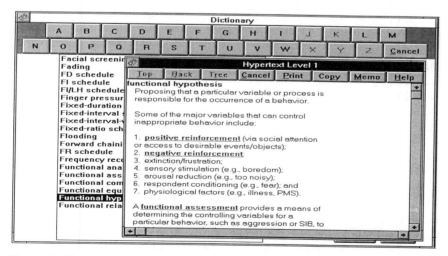

Figure 5. Example of a definition from MR-E's glossary module.

to explore the meanings of various terms and concepts and their relation-ships to one another.

Clinician's Use of MR-E Modules

MR-E's four components combine to provide clinicians with a flexible system that supports the treatment of the undesirable behaviors of persons with mental retardation. MR-E is designed to provide its users with a wide variety of information taken from human experts, the scientific literature, the practice of other clinicians, and the behavioral lexicon. As a performance support system it is not designed to replace clinicians, but rather to enhance their effectiveness, ease their tasks, and expand their competencies.

Reliability and Validity of MR-E's Consultations

A decision support system and traditional psychological assessment share many important characteristics. Each collects information in a more or less structured manner, combines the information in ways that are not necessarily intuitively obvious, and provides that information in summary form to its users. In assessments, responses to items are collected, scales scored based on empirical or logical constructions, and results presented. In DSSs, questions are answered, those answers are combined using the intelligent algorithms of the system, and suggestions are made.

Developers of psychological assessment have long attended to both the reliability and validity of their instruments. Reliability measures the con-sistency of the measure and asks a simple question: "Does the instrument return the same results time and time again or do different users obtain the same or similar results?" Validity refers to the relationship of the measure to the real world, that is, does an instrument measure what it says it measures. An assessment may be reliable and not valid. However, it cannot be valid without being reliable. To be truly useful an instrument must have both features.

Developers of DSSs have not previously addressed the similarities of their systems to more traditional assessments. In the case of MR-E, we have acknowledged this similarity and have begun the process of examining its reliability and validity in a series of studies.

Interrater Reliability

One form of reliability asks the question, "Will two people observing the same phenomena respond the same way?" In the specific case of MR-E, one asks "Will different people using the system to obtain a consultation about the same client receive substantially similar suggestions?" If not, then the consultations are based more on the raters' judgments and personalities than on the client's problems and would have little chance of being helpful.

To explore interrater reliability we first abstracted 31 case histories from the scientific literature. Four doctoral level clinicians, varying in terms of their clinical experience and their familiarity with MR-E, used those histories to independently obtain MR-E consultations. We then examined the similarities between the functional hypotheses generated by each of the clinicians for each of the cases using Kazdin's inter-observer reliability score (IOR; Kazdin, 1982, p. 54). IORs range from 0 where no agreement exists to 1 representing unanimity. Across all cases the average IOR between clinicians of different levels of clinical experience was 0.91. That is, consultations obtained by clinicians with little experience were substantially identical to those obtained by experienced clinicians. When clinicians with little experience with MR-E (at least at the start of this study) were compared with highly experienced MR-E users, the average IOR was 0.92. This indicates that essentially equivalent results are obtained using MR-E regardless of the user's level of experience with the system.

This study used analogue case descriptions and documents to MR-E's ability to provide suggestions that were more dependent on the client's clinical problems than on the user's clinical and computer experience. For a full description of this study and other findings relating to the system's interrater reliability see Hile, Campbell, Ghobary, and Desrochers (1994). Currently similar reliability studies are being conducted in clinical settings to assess MR-E's interrater reliability under real world conditions.

Validity

Validity addresses the relationship of an instrument to an external criteria, that is, "Does the assessment, or DSS, provide results that are consistent with what we know to be true?" For a DSS the most obvious external criteria are human experts. To examine this form of validity we first compared the recommendations provided by MR-E with those of three human experts. If valid, we would expect MR-E to provide suggestions that are similar to those from human experts.

The three nationally recognized experts read two fictional case descriptions providing both their judgments about the function of the particular undesirable behavior and their recommended interventions. The experts then read an MR-E consultation report for those cases and again provided their functional hypotheses and recommended interventions. The level of agreement among the three experts ranged from 0.74 to 0.79, indicating that human experts do not wholly agree with each other, a result that was not unexpected. IORs comparing each expert's evaluations with that of MR-E ranged from 0.79 to 0.93. This suggests that the three experts are more in agreement with MR-E than they are with each other. After reading the consultation reports, the IORs between the experts and MR-E increased, ranging from 0.81 to 1.0. It is interesting to note that the highest level of agreement (IOR = 1) was between MR-E and the expert on whom the system was based. The high level of agreement found in this study shows that the judgments provided by MR-E are consistent with those provided by human experts. Its consistency with individuals whom others would acknowledge as experts suggests that MR-E is capable of providing expert advice. For a more complete description of this study see Hile, Campbell, and Ghobary (1994).

Another examination of MR-E's validity involved a comparison of the advice obtained from the system with recommendations derived from the scientific literature (Hile, Ghobary, & Campbell, 1995). In this study, the MR-E's recommendations from 30 of the cases from the reliability study described above were compared with the advice offered in the published articles from which the cases were abstracted. Because clinicians often rely on scientific literature to develop new treatment approaches, this comparison examined the differential impact of two potential sources of treatment suggestions.

In this study, two individuals independently rated MR-E's consultation reports and the literature's suggestions in terms of the use of proactive or reactive approaches, their reliance on basic behavioral principles, and on the specific treatments suggested. Only a partial description of the study's results will be presented here.

Compared to the literature, MR-E typically recommended more proactive approaches, that is interventions, that occur before the behavior in question. For example, MR-E was more likely to recommend skill training to provide the individual with a prosocial alternative to their undesirable behavior. MR-E relies more on positive and negative reinforcement in its treatment suggestions compared to the reliance on punishment and extinction found in the literature. This suggests that it takes a positive rather than a punitive approach to the client. Additionally, MR-E's treatment suggestions tended to be more specific to the behavior's function than the more general approaches found in the literature. This latter difference can be seen in the recommended usage of differential reinforcement procedures. The literature more frequently recommended the differential reinforcement of other behaviors (DRO). In a DRO procedure the client is reinforced for doing anything other than the undesirable behavior. MR-E is more likely to recommend a differential reinforcement of an alternative behavior (DRA). In a DRA procedure the individual is reinforced for engaging in a prosocial behavior that has the same function as the undesirable behavior. This specificity of training should increase the impact of the behavioral intervention (Carr, Robinson, & Palumbo, 1990).

These two validity studies, in addition to the reliability study described above, support MR-E's ability to offer suggestions that are similar to human experts and more specific than those found in the scientific literature. They begin the long process of identifying MR-E's ability to adequately reflect the reality of undesirable behaviors and to identify treatments appropriate to them.

Impact

We have identified some of the reliability and validity characteristics of MR-E. However, the more compelling question is "What impact does MR-E have on its users?" To answer this question, we provided case descriptions to experienced clinicians and collected their hypotheses and treatment recommendations. They were then provided with an MR-E consultation report and their hypotheses and recommendations were again assessed (Hile, Campbell, & Ghobary, 1994).

With this protocol clinicians agreed significantly more with MR-E's recommendations on the posttest than on the pretest, with the IORs increasing from 0.88 to 0.94. Examining the specific impact on their responses, we found that the clinicians' *specificity* (their ability to identify the correct functional hypotheses) increased significantly (pretest = 0.92, posttest = 0.95). Although significant, this increase is of little clinical importance. However, the increase in clinicians' *sensitivity* (their ability to reject incorrect hypotheses) increased significantly from both a statistical and practical view point (pretest = 0.67, posttest = 0.91). MR-E's suggestions helped clinicians eliminate untenable hypotheses from consideration and allowed them to focus attention on more probable hypotheses.

Summary

MR-E provides a range of functions that support clinicians in discharging their diagnostic and treatment responsibilities. Initial studies examining its reliability and validity have showed promise and support continued development efforts. Users have been excited about the possibilities of this PSS and about adding other components (e.g., behavioral tracking and charting). Current plans for the system include moving it to a pediatric outpatient population (to eliminate problems before they become well entrenched), and developing means of more reliably updating and summarizing the literature.

The major stumbling blocks in the development of MR-E and of any future system is time and money. These systems contain a great deal of information and its collection, organization, and preparation is difficult and time consuming. Nonetheless, the rewards to the users of such a system are potentially enormous.

References

American Psychiatric Association. (1994). *Electronic DSM IV*. Washington, DC: American Psychiatric Association.

Carr, C. (1991). Performance support systems: A new horizon for expert systems. *AI Expert*, 7(5), 44–49.

Carr, E.G., Robinson, S., & Palumbo, L.W. (1990). The wrong issue: Aversive versus nonaversive treatment. The right issue: Functional versus non functional treatment. In A.C. Repp & N.N. Signh (Eds.), *Perspectives on the use of nonaversive and aversive interventions for persons with developmental disabilities* (pp. 361–379). Sycamore, IL: Sycamore Publishing.

Clancey, W.J. (1985). Heuristic classification. *Artificial Intelligence*, 27, 289–352.

Computer assisted service planning [Computer software]. (1994). Oakland, CA: PSP Information Group, Inc.

Gery, G.J. (1991). *Electronic performance support systems*. Boston, MA: Weingarten.

Goodman, H., Gingerich, W.J., & de Shazer, S. (1989). Briefer: An expert system for clinical practice. *Computers in Human Services*, 5, 53–68.

Hedlund, J.L., Vieweg, B.W., & Cho, D.W. (1987). Computer consultation for emotional crises: An expert system for non-experts. *Computers in Human Behavior*, 3, 109–127.

Hile, M.G., Campbell, D.M., & Ghobary, B.B. (1994). Automation for clinicians in the field: The validity of a performance support system. *Behavior Research Methods, Instruments, and Computers*, 26, 205–208.

Hile, M.G., Campbell, D.M., Ghobary, B.B., & Desrochers, M.N. (1993). Development of knowledge bases and the reliability of decision support for behavioral treatment consultation for persons with mental retardation: The Mental Retardation-Expert. *Behavior Research Methods, Instruments, & Computers*, 25, 195–198.

Hile, M.G., Campbell, D.M., Ghobary, B.B., & Desrochers, M.N. (1994). Reliability of an automated decision support system for behavioral treatment planning: Preliminary results from the mental retardation expert. *Computers in Human Services*, 10(4), 19–29.

Hile, M.G., Ghobary, B.B., & Campbell, D.M. (1995). Sources of expert advice: A comparison of peer-reviewed advice from the literature to that from an automated performance support system. *Behavior Research Methods, Instruments, & Computers*, 27, 272–276.

Kazdin, A. (1982). *Single-case research design: Methods for clinical and applied settings*. New York: Oxford University Press.

Michaelsen, R., Michie, D., & Baouanger, A. (1985). The technology of expert systems. *Byte*, 10, 303–312.

The Observer 3.0 [Computer software]. (1993). Wageningen, The Netherlands: Noldus Information Technology.

Ochs, E.P., Meana, M., Pare, L., Mah, K., & Binik, Y.M. (1994). Learning about sex outside the gutter—Attitudes toward a computer sex-expert system. *Journal of Sex & Marital Therapy*, 20, 86–102.

Ray, R.D. (in press). A behavioral systems approach to adaptive computerized instructional design. *Behavior Research Methods, Instruments, & Computers*.

2
Sexpert: An Expert System for Sexual Assessment, Counseling, and Treatment

Yitzchak M. Binik, Eric P. Ochs,
and Marta Meana

There are probably few associations less likely in our minds than computers and sexuality. In fact, the link between computers and sexuality in our culture has not only been deemed improbable, but, explicitly negative. The mechanization that arose with the industrial revolution has been a critical focus of two centuries of art and literature that have sought to protect the realm of affect and sensuality from the ultimate threat of the microchip. A 1970s horror film (Cammell, 1977) even had Julie Christie being impregnated by a not very user-friendly mainframe.

Despite this less than favorable environment, the idea of the computer as a self-help sex educator–counselor has now become a distinct possibility. Although the focus of our discussion will be to review our attempts to facilitate this possibility, we would also like to address issues related to the desirability and ethics of computer-assisted sex education and therapy. Finally, we will discuss our professional dilemmas resulting from being approached by companies wanting to exploit the potential commercial value of our work.

Before we began our work on Sexpert, there had been several attempts to develop computer-assisted sex education or counseling programs. Reitman (1982) developed a program to treat psychogenic impotence. As far as we are aware, this program was never formally tested and, although it was commercially marketed to the general public, it is no longer available. A second program called "Intracourse" was also developed and marketed in the 1980s (Intracorp, 1985). This program asked a standardized set of questions about sexuality, provided a report at the end based on these answers, and also included a glossary of sexual terms. No evaluation data concerning "Intracourse" are available and as far as we can determine, it is no longer for sale. Two reports (Kann, 1987; Alemi, Cherry, & Meffert, 1989) evaluated the use of computer-assisted instructional techniques to foster the growth of "responsible sexuality." Although the authors are enthusiastic about such use and adolescents seem likely to respond positively to computerized interventions, there has been little follow-up to the initial work.

Computer-Assisted Assessment and Therapy

While the above cited research was being conducted, there was an explosion of activity in computer-assisted clinical work in other areas. This activity can be crudely divided into three areas: psychological testing, diagnostic interviewing, and counseling/therapy.

Psychological Testing

At present, most psychological tests have a computer-administered version and ofter built-in scoring and interpretive modules. Even unlikely candidates such as the Rorschach have been computerized (ROR-SCAN, 1991). A variety of "shell" programs exist that can facilitate computerization of new questionnaires; and it has been our experience that an increasing number of hospitals use computers to administer and score standardized psychological tests. Much of the impetus for such computerization has been economic because it is much cheaper to buy a computer and software than to hire a psychometrist. Nonetheless, a growing body of literature (e.g., Bloom, 1992) suggests that it is only a matter of time before the validity of computer-administered testing approximates that of human administration. It is our prediction that computers will ultimately replace psychometrists and psychologists in the administration and scoring of psychological tests and that most of the standard interpretive work will also be computer generated.

Diagnostic Interviewing

Several reports suggest that computer-based interviewing is well-accepted and sometimes preferred by patients (e.g., Erdman, Klein, & Greist, 1985; McCullough, Farrell, & Longabaugh, 1986; Bloom, 1992). These reports also suggest that patients may report more symptomatology to computers than to human interviewers. Although the interpretation of these data is not currently clear, there is some reason to believe that the lack of a human presence may facilitate disclosure of socially unacceptable behavior. The continuing development of computerized interviews based on the Diagnostic and Statistical Manual of the American Psychiatric Association has fostered the growth of such interviewing. Economic forces will also probably impel hospitals to institute such systems that, if supported by validity studies, may eventually become the norm.

Counseling and Therapy

There are numerous books and reviews trying to summarize the frenetic pace of development of computerized counseling and therapy programs (e.g., Lieff, 1987; Wagman, 1988; Baskin, 1990; Bloom, 1992). These programs range in application from career counseling to cognitive therapy for depression. The standards, theoretical approaches, goals, and development platforms for these programs are extraordinarily varied. Katz (1984) reviews the available information concerning career counseling programs that have become a "necessity" for high school and university counseling advising offices in North America. Such programs provide important information efficiently and inexpensively and student response is apparently very positive. Unfortunately, there is almost no information as to whether users actually comply with the recommendations of these programs, and even fewer studies comparing computerized recommendations to those of professionals.

Bloom (1992) has comprehensively reviewed the 25 year history of research on computerized intervention. The activity in this area appears to be increasing as evidenced by symposia at recent conferences (e.g., Schneider, 1994; Miller, 1994) and new periodicals such as *Computers in Mental Health* (Ustun, 1994). It is troubling, however, that this activity has not been accompanied by the introduction of computerized intervention into standard practice. To the best of our knowledge there is no self-help therapy computer program in general use outside of the laboratory or clinics associated with its developers. One view is that it is only a matter of time before computerized intervention becomes commonplace. If such a scenario develops, it remains to be seen whether these programs, like self-help books, will be sold freely on the open market or whether, like psychological tests, they will be available only to registered professionals. Although most professionals would probably officially advocate the latter, there seems to be little interest in setting professional standards or in regulating the development and distribution of computerized clinical tools.

One necessary step in setting such standards would be therapy outcome studies comparing computerized intervention with the presumed gold standard: the clinician. Unfortunately, there are very few studies of this nature. These studies (Ghosh & Marks, 1987; Wagman, 1988; Selmi, Klein, Greist, Sorrell, & Erdman, 1990; Agras, Taylor, Feldman, Losch, & Burnett, 1990) suggest that therapy outcomes based on computerized intervention are similar to those resulting from human clinicians or self-help books. The conclusions one can draw from these studies, however, are not clear. Isaac Marks' (personal communication, July 18, 1989) conclusion was that it was not worth the effort to use computers in the treatment of agoraphobia but that a self-help book was sufficient. In a study carried out by Agras et al. (1990), a hand-held computer to treat obesity was as effective as a clinician, but neither resulted in long-term weight loss.

It is possible only to speculate about what is fueling the development of the numerous self-help therapy programs. Clearly, the success of "bibliotherapy" has encouraged clinicians to try to exploit computer technology as a way of providing potentially more individualized and more "intelligent" interventions. In addition, the financial inaccessibility of psychological care for large segments of the population has motivated the development of potentially mass market programs for home computers. Finally, there is little doubt that many developers have been motivated by the potential financial rewards of a best-seller self-help program.

Sexpert

Work on Sexpert began in 1984 as a result of a fortuitous conversation between David Servan–Schreiber, a psychiatry resident, and Irv Binik who was teaching an introductory seminar for psychiatric residents on sex therapy. After the seminar, Servan–Schreiber who had had extensive experience with artificial intelligence (AI)-based medical expert systems, approached Binik with the idea of creating an expert system for sex therapy. Although Binik initially scoffed at the idea, he ultimately became interested in the project as a way of formalizing practice in sex therapy. Binik and Servan–Schreiber were joined shortly afterward by Simon Freiwald, a computer scientist who was instrumental in creating a development environment suitable for the project.

Although the choice of sex therapy was initially a coincidence, there were some theoretical and practical justifications for creating an expert self-help system in this field. There was an already well-established self-help tradition in sex therapy including books and videos. A computer counselor could, in theory, provide the same quality of information but in a more highly individualized fashion. Moreover, interaction with a computer is potentially a more active process and therefore, we believed, more effective than reading a book or viewing a video. With the projected increase in the number of home computers and computer network users, easy access to help at minimal expense seemed likely. We hoped that such increased availability would result in early consultation that could have an important preventative function. Finally, we believed that sex therapy was relatively well-defined which would facilitate formalization of our knowledge into a "computerizable" format.

We chose a rule-based production system approach as the programming technology for Sexpert. This approach had become the standard at that time for most AI-based expert systems. Such systems are generally composed of three functional units: a knowledge base, an inference engine (i.e., a thinking mechanism), and a user interface. This technology was suitable for a variety of reasons. First, all knowledge in such systems is represented uniformly in the form of "if–then" rules. Second, these if–then rules are separate from the inference engine that controls the flow of the program, so the knowledge base can be modified or changed much more easily than more standard programs. Third, experts can usually be trained relatively easily to translate their expertise into if–then rules that can be then be organized into high level knowledge bases.

The inference engine, EXP, that Simon Freiwald constructed for us was also well suited to our needs:

1. It allowed for both backward and forward chaining control strategies that had already proved to be highly useful mechanisms for solving complex diagnostic problems.
2. It could interact very quickly with a knowledge base of several thousand rules.
3. It allowed for the dynamic construction of texts and their easy modification thus facilitating detailed control over ongoing dialogue.
4. It allowed for uncertainty and probabilistic statements in rules.
5. It worked on all the major operating systems of the time including MS-DOS, Macintosh, VAX/VMS, UNIX, and OS2, and was also easy to interface with telecommunication networks.

From the outset, our work was also directed by a set of requirements we believed were necessary for all "personal advice systems." These requirements were based on the premise that a computer must react according to user expectations of normal social discourse in counseling situations in order to create the effective illusion of an understanding and intelligent caregiver. Taking into account our experience and those of others with ELIZA and similar programs (DeMuth, 1984), we felt it was crucial to simulate the process of therapeutic dialogue (cf. Servan–Schreiber & Binik, 1989). Although we could not construct an intelligent system that would accept natural language, we could simulate this by structuring dialogue plans to follow the expectations of normal social intercourse and to present accurate feedback in natural language. The pattern feedback and dialogue we designed avoided the two extremes of human–computer interaction: a long series of questions followed by several pages of feedback; or a socially illogical set of questions that efficiently solved the diagnostic question but ignored users' feelings and expectations.

Another important requirement was that our system be able to shift focus based on users' answers rather than plod ahead trying to solve its internal goals. We also tried to construct a system that would monitor when it lacked adequate knowledge and inform the user accordingly. In addition, we required the system to allow users to backtrack and change previous answers without having to repeat the entire interaction. Finally, we believed it necessary to develop a system that could inform the user about the reasons behind a particular conclusion.

Despite our knowledge from the existing literature of the time that the average 400 rule expert system took approximately 5 person-years to develop, we naively believed that we could accomplish our task in 6 to 12 months while all working full time at other jobs. Our goal was to create an expert system that would directly interview couples, assess their sexual functioning, reach conclusions about the adequacy of this functioning, and, if necessary, lead them through a step-by-step self-help program. After several years of work, we had finished the introductory and diagnostic modules as well as those associated with the evaluation of sexual repertoire (e.g., foreplay, intercourse positions, etc.). Our initial tests suggested that there were still many errors in the diagnostic modules, but that the repertoire modules were ready for systematic evaluation. Rather than spend several more years on development without any empirical input, we decided to test those modules that appeared to be functioning well. The goals of this evaluation were to determine whether couples would interact with Sexpert and follow the program's advice.

The following dialogue illustrates a couple's interaction with a repertoire module of Sexpert. Other examples of dialogues can be found in the work of the following authors: Binik, Servan–Schreiber, Freiwald, and Hall (1988); Servan–Schreiber and Binik (1989); Binik, Meana, and Sand (1994); Ochs, Meana, Mah, and Binik (1993); and Ochs, Meana, Paré, Mah, and Binik (1994). This excerpt begins with feedback about the couple's current foreplay. Sexpert then investigates potential changes.

Although you are both somewhat satisfied with your foreplay, you agree that there is room for improvement. Since you appear to disagree a bit about an ideal length of foreplay, I'm curious to find out how far apart you really are. One possibility might be that since most of your activities involve nongenital stimulation, you might like to consider changing the pattern of your foreplay by adding some of the genitally oriented activities that I've mentioned. If you do this and make them part of your regular repertoire make sure not to neglect the nongenital activities that you're now engaging in. Let me pursue this with you a bit more.

Adam, about how many minutes does foreplay usually last?
>>>>>10

Eve, do you agree with this estimate?
>>>>>Y

You mentioned that you would like foreplay to last longer than the 10 minutes that it currently lasts, Eve. What would be an ideal length of time Eve?(in minutes)
>>>>>20

Adam, you said that you didn't want to change the length of your foreplay. Can I assume that your current duration is your ideal one?
>>>>>Y

Would you like to try some new foreplay activities or greatly increase in frequency any of your usual current foreplay activities, Eve?
>>>>>Y

OK, I hate to do this, but I'm going to have to mention all activities that we have already talked about. Eve, here are the same lists you saw before. To jog your memory, I'm going to list both the foreplay activities you said that you don't normally engage in (not in parentheses) and the ones you said that you do typically engage in (in parentheses). Please don't choose more than three new activities that you'd like to add for now. Remember that you can choose activities from more than one list.

Eve, would you like to add any of these activities?

 1: Being alone together
 2: Going out
 3: Lighting candles, playing music
 4: Dancing together
 5: Adam wearing special clothes
 6: Eve wearing special clothes
 7: Undressing each other
 8: Adam undressing Eve
 9: Eve undressing Adam
10: (Eve undressing in view of Adam)
11: Adam undressing in view of Eve
12: Taking a bath or shower together
13: Watching a romantic or erotic movie together
14: Playing or being playful with each other
15: Adam making sexually suggestive gestures or motions
16: Eve making sexually suggestive gestures or motions
17: Other mood-setting activities
18: None of the above
>>>>>1   2

How about adding any of these?
1: Talking or sharing feelings
2: Talking about sex
3: Adam talking "dirty"
4: Eve talking "dirty"
5: Eve revealing a sexual fantasy or desire
6: Adam revealing a sexual fantasy or desire
7: Other talking activities
8. None of the above
>>>>>1

OK, that makes three activities you wish to add, so I won't present any more lists. Would you like to try some new foreplay activities or greatly increase in frequency any of your usual current foreplay activities, Adam?
>>>>>N

You disagree somewhat about an ideal length of foreplay. Let's consider some possible changes to try to minimize your disagreement. Would you

like to drop or greatly reduce in frequency any of your current regular activities, Adam?
>>>>N

Would you like to drop or greatly reduce in frequency any of your current regular activities, Eve?
>>>>N

If you think it will be of any use, I can give you some feedback about foreplay activities that I think might be fun for you to try. Would you like me to do so?
>>>>Y

OK, here is my first suggestion.

Although I don't agree with the cliche "you are what you wear" there's little doubt in my mind that sexy clothes will help turn both of you on. When I talk about wearing special clothes, I don't mean just Eve. There are lots of sexy garments for men. Specialty shops have quite a selection ranging from "designer"condoms (different colors and textures) to silk and leather underwear. If you're shy about specialty shops, take your imagination shopping in any major department store. Boxer shorts are making a come-back and silk bathrobes or smoking jackets can also be extremely appealing.

One needn't spend lots of money either. Making love in the shower while the two of you are wearing cotton T-shirts can be quite a fashion show. Needless to say, sexy clothes such as negligees, garter belts, and "merry widow" corsets are widely available for women. The next time you go out to dinner you may want to skip dessert and have some "edible underwear" at home instead.

Empirical Studies

We have carried out four separate empirical studies of the introductory and repertoire modules of Sexpert involving approximately 250 individuals or couples. Three of these studies have been published (Binik, Westbury, & Servan-Schreiber, 1989; Ochs et al., 1993; Binik, Meana, & Sand, 1994; Ochs et al., 1994) and the fourth (Ochs, Meana, & Binik, 1995) is a direct extension of the previous work. Because these studies followed a similar pattern, we will summarize the major procedures and results of the research program rather than summarizing each study in detail.

Couples volunteering to participate were randomly assigned in a between groups design to interact for 20 to 60 minutes with a source of advice about their sexuality (e.g., Sexpert, a self-help book a video, a therapist etc.). Before and after this interaction, couples provided information about their attitudes toward each source of information and reported on their sexual behavior. Our two primary goals were to demonstrate empirically that Sexpert's style of interaction was engaging and positive for couples and that Sexpert would motivate behavior change.

Attitude Change. To demonstrate our first goal, we looked to the extensive social psychological literature on the measurement of attitudes. We adopted standard and well-known methodologies for assessing attitudes including direct rankings, semantic differential ratings, and multidimensional scaling. In each case, we were interested in how a computerized sex counselor would rate as compared with other sources of help or information about sexuality such as a book, video, sex therapist, doctor, friend, lover, etc. We hypothesized that initial attitudes toward a computerized sex therapist would be negative rather than neutral. Thus, Sexpert would have to overcome a negative bias in order to engage the average user. We further hypothesized that couples would dramatically and positively shift their attitudes after interaction with Sexpert.

Overall, these predictions have been confirmed. Before exposure, couples consistently rated a computerized sex counselor as the worst possible source of information or help about sex. Figure 1 illustrates these initial attitudes using simple ranking data collected in our most recent study (Ochs, Meana, & Binik, 1995). These low rankings probably reflect both our culture's unfamiliarity with the idea of a computer sex counselor as well as a knee jerk rejection of the notion of linking computers and sexuality.

Nonetheless, after a fairly short interaction with Sexpert, these highly negative attitudes shifted in a markedly positive direction. This find-

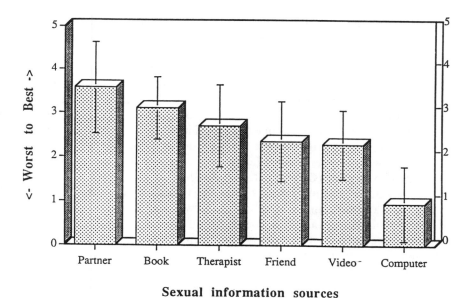

Sexual information sources

Figure 1. Average pretreatment quality rankings from Ochs et al. (1995).

ing has been replicated in all four studies. The degree of attitude shift depended on the study, on the measures used, and on the alternative source of information to which Sexpert was compared. For example, in Binik, Westbury, and Servan–Schreiber (1989), individuals, after approximately 20 minutes of interaction, rated Sexpert as highly similar to a human sex therapist. Figure 2 illustrates semantic differential data from Ochs et al. (1994) showing how subjects dramatically improved their attitudes toward computerized sex counseling immediately after interacting with Sexpert (session 2). This attitude shift remained stable over the follow-up period of 2 weeks (session 3).

Generalizing over all our studies, Sexpert was rated just as good as, if not better than, other sources of self-help such as books or videos. Interaction with a therapist, however, is still considered the ideal. Our most recent, unpublished study (Ochs, Meana, & Binik, 1995), in which we included for the first time a 1 hour session with a therapist as one of the experimental manipulations, indicated that a therapist is rated more highly than Sexpert on most measures. Nonetheless, the overall data suggest that Sexpert is on the right track in simulating therapeutic dialogue and has the ability to engage couples in positive interactions. This interpretation is confirmed by answers to open-ended questions we have collected from subjects indicating that, much to their surprise, they found Sexpert to be intelligent, humanlike, and engaging. We were also able to videotape several couples interacting with Sexpert. In viewing these tapes, it became clear to us that the richness of the couple interaction while they were responding to Sexpert is not being recorded on the keyboard and is similar in a number of respects to a therapy session.

Behavior Change. Demonstrating behavior change has proved to be a more difficult task than transforming attitudes. We have taken two methodological approaches. In the first, we used a daily self-monitoring strategy to assess changes in sexual behavior. In the second, we asked subjects during and at the end of each experiment to report retrospectively whether interaction with Sexpert resulted in behavior change (Binik et al., 1989; Ochs et al., 1995). We used the daily sexual self-monitoring scales in two studies (Ochs et al., 1993; Binik et al., 1994) to assess a variety of couple and individual sexual behaviors including frequency of intercourse, orgasm, and masturbation, as well as ratings of satisfaction with these activities and with couple communication. In neither study were we able to demonstrate any significant behavior change resulting from interaction with Sexpert or, for that matter, with any other source of information and advice.

Our experience with these instruments, however, has led us to question their validity. It became quite clear in these experiments that filling out a sexual self-monitoring form every day was itself a potent intervention that may have overshadowed our experimental manipulations. Couples

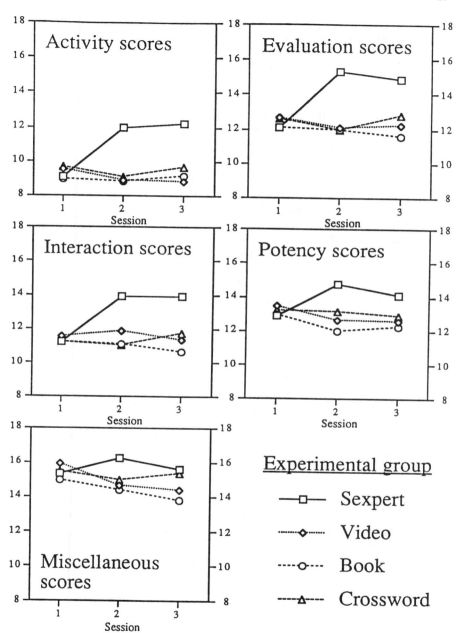

Figure 2. Changes in the ratings of the computer as a source of sexual information by each experimental group on each of the five subscales of the semantic differential over three experimental sessions.

complained about filling out these monitoring forms, especially on successive days when there was no sexual activity. In neither experiment
were we able to establish a stable baseline from which to evaluate behavior
change and, by the end of the experiment, the average rate of response
dropped for subjects in all groups.

Retrospective reports of behavior change, on the other hand, indicated
that interaction with Sexpert, videos, or books resulted in significant
behavior change as well as improved communication about sexuality,
satisfaction with the relationship, and learning about sexuality. In these
studies (Ochs et al., 1993; Binik et al., 1994), Sexpert was as successful
(or unsuccessful) at inducing behavior change as the more traditional self-
help methods and all were superior to no-treatment controls. Our most
recent study (Ochs et al., 1995) compared interaction with Sexpert to
interaction with a therapist, a video, and a crossword puzzle control. This
study suggested that a session with a therapist resulted in the highest
number of positive sexual behavior changes. Interaction with Sexpert or
exposure to a video also resulted in positive sexual behavior changes but
at a significantly lower rate than those reported in the therapist condition.
Controls reported little behavior change.

At present, there is no definitive evidence that Sexpert is effective in
inducing behavior change. We are confident, however, that if future
studies are able to remedy certain procedural and methodological problems, then such behavior change will be demonstrable. First, all of our
studies have used a maximum of 1 hour of intervention with any source of
sexual advice. This amount of time may not be sufficient to induce
reliable behavior change using any method, including a clinician. Second,
because the diagnostic and therapeutic modules of Sexpert remain
unfinished, we were not able to deal with focused problems such as
premature ejaculation or anorgasmia. We were forced, therefore, to
measure many different possible kinds of change in couples' typical sexual
repertoires. As a result, we monitored the frequency of a large range of
sexual behaviors over short periods of time. Such measurement was
probably not reliable and probably did not adequately reflect couples'
sexual lives. Finally, because we recruited paid volunteers, it was not
clear that these couples were significantly dissatisfied and therefore highly
motivated to change their sexual behavior. Further studies should recruit
couples seeking help for specific aspects of their sexual lives.

Current Status of Sexpert

At the moment, the only reasonably functioning and debugged sections of
Sexpert are the introductory and repertoire modules. The diagnostic
modules have been redesigned but not reimplemented; the therapeutic
modules have not yet been implemented. Our major difficulty in com-

pleting Sexpert has been financial. Granting agencies have shown almost no interest in funding the project for a variety of reasons: lack of confidence in the idea; low priority for sexual dysfunction research; and reluctance to fund development research once basic principles have been demonstrated.

In the course of this project, we have been approached by numerous software companies who were interested in commercializing Sexpert. Most of these companies were interested only in funding a finished product and were not willing to undertake significant development or validation costs. Several companies who considered funding development dropped the idea after their marketing studies confirmed our data that people generally considered the idea of a computer sex counselor unappealing. We did receive two offers that would have funded development; however, we turned both of these down. The first offer was contingent on us quitting our jobs, moving to another city, and devoting ourselves full time to the project. We turned the second offer down for similar reasons, but also because, had we accepted it, we felt that we would not be able to control the level of professional development. As a result, research and development concerning Sexpert is no longer continuing and there is little prospect that it will start again in the near future.

Our experiences dealing with commercial software companies forced us to directly consider the "ethics" of developing self-help software. Clearly all new interventions carry significant unknown risks and we were reluctant to "publish" Sexpert without what we considered adequate validation studies. The self-help book industry was launched without any professional standards and yet these unvalidated texts were accepted and integrated into clinical practice with little reluctance. It is only recently that professional standards have been retroactively developed (Rosen, 1981) to regulate what is already a decades-old intervention. We feel that reversing this process and pursuing outcome studies first will encourage serious development and protect the public without infringing upon freedom of speech.

Despite the fact that Sexpert will probably never be "finished," we feel that the project has been worthwhile from a variety of perspectives. We believe that we have demonstrated the feasibility of a computerized sex counselor and that it is just a matter of time before one is completed. Technological advances in the last 10 years have now made possible new features that will greatly enhance the attraction and power of such systems. For example, the easy integration of multimedia into expert systems now makes it possible to create a version of Sexpert where couples will interact with an image of a therapist that responds to them in natural language. The growth of computer networks has solved much of the problem of the delivery of self-help computer services to the home. Advances in hardware technology have erased most of the memory and programming limits with which we had to contend early in the project.

New programming approaches such as neural networks provide alternative ways of solving difficult diagnostic problems.

The diagnostic portion of the project has also confirmed our view that, to a large extent, the diagnosis of sexual problems is a social construction with large grey areas unsupported by data. It seems unlikely to us that it will be ever be possible to write a set of formal rules to define most sexual dysfunctions because such definitions are dependent on social expectations that change over time and across cultures. Modern sexual diagnostic systems such as the DSM-IV or the multiaxial problem-oriented system (Schover, Friedman, Weiler, Heiman, & LoPiccolo, 1982) indirectly acknowledge this by leaving much to the judgment of the therapist or by using arbitrary diagnostic cutoff points. The most recent diagnostic module of Sexpert deals with this necessary uncertainty by telling couples whose sexual behavior falls into these grey areas that they have to decide whether or not to consider their sexual behavior problematic. Consider for example: a 30-year-old male who fails to achieve or maintain an erection on about 15% of all attempts at intercourse; or a woman who is orgasmic with her partner about a third of the time; or a man who ejaculates after about 4 minutes of intercourse; or a woman who feels desire about once every 2 weeks. We can currently construct a set of diagnostic rules to deal with each of these-cases, but we are unlikely most of the time to insist that each of the above is or is not a problem until a couple construes it as such. Moreover, 30 years ago, the arguments or diagnostic rules we would have accepted would have been quite different.

One unexpected result of the project was our discovery that expert systems may be a highly effective training tool. A variety of trainees at our hospital spent a considerable amount of time interacting with Sexpert because it gave them the opportunity to simulate and experience a relatively large number of cases without having to actually see them. We believe that the training potential of most expert systems has been left unexploited. In addition, the existence of such systems also opens the possibility of empirically testing longstanding issues in psychotherapy research concerning the essential nature of the therapeutic alliance and the importance of nonverbal cues in diagnosis.

More than our previous research, this project forced us to confront our attitudes regarding the media. Despite, or perhaps because of, the fact that initial attitudes in the general population toward computerized sex therapy were not positive, the media exhibited a marked fascination with Sexpert. One casual interview David Servan–Schreiber gave to a local reporter in Pittsburgh in the mid 1980s was picked up by the wire services and resulted in newspaper articles appearing all over the world. Our initial reaction to this was to avoid all further contact with reporters, but articles continued to appear anyway. One the one hand, we were pleased that the media took such a positive view of our work; on the other, we were suspicious about its history of portraying sex in a sensationalistic fashion. We ultimately began to respond to requests from what we perceived as reputable sources (e.g., Software fur die Seele, 1994; McAuliffe, 1991; *The Jennie Jones Show*, 1991; *Visa Santé*, 1991) both to insure accurate portrayal of information about Sexpert and to try to raise development money for completion of the project. We did not achieve the second goal but found the media's portrayal of our work quite accurate and insightful.

Conclusion

The research conducted on Sexpert confirms that, before exposure to the program, individuals have difficulty conceiving of a computer as an adequate sex counselor and consistently rank it as the worst possible source of sexual information and advice. More importantly, however, this research strongly suggests that, once people interact with the program, their views change dramatically. One short interaction overturns a lifetime of cultural conditioning, and the computer–sexuality association becomes not only conceivable, but highly positive. What could explain such a drastic change of mind, or maybe even heart?

We might turn to the properties of the program to explain the change: its humanlike manner of discourse, its ability to address the specific issues raised by the user, and its varied information. We might also turn to a cultural notion that is easily debunked because it lies in some unfounded, sci-fi nightmare scenario where machines rob us of our humanity. It is most likely that both explanations contribute to the change of attitude we witnessed in the laboratory. The challenge, however, lies in the export of this attitude change from the laboratory to the real world.

We hope that our experience with Sexpert will provide the basis for the development of future expert systems for sexual counseling that will offer professional level advice and merit the marketing effort. In principle, a number of health promotion campaigns that have enjoyed substantial success in the past 20 years have been up against similar obstacles. Antismoking advertising continues to combat an ingrained cultural notion that smoking is an index of sophistication, attractiveness, and, for women, a liberation from gender stereotypes. The anticholesterol, antifat foods campaign must counter the hedonic forces of pleasure and convenience. Dental care, to most people an aversive experience, has also been promoted very successfully.

Although neglect of sexual functioning may not be life threatening, a healthy sex life would surely be ranked by most people as at least as important as being cellulite and cavity free. In a culture preoccupied with sexual desirability and stellar performance, the more moderate goal of healthy sexual functioning should not be such a hard sell.

References

Alemi, F., Cherry, F., & Meffert, G. (1989). Rehearsing decisions may help teenagers: An evaluation of a simulation game. *Computers in Biology and Medicine, 19*, 283–290.

Agras, W.S., Taylor, C.B., Feldman, D.E., Losch, M., & Burnett, K.F. (1990). Developing computer-assisted therapy for the treatment of obesity. *Behavior Therapy, 21*, 99–109.

Baskin, D. (Ed.). (1990). *Computer applications in psychiatry and psychology.* New York: Bruner/Mazel.

Binik, Y.M., Servan–Schreiber, D., Freiwald, S., & Hall, K.S. (1988). Intelligent computer-based assessment and psychotherapy: An expert system for sexual dysfunction. *Journal of Nervous and Mental Disease, 178*, 387–400.

Binik, Y.M., Westbury, C.F., & Servan–Schreiber, D. (1989). Interaction with a "sex-expert" system enhances attitudes towards computerized sex therapy. *Behavior Research and Therapy, 27*, 303–306.

Binik, Y.M., Meana M., & Sand, N. (1994). Interaction with a sex-expert system changes attitudes and may modify sexual behavior. *Computers in Human Behavior, 10*, 395–410.

Bloom, B.L. (1992). Computer assisted psychological intervention: A review and commentary. *Clinical Psychology Review, 12*, 169–198.

Cammell, D. (Director). (1977). *Demon Seed* [Film]. MGM/UA Home Video, New York.

Erdman, H.P., Klein, M.H., & Greist, J.H. (1985). Direct patient computer interviewing. *Journal of Consulting and Clinical Psychology, 53*, 760–773.

DeMuth, P. (1984). Eliza and her offspring. In M.D. Schwartz (Ed.), *Using computers in clinical practice* (pp. 321–327). New York: Haworth.

Ghosh, A., & Marks, I.M. (1987). Self-treatment of agoraphobià by exposure. *Behavior Therapy, 18*, 3–16.

Intracourse [Computer Software]. (1985). Miami, FL: Intracorp Inc.

The Jennie Jones Show. (August 1991). Chicago, IL: National Broadcasting Corporation (never broadcast).

Kann, L.K. (1987). Effects of computer-assisted instruction on selected interaction skills related to responsible sexuality. *Journal of School Health, 57*, 282–2897.

Katz, M.R. (1984). Computer-assisted guidance: A walkthrough with running comments. *Journal of Counseling aned Development, 63*, 153–157.

Lieff, J.D. (1987). *Computer applications in psychiatry.* Washington, DC: American Psychiatric Association Press.

McCullough, L., Farrell, A.D., & Longabaugh, R. (1986). The development of a microcomputer-based mental health information system. *American Psychologist, 41*, 207–214.

McAuliffe, K. (1991). Computer shrinks. *Self*, July, 103–105.

Miller, M.J. (Session Chair). (1994, April). *Computerized evaluation and treatment in mental health.* 1st International Conference on Computational Medicine, Austin, TX.

Ochs, E.P., Meana, M., Mah, K., & Binik, Y. (1993). The effects of exposure to different sources of sexual information on sexual behavior: Comparing a "sex-expert system" to other educational material. *Behavior Research Methods, Instruments, & Computers, 25*, 189–194.

Ochs, E.P., Meana, M., Paré, L., Mah, K., & Binik, Y.M. (1994). Learning about sex outside the gutter: Attitudes toward a computer sex-expert system. *Journal of Sex and Marital Therapy*, *20*, 86–102.

Ochs, E., Meana, M., & Binik, Y.M. (1995). Unpublished data.

Plutchik, R., & Karasu, T.B. (1991). Computers in psychotherapy: An Overview. *Computers in Human Behavior*, *7*, 33–44.

Reitman, R. (1982). Treating erection problems (Version 1.0) [Computer Software]. Woodland Hills, CA: PSYCOMP.

ROR-SCAN (Version 3) [Computer Software]. (1991). Las Vegas, NV: ROR-SCAN.

Rosen, G.M. (1981). Guidelines for the review of do-it-yourself treatment books. *Contemporary Psychology*, *26*, 189–191.

Schover, L., Friedman, J.M., Weiler, S.J., Heiman, J.R., & LoPiccolo, J. (1982). Multiaxial problem-oriented system for sexual dysfunctions: An alternative to DSM-III. *Archives of General Psychiatry*, *39*, 614–619.

Selmi, P.M., Klein, M.H., Greist, J.H., Sorrell, S.P., & Erdman, H.P. (1990). Computer-administered cognitive-behavioral therapy for depression. *American Journal of Psychiatry*, *147*, 51–56.

Servan–Schreiber, D., & Binik, Y.M. (1989). Extending the intelligent tutoring system paradigm: Sex therapy as intelligent tutoring. *Computers in Human Behavior*, *5*, 241–259.

Schneider, S. (Chair). (1994, August). *Computers and the delivery of services in health psychology*. Symposium conducted at the meeting of the American Psychological Association, Los Angeles, CA.

Software fur die Seele. (1994). *Der Spiegel*, *36*, 116–119.

Ustun, T.B. (Ed.). (1994). *Computers in mental health*. Essex, UK: Longman Group Limited.

Visa santé. [Broadcast]. (December 18, 1991). Canadian Broadcasting Corporation.

Wagman, M. (1988). *Computer psychotherapy systems: Theory and research foundations*. New York: Gordon & Breach.

3
Computerized Assessment System for Psychotherapy Evaluation and Research (CASPER): Development and Current Status

Albert D. Farrell and Leigh McCullough–Vaillant

There is a clear need within the mental health field for methods to facilitate the routine collection of treatment outcome data (Barlow, Hayes, & Nelson, 1984; Moreland, Fowler, & Honaker, 1994). Such methods could be used to address increasing concerns about the effectiveness and cost-efficiency of mental health services raised by the government and third party payers by enabling practitioners to document the effectiveness of their interventions (Banta & Saxe, 1983). By continuously tracking clients' progress during treatment, practitioners could determine if a particular treatment plan is achieving its desired goals and could implement changes as needed. In addition to examining the impact of treatment on individual cases, aggregating these data across cases could provide a basis for more naturalistic research on the effectiveness of psychotherapy outside of typical research settings. Outcome data could also be useful for administrative purposes. For example, individual practitioners could examine their relative success with different types of clients, or community mental health centers could examine the characteristics of the clients they serve.

Although there is much to be gained by collecting outcome data, there are many obstacles that have prevented this from becoming a routine practice. Most practitioners find it difficult to fit data collection, management, and program evaluation into their busy schedules. Moreover, the field has made little progress toward the development of any standardized approach to assessing outcome (Kazdin, 1992). Broad-based measures of overall client functioning may be applicable to most clients, but not sufficiently sensitive to specific treatment changes. On the other hand, tailoring measures to specific disorders may result in wide variations in the instruments selected, making data management and comparisons across clients difficult. Practitioners may also have a difficult time selecting from the thousands of assessment instruments available (Reichelt, 1984).

One promising approach to tracking progress in treatment is the assessment of target complaints, or target problems. This method asks clients to identify and rate the specific problems for which they are seeking treatment (Battle et al., 1966). Unlike standardized instruments that evaluate all clients on identical dimensions, target complaints represent a more idiographic or individualized approach that focuses on the specific concerns presented by individual clients. This approach attempts to avoid the outcome-uniformity myth or the notion that the effects of different treatments can be assessed on a single outcome dimension (Kiesler, 1971). This approach also attempts to increase sensitivity to treatment effects by assessing outcome dimensions specifically related to clients' presenting problems (Mintz & Kiesler, 1982). Although assessment of target problems appears to be a promising method, concerns have been expressed about the variation in the methods used to identify and rate target problems (Mintz & Kiesler, 1982). Target problems are typically identified during an interview by asking clients to report the specific problems they want to have changed in treatment. There are, however, no guidelines for when to group related problems together, how many problems to probe for, or the specific type of rating scales that should be used to assess target problems. Mintz and Kiesler (1982) argued strongly for the development of a standardized approach to the assessment of target problems.

Computer-based interviewing, in which clients respond directly to questions presented on a computer screen or monitor, represents a possible method for standardizing the collection of data on target problems. Several early examples of computer-based interviews were designed to identify clients' presenting problems (e.g., Angle, Johnsen, Grebenkemper, & Ellinwood, 1979; Greist, Klein, & Van Cura, 1973). Since then a number of computer-based interviews have been developed to collect general information about psychiatric and social history, and to address specific areas such as suicide risk, alcohol and drug use, sexual dysfunction, and mental status (Erdman, Klein, & Greist, 1985). This approach offers several advantages over human interviewing. Erdman et al. (1985) noted that computer interviews are: (a) reliable in that they always ask the questions they are supposed to; (b) have the potential for being less uncomfortable or embarrassing to the client because they do not respond to the client's answers to sensitive questions; and (c) provide a complete record of responses to every question. Although practitioners have been skeptical about clients' reactions to computer-based interviews, there are considerable data to indicate that clients are both capable of completing computer interviews and that they typically respond positively to them. Indeed, several studies have found that some clients prefer answering questions to the computer rather than to a human, and that under certain conditions, their responses may be more candid (Erdman et al., 1985).

This chapter describes the Computerized Assessment System for Psychotherapy Evaluation and Research (CASPER; Farrell & McCullough, 1989; McCullough & Farrell, 1989), a computer system designed to facilitate the collection of psychotherapy outcome data. CASPER includes a computer interview to collect basic information about clients' functioning, and to identify and assess the severity of their target problems. Additional modules within CASPER are used to assess these problem areas during the course of treatment and at termination. CASPER also collects client and therapist data on global measures of functioning and satisfaction with treatment. In this chapter we describe CASPER and how it can be used at different points in treatment, and present the results of several studies that have evaluated this system. We close with a discussion of some of the strengths and weaknesses of this approach.

Development of System

CASPER was modeled after the Major Problem Rating System (MPRS), a computer-based interview developed by Stevenson, McCullough, Longabaugh, and Stout (1989). The MPRS was designed to support a problem-oriented approach to record keeping and treatment by providing a standardized format for identifying and rating major problem areas. Rather than asking clients to list problems in their own words, the MPRS used a computer interview to identify their target problems. The target problems included in the MPRS were based on a coding system developed and validated for use with problem-oriented psychiatric records (Longabaugh, Fowler, Stout, & Kriebel, 1983). These problems represented the most frequently identified problem areas for a sample of over 800 psychiatric patients. The MPRS also included four or five questions designed to probe each problem area. If clients' responses to the items in a particular category suggested they were having difficulties in that area, they were asked if the target problem associated with those items was a major problem. Clients completed the MPRS using a computer terminal connected to a mainframe computer. The problems identified for each client were listed in a report, and clients were contacted by telephone after treatment and asked to rate their degree of improvement on each problem. The validity of the MPRS was established through a series of analyses that examined its factor structure and correlations with a variety of established measures (Stevenson et al., 1989).

CASPER was initially conceived as a microcomputer version of the MPRS. At the time of its development, microcomputers were just becoming widely available (McCullough, Farrell, & Longabaugh, 1984). We felt that a microcomputer-based version would facilitate the use of this system among practitioners who did not have access to a mainframe computer. By the time the first version of CASPER was completed in 1983, it differed from the MPRS in a number of other ways. The MPRS included

280 interview items and required almost an hour for most clients to complete. CASPER included 127 questions and required about 35 minutes to complete. The content validity of the specific items included in the CASPER interview was established through a content analysis of more than 25 of the most commonly used intake instruments (McCullough, Longabaugh, & DePina, 1985). CASPER also provides a more thorough assessment of target problems. For each problem identified during the interview, clients are asked to indicate how long it has been a major problem for them and to rate its severity during the past week. Consistent with Hayes and Nelson's (1986) recommendations for program evaluation, CASPER was designed to permit continuous assessment of outcome by allowing clients to rate severity and improvement for each of their target problems during the course of treatment and after completion of treatment. Finally, CASPER enables therapists to revise their clients' problem lists and rate their progress on each problem directly on the computer at any point during treatment.

CASPER has gone through two revisions since the first version was completed in 1983. The original version was· written for the Apple II microcomputer. In 1984 the first DOS version (Version 2) was developed. This version was implemented successfully at the Center for Psychological Services and Development (CPSD), an outpatient training clinic for the doctoral programs in clinical and counseling psychology at Virginia Commonwealth University, that same year. In 1988, CASPER was revised based on analyses of data from several hundred cases. This process included a content analysis of the problems clients entered in their own words at the end of the CASPER interview. Several changes were made in the content of the CASPER interview: (a) Items were added to assess satisfaction with relationships for individuals who were not married; (b) items in the interpersonal category were revised to include dimensions of interpersonal behavior described by Horowitz, Weckler, and Doren (1983); (c) questions about sexual activity were revised and a question about affectional preference was added; and (d) questions were added about concerns regarding religious beliefs and concerns about contracting a disease. Thresholds linking probe questions to target problems were also set lower to ensure that clients were asked about relevant target problems. Finally, the scale for assessing the severity of problems was changed from an 11-point scale to a 5-point anchored scale. A new rating dimension was also added to assess the extent to which clients wanted to focus on each target problem during treatment.

Using CASPER at Different Points in Treatment

CASPER was designed to enable practitioners to identify target problems and track them throughout the course of treatment. This system includes modules that provide practitioners with several methods for accomplishing this goal. In addition to the interview, there are modules for obtaining problem ratings from clients and therapists and a module that prints individualized paper-and-pencil outcome measures. This section describes how of each of these components may be used at each stage of treatment. An overview of this process is presented in Figure 1.

Intake Procedure

Use of CASPER begins by having clients complete a computer interview. This interview takes an average of 35 minutes and must be completed before any other CASPER data are collected. The interview includes 122 questions representing 18 content categories (see Fig. 2), and 62 target problems linked to these questions. Consistent with Nelson's (1981) call for realistic dependent measures, the majority of interview questions focus on the frequency of behaviors within a specified time period. For most questions, clients are asked to report the number of days in the past month in which a specific behavior occurred at least once (e.g., "About how many days in the past month have you had problems with losing your temper, or hitting or throwing things?"). Other formats include Likert-type scales, and multiple choice responses.

Clients use the keyboard to respond to items presented on the computer screen. They also have the option of skipping questions or going back to change their response to a previous question. The program checks each response to determine if it is a numeric value in the acceptable range for that question and prompts the client to reenter their answer if necessary. The computer also uses branching to determine if particular questions are relevant to a particular client. For example, clients that indicate that they are *married* or *living with someone* are asked a series of questions about their spouse or partner. Other clients are asked if they are currently involved in a relationship. Those who are in such a relationship are asked about their satisfaction with it.

Branching is also used to link interview questions to each of the 62 target problems. If a client endorses a particular pattern of responses to the interview items, they are asked if the target problem linked to those items is a major problem. Major problem is defined as "something causing you great personal distress or interfering with your daily functioning." For example, clients are asked if trouble with sleep is a major problem for them if they (a) indicate they averaged less than 6 hours of sleep per night in the past month, (b) had difficulty falling asleep or staying asleep more than four times in the past month, (c) reported early wakenings more than four times in the past month, or (d) rated their sleep as poor or very poor. Thresholds are low to ensure that clients are asked about relevant major problems.

After all of the appropriate items have been asked, clients are presented with each target problem they identified and asked to rate it on the

Intake

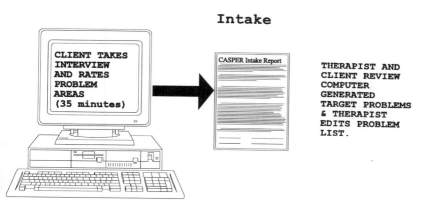

During Treatment

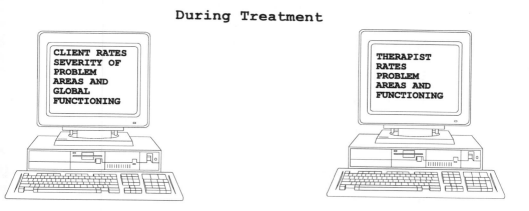

Termination and/or Followup

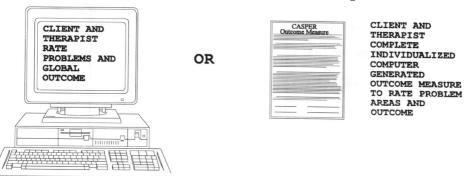

Figure 1. Use of CASPER to monitor and evaluate treatment.

1. **HEALTH AND PHYSICAL SYMPTOMS** (e.g., headaches, pains, stomach/digestive problems, energy level, days of sick leave).

2. **MOOD** (e.g., depression, anxiety, irritability, lack of feelings).

3. **THOUGHT PROBLEMS** (e.g., halucinations, racing thoughts, paranoid thoughts, memory).

4. **SLEEP** (e.g., hours, sleep difficulty).

5. **EATING BEHAVIOR** (e.g., weight gain or loss, appetite problems).

6. **CHEMICAL DEPENDENCE** (e.g., use of alchol and other drugs, extent to which use effects relationships with family, work, and health).

7. **UNWANTED REPEATED BEHAVIOR** (e.g., obsessive behaviors, anger management).

8. **SUICIDAL THOUGHTS AND BEHAVIOR**.

9. **LIFE TASKS** (work, school, housework).

10. **LEISURE TIME**.

11. **INTERPERSONAL BEHAVIOR** (e.g. assertiveness, concern about others, dependence).

12. **SOCIAL SUPPORT**.

13. **RELATIONSHIPS** (satisfaction with marriage or other relationship, children, and family).

14. **SEXUAL BEHAVIOR** (e.g., orientation, frequency, problem areas).

15. **SELF-CONCEPT**.

16. **ENVIRONMENTAL** (e.g., living situation, financial, legal).

17. **LIFE SATISFACTION**.

18. **OVERALL FUNCTIONING** (i.e., distress, socialization, ability to function).

19. **OTHER PROBLEMS NOT INCLUDED ABOVE**.

Figure 2. Outline of CASPER interview content.

following scales: (a) "About how long has the following been a major problem for you?" (1. *Less than 2 weeks*, 2. *2–4 weeks*, 3. *1–6 months*, 4. *7–12 months*, 5. *1–5 years*, 6. *5–10 years*, 7. *Over 10 years*); (b) "How much did the following problem bother you during the past week?" (1. *Not at all*, 2. *Slightly*, 3. *Moderately*, 4. *Severely*, 5. *Couldn't be worse*); and (c) "How much do you want the following problem to be focused on during your therapy or counseling?" (1. *I do not want to deal with this problem*, 2. *I want this problem to receive some attention*, 3. *I want this problem to receive a moderate amount of attention*, 4. *I want this problem to receive a great deal of attention*, 5. *I want this problem to be the main focus*). Clients are also asked if they have any additional target problems. If they answer *yes*, they can enter up to eight problems in their own words using the computer keyboard. These problems, including the clients' descriptions, are included in their data files and rated on the same dimensions as their other target problems.

At the end of the interview, clients' responses are stored in a data base system. All future data associated with each client are linked to these initial intake data. These data are also used to print a five to eight page report listing clients' answers to each interview question and their target problems, including the ratings of duration, severity, and priority for treatment.

Using CASPER During Treatment

There are several options for using CASPER to monitor progress during treatment. Clients can repeat the full interview or complete an abbreviated interview that collects ratings on therapy process and outcome, but does not include the interview items. Clients may be asked to enter the data directly into the computer or on an individualized paper-and-pencil measure. Therapists can also use either method to rate their clients' progress.

The process for completing the CASPER interview during treatment is similar to the intake process. Clients respond to the same questions and are asked to identify target problems based on their responses. After answering the interview questions, clients are again asked to rate their target problems. For any new problems that are identified, clients are asked to indicate their duration. Clients are asked to rate the severity of each of their problems using the same scale as at intake. During the course of treatment clients are asked to rate how much each problem has been focused on during treatment instead of how much they want it to be focused on. Ratings of severity and treatment focus are obtained not just for the problems they identified during the current interview, but also for any problems that were identified during previous interviews. Clients are also asked to rate their therapists on three 5-point process dimensions: "How well do you feel your therapist understood you during your most recent session?"; "How interested, concerned or involved did you feel your therapist was during your most recent session?"; and "How genuine or sincere did you feel your therapist was during your most recent session?".

As an alternative, clients can complete a short version of this interview that does not include the probes for each target problem. This version simply asks clients to rate the severity and treatment focus of each of their problems, rate their overall functioning on three global scales, and complete the three process ratings of their therapist. This reduced interview takes between 3 and 10 minutes depending upon the number of problems being rated.

To facilitate the collection of outcome data, CASPER can generate a paper-and-pencil form of the short version of the interview. This form can be printed in advance and used when it is not convenient for clients to use the computer. Unlike most paper-and-pencil measures, CASPER prints an individualized measure tailored to each individual client. This measure lists the target problems for each client and asks the client to rate each one on severity and treatment focus.

Data can also be obtained from therapists at any point during treatment. Therapists have the option of modifying a client's problem list by deleting problems they do not wish to monitor, adding problems, or entering other problems in their own words. All future assessments are based on these modified problem lists. Therapists can also enter diagnostic data and comments into their clients' data files. Finally, therapists can complete a short interview to record progress during treatment. In this interview, therapists rate their clients' functioning on each of the three global scales, and the severity of each of the clients' problem areas and how much they have focused on it during treatment. Therapists also rate their clients on three process variables: "How motivated was this client during your most recent session?"; "How resistant to interpretations or discussions of unpleasant or sensitive topics was this client during your most recent session?"; "How likeable was this client during your most recent session?". As with clients, a paper-and-pencil version of this scale is available.

Using CASPER at Termination or Follow-Up

The process for using CASPER to assess clients at the end of treatment is similar to the process used during treatment. Clients can retake the full CASPER interview or the short form. The paper-and-pencil form can be mailed to clients when they terminate unexpectedly or to collect follow-up data. Therapists can also rate clients' progress on either form. The data obtained at the end of treatment differ slightly from data collected at the earlier time points. As before, clients are asked to rate their functioning on the three dimensions and to rate their therapist on the three global process dimensions. In addition to rating each problem's severity and focus during treatment, clients are asked to rate how each problem has changed since they started treatment on the following scale: "How much has this problem changed since you started counseling or therapy?" (1. *Problem is worse now*, 2. *No change*, 3. *Problem is a little better*, 4. *Problem is moderately better*, 5. *Problem is much better*). This procedure is in line with Mintz and Kiesler's (1982) suggestion that both severity and change measures be assessed for target problems. Clients are also asked to rate their overall satisfaction with treatment on the following three scales: "How would you rate your overall level of satisfaction with the therapy or counseling you received?" (1. *Very dissatisfied*, 2. *Dissatisfied*, 3. *Neither satisfied nor dissatisfied*, 4. *Satisfied*, 5. *Very satisfied*); (b) "How would you rate the overall success of your therapy or counseling?" (1. *Not at all successful*, 2. *Somewhat successful*, 3. *Moderately successful*, 4. *Very successful*, 5. *Extremely successful*); and (c) "In general, how are you doing now compared to when you started therapy or counseling?" (1. *Worse now*, 2. *No change*, 3. *A little better*, 4. *Moderately better*, 5. *Much better*). Similarly, therapists rate clients on the three overall functioning scales, the three process measures, the three measures of overall treatment effect, and rate each clients' target problems for severity, focus during treatment, and change.

Evaluation of CASPER

CASPER has been evaluated at two sites—a university-based training clinic and a counseling center. As previously mentioned, CASPER was first implemented in 1984 as a routine part of the intake procedure at the CPSD at Virginia Commonwealth University. Data collected at the CPSD formed the basis of a study examining the reliability and validity of Version 2 of CASPER (Farrell, Camplair, & McCullough, 1987), and several studies currently in progress examining the reliability and validity of Version 3. In 1989, Version 3 of CASPER was implemented as a routine part of the intake procedure at the university counseling center at a major public university in the midwestern United States. Data from this site have been used to examine scale properties and client reactions to CASPER, and to develop a categorization scheme for classifying clients' presenting problems (Heppner et al., 1994).

Client Reactions to CASPER

Data on clients' reactions to completing the CASPER intake interview have been routinely gathered at both sites where the system has been used. Multiple-choice questions are included at the end of the interview to assess clients' prior experience with computers and their reactions to the computer interview. Responses to these questions were available from 305 clients at the CPSD and 589 clients at the university counseling center. Very few clients at either site had strong negative reactions to the interview process; less than 4% of the clients in both samples described the interview as *very unpleasant*, and about 18% described it as *somewhat unpleasant*. Interpreting these data is difficult in that we are not aware of comparable data on clients' reactions to traditional intake interviews. Nearly 80% of the clients in both samples indicated that the questions were *not at all difficult*. Most clients (85%) reported that their responses to the interview described them at least *adequately*. When asked whether they felt it was easier to answer personal questions on the computer or to a human interviewer, 26% of the CPSD clients and 37% of the counseling center clients indicated that it was *much easier* or *a little easier* on the computer; 29% of the CPSD clients and 20% of the counseling center clients indicated that it was *about the same*; and 45% of the CPSD clients and 42% of the counseling center clients reported it was *much easier* or *a little easier* to a human. In general, we have found that most clients are able to complete the CASPER interview with minimal assistance. When clients have difficulty, it is usually because of poor reading ability. Our experience is consistent with previous studies that have found little difficulty implementing computer interviews with a variety of client populations (Erdman et al., 1985).

Reliability

Several studies have examined the internal consistency of CASPER interview questions within content categories. In general, we expect only moderate internal consistency among items within categories. Interview items were selected to cover the domain within each category, but not to be redundant. Moreover, we recommend examining responses to individual interview questions rather than calculating summary scores. Farrell et al. (1987) calculated alpha coefficients assessing the internal consistency of items within each of the 13 content areas in Version 2 of CASPER. Most of these coefficients were moderately high with a mean of 0.59. Low coefficients were typically found for categories with a small number of items; the mean alpha coefficient for categories with more than 4 items was 0.69. Heppner et al. (1994) examined the internal consistency of seven CASPER categories and reported alpha coefficients ranging from 0.45 to 0.93, with a mean of 0.73. They also defined a 17-item global distress scale that had an alpha of 0.75.

Analyses have also been conducted to determine the test–retest reliability or the extent to which clients' problem lists remain stable during treatment. Burijon and Farrell (1989) investigated the stability of target problems for a sample of CPSD clients who completed the CASPER interview at three time points: (a) intake, (b) 3 weeks into treatment, and (c) 6 weeks into treatment. A total of 19 subjects completed intake and 3 week assessments, and 12 completed all three assessments. Kappa coefficients representing agreement on the presence or absence of individual client problem areas across the time points indicated considerable variability in the stability of specific target problems over time. Clients identified an average of 3.2 *new* target problems at the 3 week interview and 2.6 new target problems at the 6 week interview. Results of this study were consistent with those of Sorenson, Gorsuch, and Mintz (1985) who examined the stability of target problems obtained using a standardized interview format. These findings underscore the importance of assessing target problems continuously during treatment. Researchers and practitioners using target problems as an outcome measure need to be certain that they assess target problems frequently enough to obtain a stable problem list.

The reliability of the CASPER intake interview was also assessed by comparing the target problems identified by CASPER to problems identified by intake clinicians who independently completed a problem checklist (Farrell et al., 1987). Results of this study indicated that clients reported nearly three times as many problems on the computer interview than the clinicians reported on the checklist. Clients identified an average of 9.4 target problems (SD = 6.9) compared to an average of 3.4 (SD = 3.9) identified by intake clinicians. Kappa coefficients representing the agreement between CASPER and the intake clinicians on the presence or absence of individual target problems were generally low. Farrell et al. attributed this low rate of agreement to several factors including differences in perspective between clients and therapists, and the use of an unstandardized intake interview rather than a more structured format. These findings parallel those of other studies that have reported a tendency for clients to report a greater number of problems during computer interviews (Angle et al., 1979; McCullough, 1981). Whether this represents a more complete picture of clients' presenting concerns or a tendency for clients to overreport problems is not clear. In either case, this suggests that computer interviews provide a more conservative approach by presenting a longer list of problem areas that practitioners can then narrow down to the key problem areas to be focused on in treatment.

Validity

The validity of CASPER data collected at intake was investigated by Farrell et al. (1987) who examined correlations between CASPER interview data and several concurrent measures including the Symptoms Checklist-90 (SCL-90; Derogatis, 1977) and the Minnesota Multiphasic Personality Inventory (MMPI). To determine the validity of CASPER as an overall measure of functioning, several global indices were calculated from the target problems data for each client. In general, the number of problems showed the strongest relationships with measures of global functioning on the SCL-90 and MMPI. These correlations were all significant and ranged from 0.45 to 0.54. The validity of the target problem summary indices was also supported by the pattern of correlations between these indices and the MMPI validity scales. In particular, none of these indices was significantly correlated with the Lie scale of the MMPI. This suggests that endorsement of target problems was not influenced by social desirability. Farrell et al. (1987) also examined the validity of individual severity ratings for 21 of the problem areas assessed on CASPER by correlating these ratings with relevant scales on the SCL-90 and MMPI. A total of 31 of the 37 correlations calculated were significant at $p < 0.05$. CASPER also demonstrated good discriminant validity in that these correlations were generally much higher than correlations between measures of unrelated target problems.

Further support for the concurrent validity of CASPER was found in a recently completed study of 289 outpatients who completed Version 3 of CASPER, the Beck Depression Inventory (BDI; Beck, Ward, Mendelson, Mack, & Erbaugh, 1961) and the Brief Symptom Inventory (BSI; Derogatis & Spencer, 1982) at intake (Farrell, 1995). Correlations between measures of overall functioning derived from the CASPER interview and measures of overall functioning on the BSI were all moderately high and significant at $p < 0.001$. As in previous research, the strongest correlations were with the number of problems identified by CASPER. Clients identified an average of 13.6 problems (SD = 9.29). This index correlated at 0.74 with the Global Severity Index of the BSI and 0.63 with the BSI Positive Symptom Total. Severity ratings for specific problem areas on CASPER were also significantly correlated with corresponding scales on the BSI and with the BDI. Particularly strong correlations were found between ratings of five CASPER major problems related to depression and the BDI. These ranged from 0.32 to 0.52, with a median value of 0.48.

Discussion

CASPER was designed to address the need for methods to facilitate the routine collection of clinical outcome data. Use of a computer interview provides an efficient method for collecting these data that requires minimal time from practitioners and provides a standardized approach that can be used across different sites. The equipment needed to run this system, an IBM-compatible microcomputer and printer, is already in the office of most practitioners (Farrell, 1989), making this system easily incorporated into a variety of settings ranging from offices of individual practitioners to community mental health centers. The system offers options for collecting data at different points in treatment. Intake data include information about clients' functioning across a broad range of areas, their specific presenting problems, the severity of these problems, and the extent to which they wish to focus on them in treatment. During the course of treatment, this system provides an efficient method for monitoring changes in the severity of these problems and the extent to which they are being focused on in treatment from the perspective of both client and therapist. Within this system, therapists have the flexibility of selecting the problems they wish to monitor during treatment. After treatment, this system makes it possible to collect data from clients and therapists on their perceptions of improvement in overall functioning and in specific target areas, and their overall satisfaction with treatment. This system represents an idiographic approach to assessment in that it individualizes the outcome criteria to each client. This addresses some of the concerns about nomothetic approaches that focus on a single problem rather than addressing all of a client's problems (Persons, 1991). Unlike most idiographic approaches, however, it employs a standard set of target problems that makes it possible to aggregate these data across different clients. These data could be used for a variety of clinical, administrative, training, and research purposes.

CASPER data collected at each stage of treatment could have considerable clinical value. The intake report provides a broad-based assessment of functioning in specific areas. Collecting and recording this information within a traditional clinical interview would be tedious and time consuming. Practitioners could make more efficient use of their time by using the information provided by the CASPER intake report as a starting point for a more focused interview of their clients' current concerns. Therapists could then modify their clients' problem lists to include the specific areas they wish to focus on during treatment. Monitoring progress on these problems could help practitioners determine if their interventions were having the desired impact and enable them to make changes when needed. By closely monitoring outcome, practitioners would be constantly challenged to improve their delivery of services, test their theoretical systems, and decide upon better treatment strategies (Hayes & Nelson, 1986). Moreland et al. (1994) argue for the importance of collecting outcome data throughout the course of treatment to help practitioners determine when it is appropriate to terminate treatment. They suggest that CASPER, or a system like it, could ultimately lead to a more objective basis for clinical decision making and for documenting the effectiveness of services. McCullough–Vaillant and Vaillant (in press) have used the target problems approach to monitor treatment progress every five sessions. Working closely with patients to assess changes in presenting problems assists clinicians under the demands of managed care to keep focused and actively working toward change.

There is also much to be gained by aggregating data across clients. Individual practitioners or clinic directors could use the target problems data collected by CASPER at intake to construct profiles of the clients they serve. For example, CASPER data collected at the counseling center referred to earlier, were used to construct a profile of the demographic characteristics and most frequent presenting problems for clients seen within a specific academic year. These data were prepared to help document the serious need for services among their student body. By identifying the types of problems for which clients are seeking treatment and examining changes in these patterns over time, administrators can determine the resources needed to tailor their services to the changing needs of their client population. Collecting outcome data adds to the possibilities. Such data can be used to determine the overall effectiveness of a facility, to examine the relative effectiveness of different options for delivering services (e.g., group versus individual treatment), or to examine the effectiveness of services for clients with particular presenting problems. These data could also be linked to other client data to address a variety of important issues. For example, linking outcome data and client characteristics to data on the number of sessions for a particular type of treatment could be used to determine the average length of treatment for a specific presenting problem. More refined analyses could identify client variables that suggest the need for a more extended treatment approach. This approach would be more empirically driven and sensitive to client characteristics than rigid systems that specify a fixed number of sessions for specific disorders.

CASPER could also be useful during training. We have used CASPER in the training clinic for the doctoral programs in clinical and counseling psychology at Virginia Commonwealth University since 1984. Clients complete both the CASPER interview and an interview with a practicum student. This provides supervisors the opportunity to review students' impressions of a case against an independent source of data. Students can also review the CASPER report to identify areas they may have missed during their intake interviews. In 1988 we started using CASPER to routinely collect outcome data independently from clients and practicum students. This provides students with early exposure to a system that documents treatment outcome and provides them with feedback from their clients. One interesting finding from these data has been that clients' ratings of treatment outcome have been significantly more positive than students' ratings. It is not clear whether this finding would generalize to other groups of therapists, or whether students tend to underestimate the impact of their interventions.

Data provided by a system like CASPER could also be used for a variety of research projects. One of the real benefits of this approach is that it would provide a basis of conducting research in a wide range of settings. Parloff (1984) has criticized much of the psychotherapy literature for being "drawn from a limited data base that is unrepresentative of forms of treatment used in practice, of patients commonly treated, and of fully trained therapists" (p. 95). CASPER could facilitate the collection of data in more typical psychotherapy settings and improve the external validity of this research. In a previous paper (McCullough, Farrell, & Longabaugh, 1986) we suggested the possibility of creating a national network of clinics and independent practitioners that could pool their data for a large-scale study on psychotherapy. Such a study could be of considerable value to the field. We know very little about the actual practice of psychotherapy outside of research settings. Conducting experimental research in such settings is problematic because of the lack of adequate control over many threats to internal validity (e.g., nonrandom assignment to treatments, absence of control groups, unstandardized treatment protocols). However, as Hayes and Nelson (1986) have argued, there are different levels of evaluation. Routinely collecting outcome data from applied settings may not permit controlled research designs, but these data could still provide a basis for conclusions about the relative effectiveness of different treatment approaches as they are implemented in applied settings. Moreover, research in these settings does provide a basis for important descriptive research. For example, norms could be determined for such things as the frequency of various presenting problems in different settings, and the number of sessions and relative success rates for treatment of different problems. Identifying meaningful clusters of target problems assessed by CASPER could provide a basis for examining interactions between client characteristics and outcome (Heppner et al., 1994). Linking these data to other data on variables such as diagnosis or therapist experience and orientation could provide unprecedented opportunities for applied research. We see this system as one means to facilitate Barlow's (1981) vision of increasing practitioners' involvement in research.

Although CASPER appears to be a very promising tool for facilitating the routine collection of outcome data in applied settings, additional work is needed before this system will be ready for dissemination. In particular, the validity studies conducted thus far have focused on the validity of CASPER as an intake measure. Further research evaluating CASPER as a measure of change is currently in progress using a sample of CPSD clients. This work will need to be completed before CASPER can be relied upon to measure outcome. Our research to date has also been restricted to clients in two specific settings—a university-based training clinic and a university counseling center. Further research is needed to examine the reliability and validity of CASPER with other client populations. We are attempting to recruit other facilities to serve as pilot sites for CASPER. Participating sites will be given use of the CASPER system in exchange for providing us with data we can use to evaluate our system.[1] We are also planning to develop a fourth version of CASPER to

---

[1] Individuals interested in participating in the pilot testing of CASPER should contact Albert D. Farrell, Ph.D., Department of Psychology, P.O. Box 842018, Virginia Commonwealth University, Richmond VA 23284-2018. Electronic mail may be sent to afarrell@cabell.vcu.edu.

take advantage of the increased computing power of current computers. This system is being designed to be compatible with a data base package to make it easier to work with aggregated data. This system should automate the process of generating routine reports (e.g., end of the year summaries) and enable the system to respond to queries for specific information (e.g., "How many single male clients between the ages of 25 and 35 reported problems with depression?").

Although the system we developed appears very promising, it also has a number of limitations. First, the data included in CASPER is based on either client or therapist report. Although these are the typical sources of data on outcome, both perspectives are subject to bias. Ideally, this information should be supported by other data such as behavioral observations, reports from significant others, or ratings by independent observers. Unfortunately, such data may be difficult to collect on a routine basis. Ultimately, self-report must be an important component of any system for evaluating outcome. As Tasto (1977) noted, clients seek treatment when they feel they have a problem and choose to terminate treatment when they feel they no longer have a problem. A second weakness in this system is that it does not record information about the treatment process. Our original intention was to include a mechanism for recording the specific interventions therapists employed in each session. In working on a treatment manual we were unable to reach a successful compromise between a manual comprehensive enough to include meaningful codes, yet brief enough to actually be used. Practitioners and researchers interested in relating process and outcome data might consider using a separate system for recording the specific therapy process variables they are interested in and using CASPER to track outcome. Finally, the data provided by CASPER are descriptive and not tied to a specific theoretical framework. However, we believe that a descriptive approach, well anchored in content validity, is the most appropriate starting point for building a more comprehensive theory and is most likely to appeal to the broadest range of therapists.

Our goal in developing CASPER was to provide a model for how computer technology could be used to facilitate the routine collection of outcome data on mental health services. We recognize that we are in the very early stages of this process and hope that others will work toward developing more sophisticated systems. Advances in computer technology during the next decade have the potential for having a dramatic impact on the mental health field (Farrell, 1991, in press). This potential will not, however, be realized unless practitioners embrace these advances. As Greist, Klein, Erdman, & Jefferson (1983, p. 181) so aptly put it more than a decade ago:

> It is time to proceed vigorously with the tools at hand. We are very much at the same stage as aviation in the 1920s when it was developing and evaluating many different airframes, engines and instruments. In time this process

will yield the standardization in design, construction, and use of clinical computing programs that has made modern air travel so swift, safe and economical.

References

Angle, H.V., Johnsen, T., Grebenkemper, N.S., & Ellinwood, E.H. (1979). Computer interview support for clinicians. *Professional Psychology, 10,* 49–57.

Banta, D.H., & Saxe, L. (1983). Reimbursement for psychotherapy: Linking efficacy research and public policymaking. *American Psychologist, 38,* 918–923.

Barlow, D.H. (1981). On the relation of clinical research to clinical practice: Current issues, new direction. *Journal of Consulting and Clinical Psychology, 49,* 147–155.

Barlow, D.H., Hayes, S.C., & Nelson, R.O. (1984). *The scientist practitioner: Research and accountability in clinical and educational settings.* Elmsford, New York: Pergamon.

Battle, C.C., Imber, S.D., Hoehn–Saric, R., Stone, A.R., Nash, E.R., & Frank, J.D. (1966). Target complaints as criteria of improvement. *American Journal of Psychotherapy, 20,* 184–192.

Beck, A.T., Ward, C.H., Mendelson, M., Mack, J., & Erbaugh, J. (1961). An inventory for measuring depression. *Archives of General Psychiatry, 4,* 561–571.

Burijon, B.N., & Farrell, A.D. (1989, November). *Reliability of a computer interview for identifying outpatient target complaints.* Paper presented at the annual convention of the Association for Advancement of Behavior Therapy, Washington, DC.

Derogatis, L.R. (1977). *The SCL-90 manual I: Scoring, administration, and the procedures for the SCL-90.* Baltimore: Clinical Psychometric Research.

Derogatis, L.R., & Spencer, P.M. (1982). *Administration and procedures: BSI manual I.* Baltimore, MD: Clinical Psychometric Research.

Erdman, H.P., Klein, M.H., & Greist, J.H. (1985). Direct patient computer interviewing. *Journal of Consulting and Clinical Psychology, 53,* 760–773.

Farrell, A.D. (1989). The impact of computers on professional practice: A survey of current practices and attitudes. *Professional Psychology: Research and Practice, 20,* 172–178.

Farrell, A.D. (1991). Computers and behavioral assessment: Current applications, future possibilities, and obstacles to routine use. *Behavioral Assessment, 13,* 159–179.

Farrell, A.D. (1995). *Reliability and validity of a revised version of the Computerized Assessment System for Psychotherapy Evaluation and Research.* Manuscript in preparation.

Farrell, A.D. (in press). The influence of technology on mental health services. In T.R. Watkins & J.W. Callicutt (Eds.), *Mental health policy and practice today.* Newbury Park, CA: Sage.

Farrell, A.D., & McCullough, L. (1989). *User's Manual for the Computerized Assessment System for Psychotherapy Evaluation and Research Version 3.1* [Computer program manual]. Richmond, VA: Department of Psychology, Virginia Commonwealth University.

Farrell, A.D., Camplair, P.S., & McCullough, L. (1987). Identification of target complaints by computer interview: Evaluation of the Computerized Assessment System for Psychotherapy Evaluation and Research. *Journal of Consulting and Clinical Psychology*, *55*, 691–700.

Greist, J.H., Klein, M.H., Erdman, H.P., & Jefferson, J.W. (1983). Clinical computer applications in mental health. *Journal of Medical Systems*, *7*, 175–185.

Greist, J.H., Klein, M.H., & Van Cura, L.J. (1973). A computer interview for psychiatric patient target symptoms. *Archives of General Psychiatry*, *29*, 247–253.

Hayes, S.C., & Nelson, R.O. (1986). Assessing the effects of therapeutic interventions. In R.O. Nelson & S.C. Hayes (Eds.), *Conceptual foundations of behavioral assessment* (pp. 430–460). New York: Guilford.

Heppner, P.P., Kivlighan, D.M., Jr., Good, G.E., Roehlke, H.J., Hills, H.I., & Ashby, J.S. (1994). Presenting problems of university counseling center clients: A snapshot and multivariate classification scheme. *Journal of Counseling Psychology*, *41*, 315–324,

Horowitz, L.M., Weckler, D.A., & Doren, R. (1983). Interpersonal problems and symptoms: A cognitive approach. *Advances in Cognitive-Behavioral Research and Therapy*, *2*, 81–106.

Kazdin, A.E. (1992). *Research design in clinical psychology* (2nd ed.). New York: Macmillan.

Kiesler, D.J. (1971). Experimental designs in psychotherapy research. In A.E. Bergin & S.L. Garfield (Eds.), *Handbook of psychotherapy research and behavioral change* (pp. 36–74). New York: Wiley.

Longabaugh, R., Fowler, R., Stout, R.L., & Kriebel, G., Jr. (1983). Validation of a problem-focused nomenclature. *Archives of General Psychiatry*, *40*, 453–461.

McCullough, L. (1981). The Major Problem Checklist. *POST Newsletter*, *3*(1) (Available from Butler Hospital, Providence, RI).

McCullough, L., & Farrell, A.D. (1989). *The Computerized Assessment System for Psychotherapy Evaluation and Research Version 3.1* [Computer program]. Richmond, VA: Authors.

McCullough, L., Farrell, A.D., & Longabaugh, R. (1984). The making of a computerized assessment system: Problems, pitfalls and pleasures. In M.D. Schwartz (Ed.), *Using computers in clinical practice: Psychotherapy and mental health applications* (pp. 173–183). New York: Haworth Press.

McCullough, L., Farrell, A.D., & Longabaugh, R. (1986). The development of a microcomputer-based mental health information system: A potential tool for bridging the scientist-practitioner gap. *American Psychologist*, *41*, 207–214.

McCullough, L., Longabaugh, R., & DePina, C. (1985). An index of items in the assessment of psychosocial functioning. *Psychological Documents*, No. 2708, 26.

McCullough–Vaillant, L., & Vaillant, G. (in press). Individual psychodynamic psychotherapy. In A. Tasman, J. Kay, & J. Lieberman (Eds.), *Psychiatry*. Orlando, FL: W.B. Saunders.

Mintz, J., & Kiesler, D.J. (1982). Individualized measures of psychotherapy outcome. In P.C. Kendall & J.N. Butcher (Eds.), *Handbook of research methods in clinical psychology* (pp. 491–543). New York: Wiley.

Moreland, K.L., Fowler, R.D., & Honaker, L.M. (1994). Future directions in the use of psychological assessment for treatment planning and outcome assessment: Predictions and recommendations. In M. Maruish (Ed.), *Use of psychological testing for treatment planning and outcome assessment* (pp. 581–602). Hillsdale, NJ: Erlbaum.

Nelson, R.O. (1981). Realistic dependent variables for clinical use. *Journal of Consulting and Clinical Psychology*, *49*, 216–219.

Parloff, M.B. (1984). Psychotherapy research and its incredible credibility crisis. *Clinical Psychology Review*, *4*, 95–109.

Persons, J.B. (1991). Psychotherapy outcome studies do not accurately represent current models of psychotherapy: A proposed remedy. *Journal of Consulting and Clinical Psychology*, *46*, 99–106.

Reichelt, P.A. (1984). Location and utilization of available behavioral measurement instruments. *Professional Psychology: Research and Practice*, *14*, 341–356.

Sorenson, R.L., Gorsuch, R.L., & Mintz, J. (1985). Moving targets: Patients' changing complaints during psychotherapy. *Journal of Consulting and Clinical Psychology*, *53*, 49–54.

Stevenson, J., McCullough, L., Longabaugh, R., & Stout, R.L. (1989). The development of an individualized, problem-oriented, psychiatric outcome measure. *Evaluation and Health Professions*, *12*, 134–158.

Tasto, D.L. (1977). Self-report schedules and inventories. In A.R. Ciminero, K.S. Calhoun, & H.E. Adams (Eds.), *Handbook of behavioral assessment* (pp. 153–193). New York: Wiley.

4

Computer-Assisted Assessment, Psychotherapy, Education, and Research

Richard A. Weaver, Jeffery E. Sells, and Phillip W. Christensen

Fourteen years after the introduction of the IBM PC it is clear that microcomputer power is here to stay and that it will only get better and cheaper. The local area network with a computer on everyone's desk will soon be the de facto standard. For the mental health professional the personal computer will be as fundamental as the stethoscope and CT scanner are for the physician.

The increasing emphasis on efficiency and cost effectiveness within the mental health arena calls for organized initiatives to harness one of the most powerful tools of the 20th century. This drove the CAPER project, directed by the authors, at the Salt Lake City VA Medical Center. Salt Lake City, Utah. CAPER, Computer-Assisted Assessment, Psychotherapy, Education, and Research, was developed with the objective of collecting, in an integrated software package, clinical and administrative tools to make mental health practitioners more efficient and to increase the quality of care provided. In this chapter we will describe the guiding principles of CAPER, the development tools used, features included, and future development directions.

Design Considerations

Standard User Interface

Commercial software companies recognize that a distinctive, yet consistent "look and feel" is an important product selling point. By standardizing on the Windows environment and the Visual Basic programming language, CAPER programs behave like standard Windows programs. The increasingly object-oriented design of Visual Basic permits easy integration of home-grown code with the latest products of the industry's skilled programmers, giving locally developed programs the same polish of commercial products. The pull-down menus, command buttons, list boxes, word processors, spell checkers, data base engines, connectivity, and graphics expected by the Windows user are implemented as "standard equipment" in CAPER.

CAPER menus take the form of lists, a convention that is used extensively. An "Everything" menu presents the clinician with a list of everything CAPER offers. The clinician launches a menu item by double clicking with a mouse. Clicking on a "Details" button provides a brief description of that item on a Windows Help screen. No matter how many applications are added to CAPER, all are accessible from this menu.

A "Subsets" menu organizes CAPER items according to primary content and makes them easier to find. If a user clicks on "mood" for example, the computer will display a subset of all CAPER items that relate to the assessment and treatment of mood problems.

A "Popular" menu shows 18 graphical buttons representing the more frequently used CAPER items. The clinician launches an item with a single click of the mouse. Popular items include psychological tests such as the Minnesota Multiphasic Personality Inventory-2 (MMPI-2) and paperwork aids such as the Treatment Planner, the Report Writer, and the Progress Note Writer.

User-friendly, context-sensitive Windows help is available whenever the clinician presses the F1 key, furnishing information that relates specifically to the task of the moment. This feature permits the designers to "look over the clinician's shoulder" and give expert tips on how best to use the system.

Common Data Base

One vexing problem when using computerized psychometric instruments from several publishers is that the gathered data end up being stored in different and incompatible data bases, complicating data retrieval and analysis across instruments. CAPER solves this by interfacing all instruments it presents to a single data base format, allowing clinicians to perform standard queries of any data available for a patient. Progress notes, reports, treatment plans, and all psychological tests for a patient can be listed on a single screen, ready for retrieval at the click of a button. The common data base produces usage statistics on all instruments at once, and allows progress notes and treatment plans to be integrated in ways impossible with paper records.

The CAPER experience suggests that commercial test publishers should consider establishing common formats for storing test data generated by their various instruments and employ a standard menuing system for launching them. This would create an incentive to buy additional instruments from such publishers. It would facilitate integrating new purchases into established user environments and reduce the training cost of acquiring new software capability.

Security Features

Security in mental health computing is vital, particularly on a network. CAPER employs a two-level password registration process that conforms with Department of Veterans Affairs data security standards. Every CAPER session is tied to a specific user, and all data updates and accessions are logged permanently, establishing responsibility and permitting the tracing of any security breaches.

Assigned privileges establish what users can do within CAPER. For example, only network managers may manage passwords and perform data base compaction and repairing. Clinicians are privileged to administer and interpret specialized tests only after demonstrating proficiency in using them. More general instruments such as patient history interviews can be designated as available to any clinical staff.

CAPER security logic prevents launching an item from a menu without the user holding valid privileges. This is helpful when CAPER interacts with patients. When a patient finishes a sequence of tests, for example, the computer prevents further action until staff authorizes it with a password.

CAPER includes instruments that produce scores and interpretations that are generally suitable for patients to read. Clinicians may configure CAPER to determine whether or not the computer will display test scores and interpretations to patients after they complete tests versus requiring retrieval at a later time.

Customizability

Personal computers owe some of their popularity to allowing users to individualize their computing environments. We have made it easy for clinicians to personalize CAPER to increase their comfort with the software. Initialization files allow setting and saving preferences from session to session. These include whether the introductory logo appears, how patients are allowed to view test results, spell checking, progress note formats, font sizes, output footers, and categories of items that appear in the Subsets menu described earlier.

Clinicians often like to combine tests into a custom test battery. CAPER lets the user select and name test batteries. This battery is attached to the user's CAPER environment, and is available at subsequent sessions with a button click.

We have tried to write *general* programs to drive user-customizable content files. For example, the Report Writer processes templates that can be modified to reflect the discipline or approach of an individual clinician. The Treatment Planner operates on content files that can be modified with a simple text editor or one's favorite word processor to fit the needs of a specific treatment team or locality. A unitary "test driver" currently handles more than 85 true/false and multiple choice tests and makes it a relatively simple matter to add new instruments to CAPER menus.

CAPER Puts Clincians First

Some clinicians complain that computer systems emphasize administrative needs over clinical functionality. CAPER attempts to meet clinician needs by giving caregivers something in return for their efforts: practical help preparing treatment plans and reports, chart-ready test data, patient education material, reference materials that can save a trip to the library, and checklists to build treatment contracts with patients and training contracts with students. Many of the CAPER exercises produce output that clinicians can give directly to their patients.

Administrative needs remain important. In a clinically oriented system most administratively important data can be collected unobtrusively in the background, tracking and summarizing workload in a format helpful to program managers and administrators. For example, when a clinician selects scheduled treatment interventions in the treatment planner, CAPER records these and generates rosters of patients who should attend those activities. Likewise, querying the data base for psychological tests administered, or the progress notes written in clinic during a specified time period is readily accomplished, and is a helpful quality management tool.

Encourage Research

CAPER's R stands for research. The common data base makes it easy to establish local norms for psychological tests, a useful refinement unavailable in most settings. Outcome research can be embedded in a treatment program by including appropriate measures in the initial and final test batteries. Correlating outcomes, diagnosis, length of stay, and treatment modalities is a straightforward process because these variables are available from the production data base.

With all users on a network contributing to the same data base, it does not take long to generate a critical mass of instrument-specific data that can be used to answer meaningful research questions.

CAPER Features

Assessment Tools

CAPER began as a small collection of assessment tools such as the MMPI, the Millon Clinical Multiaxial Inventory (MCMI) and the Beck

Depression Inventory. Now, nearly 100 instruments, with both clinical and patient education components, are available from the CAPER menus, *all* linked to a common data base.

The Department of Veterans Affairs maintains national contracts with many commercial publishers of psychological tests for computer testing and pays royalties based on accumulated usage statistics. Many instruments are covered by the contract, and CAPER administrators report usage to the main computer at appropriate intervals. Other fee schedules are directly negotiated with test publishers. For example, an annual fee is paid to The Psychological Corporation for permitting CAPER to electronically store the Wechsler Adult Intelligence Scale (Revised) tables.

In addition to traditional testing instruments, CAPER includes patient-oriented exercises that patients may take as "homework" assignments and from which they receive output in lay language to be discussed in classroom or therapy sessions. Instruments patients like include those that help them learn more about themselves, and cover such topics as accepting others, liking people, pleasant events, and self-actualization. Many of these instruments have appeared in refereed journals and are readily interpreted in a manner suitable for patient consumption. Permission to use these instruments is not difficult to obtain.

The CAPER software administers and scores tests and saves patient responses to the data base. If a clinician wishes to retrieve a test at a later date, the software rescores the test from the patient's original responses. Computer scoring allows clinicians to perform analyses that would be impossible using paper-and-pencil administrations. For example, if a clinician wanted to see how a patient earned a particular score on the Sc scale of the MMPI-2, he or she could click the button representing the scale and see the Sc scale items, the patient responses, and whether or not the responses contributed to the scale score.

CAPER automatically generates a score and/or an interpretation in one form or another for every test and exercise. In addition, clinicians may attach an annotation to any interpretation. Annotations range from simple comments to elaborations on a standard interpretation. These are unlimited in length, kept in the data base, and are permanently attached to any screen or printer output. This feature lets clinicians develop a report from *within* any CAPER test or exercise, without having to use the CAPER Report Writer or a nonintegrated word processor.

Reference Materials

Visual Basic includes a Windows Help Compiler that produces the context-sensitive help files discussed earlier. Windows Help can also be used to create hypertext reference materials, navigable with mouse or keyboard, that can tie to other Visual Basic applications. If a clinician wants to read material discussing how to assess suicidality, for example, he or she might click on the highlighted words "suicide protocol" and the material will be displayed on the screen. The Help Compiler allows the design of a professional-looking reference system that can manage megabytes of topical material. The reference materials are actually produced with a word processor and then processed by the Help Compiler for display by Windows Help. Windows Help is present on every computer that runs CAPER. There are no additional programs to purchase or run-time fees to pay.

There is a long way to go in developing reference materials, but the structure is in place. CAPER began using materials that would augment the interpretation of psychological tests. When a clinician administers the MCMI-II, for example, he or she can click on a button and instantly review profile interpretations available in the literature. Standard Windows editing features allow clinicians to copy and paste these materials into test interpretation screens or into the formulation section of the Report Writer (see below).

The ease with which reference materials are accessible by computers suggests that commercial test publishers could distribute more than just administration and scoring programs. Administration and scoring programs could provide a gateway into reference materials that cover everything there is to know about the tests, including the test bibliographies, summaries of research literature, interpretation aids, the test manual, and an electronic catalog of other instruments offered by the publisher. All of these can be set up by the Help Engine and distributed with the test at minimal expense. Support materials substantially increase the value of psychological tests, establish the publisher as a more comprehensive solution provider, and may give publishers a chance to sell updates.

Soon most new computers will include CD ROM players. When this happens, it may be more cost effective for publishers to put everything they offer on one disk, including reference materials, and allow users to install the items they wish to purchase by giving them installation codes in a separate cover letter or over the phone.

Other reference materials now supported in the CAPER system include excerpts abstracted from lay books to provide lecture notes for psychoeducational classes. Various protocols have been written to cover suicide, violence, and involuntary commitment potential. Bibliographies of major tests such as the MMPI are available at the click of a button. We are putting Medical Center policy and procedure materials into the reference system. Very few of us could normally put our fingers on the Bomb Threat Policy, for example, but if the policy were part of the CAPER Reference materials, it would be far more accessible and more likely to be used in a real emergency. Scanners can be used to translate printed materials into electronic form. All reference materials are accessible from a CAPER pull-down menu.

Anyone who writes a paper, completes a research project, or prepares useful clinical or educational material may add the work to the CAPER reference materials. This allows electronic publishing without the overhead of printing and distribution.

The current Help Engine allows some degree of communication with CAPER applications. For example, a clinician reading help for the Beck Depression Inventory can click on a specially formatted hypertext reference and start the test itself. The Windows 95 Help Engine will be more powerful (Simon, 1995) than the current version, and will include full-text searching, multimedia capabilities, multilevel outlines, and drag/drop and copy/paste services to transfer help materials into other applications, as well as the ability to set up very clever tutorials by allowing applications to communicate with the Help Engine.

Other Tools

Our primary interest with CAPER was to harness computer power to make the professional life of the mental practitioner more productive. Below are brief descriptions of some of the items that are currently part of the system.

Treatment Planner. The CAPER Treatment Planner (Weaver et al., 1994) is based on the notion that 80% of the content of most treatment plans is similar across clinicians and diagnoses and can be captured in the form of word, phrase, and sentence lists. The Treatment Planner organizes files of prewritten material into four lists of problems, manifestations, goals, and interventions. These text files can be customized by a treatment site or by an individual clinician. Clinicians proceed through the four lists, selecting items that apply to a patient, modifying items when appropriate, and adding entirely new items as necessary to produce an individualized plan. The computer assembles the material the clinician has selected and displays it on a preview screen where it can be fine-tuned and edited prior to printing. The printed output includes treatment plan update sheets, a patient copy of the plan with a schedule of interventions, rosters of patient/intervention assignments, and descriptions of each intervention.

Report Writer. CAPER's Report Writer operates on a series of core templates that model basic content for several mental health disciplines and subject areas. The Report Writer processes these templates, shows report headings as buttons at the top of the screen, and displays the content for these headings in the form of lists. The clinician selects material from the lists that applies to a patient, and modifies it as appropriate. As with the Treatment Planner, the assembled material can be previewed on the screen and the clinician can continue editing. In essence, the Report Writer allows the clinician to collect data rapidly using a list-selection process and then hands the report back to the clinician to write the summary statements (e.g., problem and formulation) that require human clinical judgment that cannot be prewritten. Both clinician and patient may cooperate in writing a report by sitting together at a desk and selecting and editing items from the lists. Patients enjoy this collaborative approach because it keeps them in the assessment loop and allows them to see what is written about them.

The Report Writer is closely integrated with other CAPER features. While working on the mental status section, for example, a clinician wondering about the extent of a patient's depression can click on a menu, administer the Beck Depression Inventory to the patient, get the score and interpretation, and copy them into the report.

Progress Note Writer. Clinicians can write progress notes on one or several patients in separate windows that are tiled or cascaded on the screen. Each clinician can define templates and choose the appropriate one prior to writing a note. An integrated template manager allows for creating, viewing, editing, renaming, and deleting templates, all of which are stored in the CAPER data base. Old notes for a particular patient or for a group of patients can be reviewed. A clinician writing group therapy notes who wants to include common information in the notes for several patients, can write the information once and copy it to the other notes, all of which are visible on the screen. Standard cut, copy, and paste operations are available as is spell checking. If a clinician wants to review a patient's treatment plan while writing a note, he or she may click on the "Show treatment plans" button and examine the plans in a secondary window on the screen. Notes can be printed on plain paper or directly on preprinted progress note forms complete with time and data stamps in the margins.

Finger-Tapper. The relative speed of finger tapping between dominant and nondominant hands is a useful neuropsychological measure of potential brain impairment. The CAPER Finger-Tapper allows any computer to become a tapping instrument. Patients tap on the space bar and the computer controls all timing and rest periods and graphically displays the results.

Muscle Fatiguer. The Muscle Fatiguer is an experimental instrument developed as a possible noninvasive measure of the motor neuron fatigue common in such diseases as myasthenia gravis. By measuring the rate at which finger tapping speed declines over time, we hope to be able to quantify neuronal fatigue. Patients tap on the space bar as rapidly as they can for 60 seconds. The fatigue rate can be graphed in from 1 to 5 second increments.

Premorbid IQ Estimator. The literature contains several regression equations designed to estimate premorbid IQ based on such demographic factors as education, profession, and area of residence. The IQ estimator fills in as much of a patient's demographic information as it can from the data base and the clinician supplies the rest. The program will then calculate several estimates of premorbid IQ using the regression equations for which it has complete information.

Wechsler Adult Intelligence Scale (Revised) Analysis. Clinicians enter raw scores for each of the 11 subtests and the computer calculates scaled scores, age-scaled scores, percentiles, reliabilities, standard errors, and factor scores.

Other CAPER programs include a stopwatch especially suited for timing patient performance on the Wechsler Adult Intelligence Scale (Revised), and a standard score generator that will produce standard scores and percentiles for distributions with specific means and standard deviations.

Patient Exercises

Mental health practitioners are good at collecting information from patients and building fat charts. One of our interests with CAPER has been to provide patients with the means to build their *own* charts, called Patient Workbooks, to use throughout their treatment program and to take home with them when discharged. A Workbook Generator lets patients define a personalized workbook where they can collect output from various patient exercises. The clinician and the patient select worksheets from the available possibilities and assemble a patient-customized workbook. Worksheets include such pages as a cover sheet, a progress note form to be used by patients, a pro and con decision-making form, and a patient-identified goals sheet.

The aphorism exercise is a collection of several hundred old sayings or aphorisms that we have gathered over the years that capture essential ideas and images that can be useful in psychotherapy. These are sorted into 25 categories that represent facets of psychological health. Patients first take a questionnaire that measures how they perform in each of these 25 areas. They then explore the aphorism collection to find ideas to help them in problems areas. The aphorisms provide a fertile hunting ground for patients to locate the words and images that express their struggles and provide them with new frameworks for conceptualizing solutions. CAPER, of course, will print copies of any aphorism a patient likes.

Other patient exercises include patient-generated problem lists, drills on healthy vs. unhealthy self-talk, and quizzes on material presented in psychoeducational classes. These exercises appeal particularly to clinicians who use cognitive behavioral and self-instructional speech strategies in their treatment approaches.

Electronic Record

CAPER stores all test data, progress notes, treatment plans, reports, and patient and staff information in a single Microsoft Access data base. The CAPER Data Base Manager supports user-developed queries of all these elements. For example, clinicians may request a list of testing activity organized by patient ID, test name, and date. Clinicians highlight the test they wish to retrieve, click on the "Retrieve" button, and the computer rescores the test and presents the results on the screen. Clinicians may ask for a summary of all activity that has occurred on CAPER, show lists of tests that patients have not yet completed, restart unfinished tests, enter demographic data on new patients, register new clinicians, change access and verify codes, and display a master patient data sheet that shows everything in the data base on a particular patient. The master data sheet allows the clinician to see, on a single screen, lists of progress notes, treatment plans, reports, and testing that are available for a patient and clicking on the appropriate list will retrieve the information.

The potential of electronic records to organize the mental health practitioner's information-intensive workplace is enormous and sure to expand during the next few years in many organizations. At present there are many ways to design an electronic record but few standards. This is another area test publishers should examine: establishing standards that would give their offerings a competitive edge in the modular, "clinical component-ware" environment that CAPER exemplifies. Accounts receivable, insurance collections, and patient visits are other portions of a comprehensive electronic record and management information system that would be attractive to modularize to meet specific needs. For example, office management software abounds, but few of these systems operate in the background, collecting data as the patients and clinicians pursue clinical activities.

Future Directions

CAPER continues to expand, driven by its users and developers. Clinicians identify tests that they would like to use and ask us to include them. We try to accommodate these if we can obtain appropriate permissions for copyrighted materials. New ideas occur daily to the developers, who are also practicing clinicians. There does not seem to be any end in sight to finding new ways to use computers to assist mental health clinicians.

The most important issue facing CAPER developers relates to establishing appropriate data links to external patient data bases. What is required is a smooth, fast, and seamless gateway to VA's Decentralized Hospital Computer Program (DHCP) data base, the backbone of computer applications throughout the VA system. The VA has a huge commitment to DHCP. It is the foundation of its developing electronic record and the VA is not likely to abandon it. One of the most stringent tests of CAPER's flexibility will be the ability to link its user-friendly features and intuitive graphical interfaces to the power and depth of medical center and national data bases.

The key is learning how to capitalize on the strengths of both the DHCP with its rich data structures and of the personal computer that is setting the world on fire. The Department of Veterans Affair's has recently made linkage of DHCP, personal computers, commercial sofeware, and high-speed wide area networking a top priority. One idea is that microcomputer workstations, running programs like CAPER written in Visual Basic or some other language, will serve as a graphical "front end" to the DHCP. These systems will collect information from clinicians and patients and send it to the DHCP for storage in defined data structures where it will be available to other DHCP users and processes. Personal computers in turn will request data from the DHCP, populate local data structures, and manipulate and return the data to the DHCP. Ideally, this client/server arrangement will be transparent to the computer user.

There are obviously many details to be worked out, but the concept of personal computer and "mainframe" communication is well-established. It is only a matter of time before communication links between personal computers and the DHCP will be standardized, opening DHCP to the infusion of energy and vitality that characterize the personal computer world. We put mainframe in quotes in this paragraph because the main computer of the Salt Lake City Medical Center actually consists of a cluster of four DEC Alpha microcomputers small enough to fit on a single desktop. The distinction between mainframe and personal computer is becoming less clear every day.

For mental health sites that do not need to overcome the challenge of interfacing with an established data base, the combination of Visual Basic and Microsoft Access tools described in the technical section offers a wealth of development and customization opportunities with very few limitations.

Technical Information

Programming Languages

CAPER relies on two primary programming tools: Microsoft Visual Basic and Microsoft Access. All CAPER programs are written in Visual Basic, arguably the most successful programming language that Microsoft, Inc.

has ever produced and well-suited to developing the applications mental health professionals require. With its rich supply of third party controls (additions to the Visual Basic programming language), Visual Basic can address virtually any programming situation. It is powerful, easy to use, and Microsoft will see to it that it continues to grow in capability along with the Windows and Windows NT operating systems.

A unique advantage of Visual Basic is its full integration with the Microsoft Access data base engine. Visual Basic serves as both primary programming *and* data base manipulation language. At present most CAPER data base manipulations originate from within the Visual Basic applications themselves using standard application interfaces. All data, ranging from log-on statistics to test scores to patient records are managed by CAPER Visual Basic applications using the integrated Access data base management system.

Anyone with a copy of Microsoft Access and the appropriate security codes can open CAPER's data base and manipulate it with the full power of Access. This allows administrators to query the data base on an ad hoc basis and ask questions that have not been hard-coded into CAPER. Furthermore, data entry screens can be designed so that Microsoft Access itself becomes a door into the data base allowing further expansion and elaboration of the built-in data structures. The extensive security features of Microsoft Access, including data base encryption, permit confident protection of sensitive patient information.

Depending upon how well we are able to merge with the DHCP, Microsoft Access may provide the tools needed to present the user with a complete patient record, allowing integrated mental health service delivery in inpatient, outpatient, and community settings. Another advantage of using Visual Basic and Access is the natural migration path it offers to the client–server architecture of Microsoft's SQL Server system. Microsoft provides the tools necessary to convert all or part of an Access data base to the SQL Server platform.

Computer Equipment

CAPER runs on IBM compatible platforms ranging from 386 MHz machines to complex networks with multiple Pentium workstations. A 386 is adequate for administering psychological tests or writing progress notes, but 486 class machines are better for data base queries. Obviously, the faster the equipment, the more responsive the system will feel and the more enjoyable it will be to work with.

The present CAPER system requires approximately 13 megabytes of hard disk space. The programs and content files are relatively small, but Visual Basic requires many supporting files in the form of dynamic link libraries and Visual Basic extensions. The royalty-free run-time version of Microsoft Access requires 2 megabytes of disk space. The complete

CAPER system is installable using standard Windows setup routines and requires four high density diskettes.

Summary

This chapter describes the work of the CAPER developers at the Salt Lake City VA Medical Center. At present there are many such groups working in many directions and yet all have something to offer. How long this will be the case is uncertain. As organizations come to recognize the significant benefits of software interconnectivity, we expect that a market shaped by this important need will grow. The key factors that we anticipate will determine the future of the CAPER initiative are:

1. how helpful its software is for users,
2. how well it meshes with national VA initiatives, and
3. how well it keeps up in a rapidly changing computer industry.

Whatever the outcome, it has been a stimulating and challenging process to discover new ways to coax these remarkable machines into making clinical work more efficient and effective.

References

Simon, B. (1995). Taking windows help to the limit. *PC Magazine, 14*, 233–237.
Weaver, R.A., Christensen, P.W., Sells, J., Gottfredson, D.K., Noorda, J., Schenkenberg, T., & Wennhold, A. (1994). *Hospital and Community Psychiatry, 45*, 825–827.

5
Computerized Psychiatric Assessment in Outpatient Practice
Edward A. Workman

The clinical use of personal computers is not particularly new to the behavioral sciences in general and to mental health areas in particular. Psychology clinicians and researchers, perhaps having been introduced to large minicomputers for research purposes during graduate school, have been using computers for the administration and scoring of questionnaires since the early to mid 1980s. Computers are well-established technology in that field. Unfortunately, early work done by psychiatrists in the development of computerized assessment systems (e.g., Greist, Van Cura, & Kneppreth, 1973) has only recently been recognized and accepted in the discipline. In fact, in a recent issue of *Psychiatric Clinics of North America*, Dunner (1993), in a discussion of the use of computerized assessment, stated that, "It is not inconceivable that clinicians in the next decade will be interviewing their patients for diagnosis using a computer driven structured interview . . . Although this notion may seem fanciful in today's clinical setting, the interest of third party payers in obtaining the most effective treatment . . . may drive the clinical system toward a model similar to what has been discussed." Although it is probably accurate that the use of computerized assessment may seem "fanciful" to many psychiatric clinicians, the reality is that growing numbers of psychiatrists are already using or thinking about using computers to enhance their clinical efficiency and efficacy.

Attesting to this growth is a recent complete issue of *Psychiatric Annals* (January 1994) devoted to the use of computers in psychiatry. A wide array of articles very clearly demonstrated that psychiatrists' interest in computerization is expanding, and their interest is not just confined to billing programs (as was the case historically).

Acknowledgment is given to Drs. Joe Yazel and Delmar Short, both of the University of Virginia School of Medicine Department of Psychiatric Medicine, and the VA Medical Center at Salem, VA, for their comments on initial drafts of this chapter.

The purpose of this chapter is to describe a useful clinical approach to psychiatric computing, involving computerized psychiatric assessment. We cover the concepts of computerized psychiatric assessment for initial evaluation as well as follow-up assessment, and describe the use of actual psychiatric computing assessment labs in two different University of Virginia residency training settings. Case studies will be presented that exemplify the clinical value of computerized assessment. Finally, we very briefly discuss the growing use of expert systems to integrate artificial intelligence logic circuits with data derived from computer administered and scored questionnaires and interviews.

Basics of Psychiatric Computing Systems

There are two basic configurations for the clinical use of computerized assessment in psychiatry. First, computer administered and scored questionnaires can represent an integral part of the initial diagnostic evaluation, assisting in the validation of information obtained directly by the psychiatrist in the context of a traditional psychiatric interview. Second, computerized assessment can be used in follow-up to assess the efficacy of psychotherapeutic or pharmacotherapeutic (or combined) interventions.

Questionnaires administered by a computer are generally administered via a questionnaire driver program. However, spreadsheets and data bases can also be configured to present questions to patients and record their responses, and eventually score and report on their responses. However, the most straightforward way of administering questionnaires to patients involves the use of questionnaire drivers. Several driver programs are available including three generations of programs produced by Psychometric Software Incorporated (Rainwater, 1984, 1992). The Psychometric Software programs include Quest-Mate, Q-Fast, and Test-Make that are subsequent generations of questionnaire driver programs. A questionnaire driver program is also available from Mental Health Connections, entitled The Computer Administered Interview Driver (Department of Psychiatry, University of Wisconsin, 1993). There are also a number of relatively simple to use questionnaire driver programs available as Shareware. An example is the Tharp and Miller (1992) Generic Questionnaire Driver Program available on several bulletin board systems as a Shareware program. It is also possible to use simple languages such as Basic, Q-Basic, and Visual Basic to write one's own questionnaire driver programs.

The commonality across the vast majority, if not all, questionnaire driver programs is the ability to insert into the series of computer screens, whatever questions the psychiatrist wants to present to the patient. The patient responds to each question with either a yes/no or Likert-type (*sometimes*, *always*, *never*, etc.) response. Responses are tallied and scored by the program and a report is generated for review/analysis by the psychiatrist. This type of system allows the administration of questionnaires that are standardized (Beck Depression Inventory) as well as "homemade" questionnaires that allow the psychiatrist to present his/her own specialized questions to the patient via computer. The time efficiency of such a procedure should be obvious. Also, at our research and practice sites we have found that patients are highly receptive to computer administered questionnaires, and actually look forward to using the computer on repetitive office visits.

Prior research has also addressed the issue of patient satisfaction with computerized assessment, and the validity of computerized assessment vis-à-vis paper-and-pencil traditional measures. Rosenfeld, Reuvren, Anderson, Kabak, and Greist (1992) found that a computerized version of the Yale/Brown Obsessive Compulsive Scale (YBOCS) was well understood and well liked by subjects, and there was no preference for the clinician administered versus computer administered versions of the scale. Furthermore, a regression analysis of validity indicated that the computer and clinician administered YBOCS were highly concordant.

Hinkle, Sampson, and Radonsky (1991) found that computerized and paper and pencil versions of detailed problem checklists had a Pierson Product Moment correlation coefficient of +0.89. This indicates that the vast majority of variance in the two instruments is common variance: That is, they are measuring the same thing. Greaud and Green (1986) and Harrell and Lombardo (1984) have separately compared the relationship between computer and paper-and-pencil administered versions of commonly used psychological and psychiatric measures. These studies very clearly indicate the equivalence of computer and paper-and-pencil forms in terms of reliability and validity.

The bulk of research to date underscores Butcher's (1987) assertion that computer-assisted testing is more economical, efficient, and objective than traditional methods. It is clearly more economical to have computer administered and scored questionnaires than it is to take up office staff time, or even clinician time doing these "machine" tasks. The efficiency of this procedure is without question. The objectivity of computer-assisted assessment is probably no different from that of paper-and-pencil assessment as items from a questionnaire are being administered in the exact same manner each time to every patient. However, when a clinician administers an interview, it is well established that tone of voice, body language, and other situational factors can have a major impact on the expectational set of the patient (Othmer & Othmer, 1994). Such is not the case with either computer administered questionnaires or paper-and-pencil questionnaires. Thus, computer administered interviews and questionnaires have distinct advantages over more traditional assessment modes.

It should be understood that we do not advocate assessment only via computer administered instruments, to the exclusion of direct clinician assessment. The computer can be used to administer instruments that would otherwise take up valuable clinician or staff time, and can score such instruments in a much more efficient manner. But, some assessment components should always involve direct assessment by the clinician, such as the psychiatric interview. Clearly, information can be gleaned from the psychiatric interview performed directly by the psychiatrist that could never be obtained via either a computer or paper-and-pencil administered questionnaire (e.g., subtle information regarding the patient's emotional tone, use of language, and ocular and other motor movements that have emotional significance). Thus, computer administered interviews and questionnaires should be seen as an *addition* to the traditional assessment involving direct psychiatric interviewing.

The Computerized Psychiatric Assessment Laboratory

Initial diagnostic work-ups in most residency training programs involve a psychiatric interview, a medical examination (including a neurological examination), and the administration of various questionnaires (e.g., The Symptom Checklist-90 revised, Minnesota Multiphasic Personality Inventory-2, Personality Assessment Inventory, Beck Depression Inventory, etc.). As will be seen in subsequent sections that describe the Computerized Psychiatric Assessment Laboratory we have developed at the University of Virginia, a personal computer (PC) can be used to administer parts of the psychiatric interview (such as basic medical history, medication history, history of side effects, as well as other aspects of the interview). The PC can also be used to administer whatever objective personality tests or other questionnaires the clinician may be interested in. For example, at the University of Virginia's Residency Training sites (more fully described in later sections), we have developed an initial assessment battery that consists of traditional psychiatric interviewing, medical and neurological exams, and computer administered/scored versions of several widely used instruments such as the Personality Assessment Inventory, Personality Diagnostic Questionnaire-Revised (Hyler, 1994), Symptom Checklist-90 (SCL-90), Symptom Questionnaire (SQ), Beck Depression Inventory, and the Sheehan Anxiety Scale (Workman, 1993). Follow-up assessments involve serial administration of portions of the initial evaluations that allow the clinician to assess progress in a maximally efficient and objective manner, an increasingly common necessity in the managed care environment (Workman & Tellian, 1994).

Basic Setup Equipment

The basic equipment configuration used in our residency program for the purpose of computerized outpatient psychiatric assessment involves a PC workstation. The specifics vary from site to site but commonly involve an IBM clone PC with at least a 286, and usually a 386 or 486 CPU, a hard drive with at least 40 megabytes (MB) of space, and at least 1 MB of random access memory (RAM; 4 MB is preferred). Each computer is attached to either a laser jet or 24 pin dot matrix printer. Some sites are fortunate enough to have 486 processors with 4 to 8 MB of RAM and hard drives in excess of 200 to 400 MB of space. Some workstations have color screens. We have noticed no patient complaints against the monochrome screens, although patients do tend to make comments about some of the colored screens being nice to look at. The questionnaire driver software used at each site varies and includes programs such as those described above. Some questionnaires, such as the Personality Assessment Inventory, require that a program be purchased from the company that distributes it on a disk allowing 25 users. SCL-90 is available from Mental Health Connections for unlimited uses, and the revised version is available for computer administration from National Computer Services (which also distributes the Minnesota Multiphasic Personality Inventory-II, MMPI-II, etc.).

Office/Clinic Procedures

Very simply, residents or office staff orient patients initially to the computer, explain the purpose of computerized assessment, and get each patient started on that portion of the initial evaluation administered by computer (all patients receive computerized assessment via the SCL-90, SQ, and site-specific questionnaires that assess dangerousness, psychosis, medical history, psychiatric history, and medication reaction history. Selected patients might receive additional measures as needed, such as the Personality Assessment Inventory, Basic Personality Inventory, Yale-New Haven Pain Questionnaire, or the MMPI). The resident or office staff member is available for problems patients might encounter, but our surveys indicate that their assistance is seldom needed after the first 2 to 3 minutes of patient orientation. After each questionnaire is completed and printouts of results are obtained, the information is placed in the patient's chart. The chart is then given to the attending psychiatrist who conducts the initial psychiatric interview and medical and neurological exams. Computer administered and scored questionnaire data are thus integrated into a traditional psychiatric evaluation. It not only saves time, but provides much more clinical data than the average psychiatrist could hope to have at his/her disposal on the initial evaluation.

When patients return for follow-up, two questionnaires are administered and scored via the computer. The first involves a questionnaire entitled Medcheck that the author developed to measure side effects of psychotropic medications as well as intentions of self harm (i.e., suicidality) and psychosis. This very simply entailed inserting the questions ordinarily asked about side effects (or suicidality, etc.) into a questionnaire driver. The computer, rather than the clinician, now asks the questions. Positive or otherwise worrisome responses to side effect or suicidality items are flagged by the computer so that the psychiatrist can ask more detailed questions about these areas of concern. The second questionnaire that is administered on follow-up is a repeat of one of the questionnaires from the initial evaluation, the SQ (Kellner, 1987). We began using this questionnaire on a paper-and-pencil basis several years ago and then inserted it into various questionnaire driver systems so that it could be administered, scored, and results reported/printed by computer. The questionnaire is widely used for evaluation of psychiatric treatment effects, and has been widely recommended particularly for use as a measure of psychopharmacological treatment efficacy (Workman, 1993; Fava, Kellner, Lisonsky, & Park, 1986; Molnar, Fara, Zielezny, & Sprinks, 1987).

Computerized SQ

The full SQ, consisting of 92 yes/no or true/false items is presented in Figure 1. The scoring of both the pathology and well-being scales is shown in Table 1. This information is presented because the author is convinced that this is one of the most useful objective measurement instruments available in psychiatry, and is highly adaptable to computer administration and scoring, as we have rather clearly demonstrated in our residency training sites. Aside from the fact that this is a widely used and recommended scale for the measurement of psychiatric treatment effects, we selected this scale initially because is has both psychopathology and well-being scales. As you will notice, there are four psychopathology scales including depression, anxiety, anger-hostility, and somatic symptoms. There are also four well-being scales that include contentment, relaxation, friendliness, and somatic well-being. We used this scale initially, in part, because our team felt strongly that psychiatric treatment not only diminishes pathology but improves functioning; and the well-being scales, in our opinion, and that of other researchers, appear to measure factors that are important in improved functioning.

Several statements should be made about the scoring of this instrument. The administration by computer is straightforward; each item is simply presented by the computer (after it has been input into the questionnaire driver). Scoring is shown in Table 1. As can be seen by the instructions, the letter preceding each item number indicates that one point is received for scoring in the indicated direction (Y for yes, N for no, T for true, F

The Symptom Questionnaire.

NAME _____
DATE _____

Please describe how you have felt DURING THE PAST WEEK/TODAY and make a small check mark like this: ✓
For example, the word NERVOUS is on the first line: If you have felt nervous, check YES like this: ⟨YES⟩ NO.
If you have *not* felt nervous, check NO like this: YES ⟨NO⟩.
A few times you have the choice of checking either TRUE or FALSE.
Do not think long before answering. Work quickly!

1. Nervous	YES	NO	49. Terrified	YES	NO
2. Weary	YES	NO	50. Feeling of courage	YES	NO
3. Irritable	YES	NO	51. Enjoying yourself	YES	NO
4. Cheerful	YES	NO	52. Breathing difficult	YES	NO
5. Tense, tensed up	YES	NO	53. Parts of the body feel numb		
6. Sad, blue	YES	NO	or tingling	YES	NO
7. Happy	YES	NO	54. Takes a long time to fall asleep	YES	NO
8. Frightened	YES	NO	55. Feeling hostile	YES	NO
9. Feeling calm	YES	NO	56. Infuriated	YES	NO
10. Feeling healthy	YES	NO	57. Heart beating fast or pounding	YES	NO
11. Losing temper easily	YES	NO	58. Depressed	YES	NO
12. Feeling of not enough air	TRUE	FALSE	59. Jumpy	YES	NO
13. Feeling kind toward people	YES	NO	60. Feeling a failure	YES	NO
14. Feeling fit	YES	NO	61. Not interested in things	TRUE	FALSE
15. Heavy arms or legs	YES	NO	62. Highly strong	YES	NO
16. Feeling confident	YES	NO	63. Cannot relax	TRUE	FALSE
17. Feeling warm toward people	YES	NO	64. Panicky	YES	NO
18. Shaky	YES	NO	65. Pressure on head	YES	NO
19. No pains anywhere	TRUE	FALSE	66. Blaming yourself	YES	NO
20. Angry	YES	NO	67. Thoughts of ending your life	YES	NO
21. Arms and legs feel strong	YES	NO	68. Frightening thoughts	YES	NO
22. Appetite poor	YES	NO	69. Enraged	YES	NO
23. Feeling peaceful	YES	NO	70. Irritated by other people	YES	NO
24. Feeling unworthy	YES	NO	71. Looking forward toward the		
25. Annoyed	YES	NO	future	YES	NO
26. Feeling of rage	YES	NO	72. Nauseated, sick to stomach	YES	NO
27. Cannot enjoy yourself	TRUE	FALSE	73. Feeling that life is bad	YES	NO
28. Tight head or neck	YES	NO	74. Upset bowels or stomach	YES	NO
29. Relaxed	YES	NO	75. Feeling inferior to others	YES	NO
30. Restless	YES	NO	76. Feeling useless	YES	NO
31. Feeling friendly	YES	NO	77. Muscle pains	YES	NO
32. Feeling of hate	YES	NO	78. No unpleasant feelings in head		
33. Choking feeling	YES	NO	or body	TRUE	FALSE
34. Afraid	YES	NO	79. Headaches	YES	NO
35. Patient	YES	NO	80. Feel like attacking people	YES	NO
36. Scared	YES	NO	81. Shaking with anger	YES	NO
37. Furious	YES	NO	82. Mad	YES	NO
38. Feeling charitable, forgiving	YES	NO	83. Feeling of goodwill	YES	NO
39. Feeling guilty	YES	NO	84. Feel like crying	YES	NO
40. Feeling well	YES	NO	85. Cramps	YES	NO
41. Feeling of pressure in head			86. Feeling that something bad		
or body	YES	NO	will happen	YES	NO
42. Worried	YES	NO	87. Wound up, uptight	YES	NO
43. Contented	YES	NO	88. Get angry quickly	YES	NO
44. Weak arms or legs	YES	NO	89. Self-confident	YES	NO
45. Feeling desperate, terrible	YES	NO	90. Resentful	YES	NO
46. No aches anywhere	TRUE	FALSE	91. Feeling of hopelessness	YES	NO
47. Thinking of death or dying	YES	NO	92. Head pains	YES	NO
48. Hot tempered	YES	NO			

DO NOT WRITE BELOW THE LINE[1]

A _____   D _____   S _____   H _____   T _____

S _____   DS _____   SS _____   HS _____

R _____   C _____   SW _____   F _____

This copy of the Symptom Questionnaire (SQ) is reduced in size and is not suitable for scoring with a stencil. The original form of the SQ, a score-sample form, and translations of the SQ are available from the author. The abbreviations for scale and subscale scores are as follows: A = anxiety; AS = anxiety symptoms; C = contented; D = depression; DS = depressive symptoms; F = friendly; H = hostility; HS = hostility symptoms; R = relaxed; S = somatic; SS = somatic symptoms; SW = somatic well-being; T = total stress score.

Figure 1. The Symposium Questionnaire (Reprinted with permission, *Journal of Clinical Psychiatry.*)

for false). An example is given in Table 1 involving the Anxiety Scale items 1, 5, and 8. If the patient responds yes to either of these items then 1 point is scored for each "yes." On the other hand, for items 9, 16, and 50, a score of "no" is given 1 point. Items with asterisks (*) to the left of

Table 1. Scales and Subscales of Symptom Questionnaire

	Anxiety		Somatic
Y	1. Nervous	*N	10. Feeling healthy
Y	5. Tense, tensed up	T	12. Feeling of not enough air
Y	8. Frightened	*N	14. Feeling fit
*N	9. Feeling calm	Y	15. Heavy arms or legs
*N	16. Feeling confident	*F	19. No pains anywhere
Y	18. Shaky	*N	21. Arms and legs feel strong
*N	23. Feeling peaceful	Y	22. Appetite poor
*N	29. Relaxed	Y	28. Tight head or neck
Y	30. Restless	Y	33. Choking feeling
Y	34. Afraid	Y	41. Feeling of pressure in head or body
Y	36. Scared	Y	44. Weak arms or legs
Y	42. Worried	*F	46. No aches anywhere
Y	49. Terrified	Y	52. Breathing difficult
*N	50. Feeling of courage	Y	53. Parts of the body feel numb or tingling
Y	54. Takes a long time to fall asleep		
Y	59. Jumpy	Y	57. Heart beating fast or pounding
Y	62. Highly strung	Y	65. Pressure on head
T	63. Cannot relax	Y	72. Nauseated, sick to stomach
Y	64. Panicky	Y	74. Upset bowels or stomach
Y	68. Frightening thoughts	Y	77. Muscle pains
Y	86. Feeling that something bad will happen	*F	78. No unpleasant feelings in head or body
Y	87. Wound up, uptight	Y	79. Headaches
*N	89. Self-confident	Y	85. Cramps
		Y	92. Head pains

	Depression		Anger-Hostility
Y	2. Weary	Y	3. Irritable
N	4. Cheerful	Y	11. Losing temper easily
Y	6. Sad, blue	*N	13. Feeling kind toward people
*N	7. Happy	*N	17. Feeling warm toward people
Y	24. Feeling unworthy	Y	20. Angry
T	27. Cannot enjoy yourself	Y	25. Annoyed
Y	39. Feeling guilty	Y	26. Feeling of rage
*N	40. Feeling well	*N	31. Feeling friendly
*N	43. Contented	Y	32. Feeling of hate
Y	45. Feeling desperate, terrible	*N	35. Patient
Y	47. Thinking of death or dying	Y	37. Furious
*N	51. Enjoying yourself	*N	38. Feeling charitable, forgiving
Y	58. Depressed	Y	48. Hot tempered
Y	60. Feeling a failure	Y	55. Feeling hostile
T	61. Not interested in things	Y	56. Infuriated
Y	66. Blaming yourself	Y	69. Enraged
Y	67. Thoughts of ending your life	Y	70. Irritated by other people
*N	71. Looking forward toward the future	Y	80. Feel like attacking people
Y	73. Feeling that life is bad	Y	81. Shaking with anger
Y	75. Feeling inferior to others	Y	82. Mad
Y	76. Feeling useless	*N	83. Feeling of goodwill
Y	84. Feel like crying	Y	88. Get angry quickly
Y	91. Feeling of hopelessness	Y	90. Resentful

The letter before the number indicates the response that scores one (Y = Yes; N = No; T = True; F = False). For example, in the Anxiety Scale, Items 1, 5, and 8 score 1 if the response is "YES," and Items 9, 16, and 50 score 1 if the response is "NO." Items with an asterisk belong to the well-being subscales.

The *Journal of Clinical Psychiatry*, 1987, *48*, pp. 268–274. Copyright 1987 by the Physicians Postgraduate Press. Reprinted by permission.

the scoring direction are well-being subscale items. For example, under the Anxiety Scale, items 9, 16, 23, 29, 50, and 89 are relaxation subscale items. Items without asterisks are anxiety subscale items. Under the Depression Scale in Table 1, items without asterisks are depression items; items with asterisks to the left of the scored response are contentment subscale well-being items. The same is true for the Somatic Scale (with asterisk items indicating somatic well-being) and the Anger-Hostility Scale (items that have asterisks indicate friendliness with anger-hostility indicated by items without asterisks).

As described above, our initial evaluations include a variety of measures, including the SQ. Although the SQ has not been found particularly useful by our team for initial differential diagnosis (we use Diagnostic and Statistical Manual of Mental Disorders, DSM-IV criteria-based diagnoses), it is extremely useful in monitoring the strength of pathological and well-being states over time, as the patient is treated. For example, a patient with major depression in almost all cases will have elevated scores on the SQ Depression Scale (as will a patient with dysthymia or bipolar depression). We utilize T scores (with a mean of 50 and standard deviation of 10) for the computer scoring of our SQ, and we monitor subsequent depression (as well as other scales) T scores after we start treatment. Our goal is to drive pathology scale T scores well below 70 ("normal" $\cong$ 40–60). Of course, we do not ignore what patients tell us in the exam room, focusing only on this SQ data base. In fact, we integrate the SQ data into the interview and encourage residents to learn to do this by going over elevated scales or worrisome items with the patient to make sure the patient understands what the item(s) means and to validate the patient's report directly. In the next section we will examine how this system is used in widely different sites associated with our residency training program.

Private Practice Sites

Several clinic sites are affiliated with the University of Virginia Psychiatric Medicine Program and allow for resident rotations in PGYIII and IV (postgraduate years three and four). One particular site, which is associated with the author's practice, has a rather extensive computerized assessment laboratory for the purpose of patient assessment. This laboratory consists of a room in a suite of offices with three computers separated by carrells. All are attached to a printer. Three patients can be assessed simultaneously, and then an office staff member can switch the printer to accept data feeds from whichever computer is to generate printed material on a patient. Frequently two and three patients are being assessed at a given point in time. All three computers have questionnaire drivers that administer initial and follow-up questionnaires as described above. In this site, the specific type of assessment varies depending on the referral problem of the patient, but typically includes computer administered and scored versions of the SQ, Beck Depression Inventory, various anxiety scales, the SCL-90, and either the Personality Assessment Inventory or the MMPI. Patients also complete an initial computerized evaluation that asks detailed questions about prior medications, prior side effects, and past medical history. A separate room is available for patients who are uncomfortable sitting near other patients while completing computer administered items (although computer screens are separated as indicated). This room doubles as an exam room and is equipped with a 486 PC that has available all of the computerized assessment tools found on the three computers in the primary computerized assessment lab.

Once a patient has completed the computerized portion of the assessment, which is monitored by office staff members (who are available to assist with problems, reading difficulties, confusion, etc.), the assessment results are printed out and placed in a chart. The patient then sees the attending psychiatrist or resident. This sequence of events allows the psychiatrist to have a great deal of pertinent data about the patient prior to any interview or examination. The psychiatric interview can thus be streamlined to focus on the areas of difficulty indicated by both the patient's complaints and indications from computer assisted assessment results. We find that this arrangement optimizes time efficiency. In addition, the utilization of computerized assessment ensures that critical areas are not overlooked. The computer, for example, always asks about comprehensive aspects of past medical history, always asks about most possible side effects of prior psychotropic and other medications, and always asks about substance abuse, suicidality, and homicidal tendencies. The computer never gets hurried and forgets to ask about something of potential importance.

When patients are followed up, generally 2 weeks after their initial visit, they have usually been started on a psychotropic medication. In the first and subsequent follow-up visits the patient completes Medcheck (described above) and SQ via the computer. Medcheck, as noted, involves a detailed computer presentation of questions about side effects and suicidality. The side-effect categories include orthostasis, cardiovascular effects, anticholinergic effects, gastrointestinal effects, motor system side effects (extrapyramida syomptoms [EPS], tardive dystcinesia [TD]) signs and symptoms), and various miscellaneous groups of side-effect items. In addition, we have developed and added sets of computer items that assess patient compliance, psychotic thought processes, as well as suicidality. The second instrument administered to and scored (both via computer) for all patients in follow-up is the SQ. We monitor SQ scale score changes rather closely and use these changes, along with discussions with patients about effects of interventions, to make major clinical decisions. This process can best be articulated by describing two actual cases from the private practice setting.

Case 1

This patient is a 37-year-old white female who works in a technical specialty and has a college degree. She is the mother of two children, and reports having had episodes of depression on and off for the past 4 or 5 years. Her most recent episode of depression has lasted for approximately 8 weeks and she met full DSM-IV criteria for major depression without psychotic features. Her initial SQ depression scale T score was 102, which is significantly elevated, and accurately reflects the intensity of her depression as indicated by other aspects of the initial evaluation. Her contentment score, however, was extremely low at a T score of 12 (remember the mean of T scores is 50 and the standard deviation is 10). This patient was started on an SSRI (selective serotonin reuptake inhibitor) in part because she reported that her sister had responded extremely well to this agent approximately 1 year ago and was still in remission. Over a period of 2 months, the patient's SSRI dosage was titrated up. as her T score on depression slowly but progressively decreased toward the normal range. Although we routinely integrate pharmacotherapy and brief behavioral psychotherapy in our treatment of patients, psychotherapy was not a major component of this patient's treatment because her insurance carrier would not preapprove its use and the patient wanted to limit costs. Psychopharmacology was the major treatment modality. At 3 months follow-up, the patient had a depression T score of 68 (which is down dramatically from her initial level), and reported being much improved with better energy, better sleep, improved interest, and brighter mood. However, she reported that she still had much discontentment from the way her life was going and her failure to live up to her own expectations. This was congruent with a contentment score that had increased only to 24. On the basis of the patient's self-report and SQ contentment score, in clinical juxtaposition with documented partial SQ depression score improvements, it was decided (and approved by the carrier) that a series of four to six cognitive psychotherapy sessions with one of our team psychologists would be appropriate. The patient was referred, started in cognitive psychotherapy for 1 hour weekly sessions, and continued on her medication and in follow-up. The patient's depression T score over the next 2 months progressively decreased to 54, and her contentment T score increased to 46 (both within the normal range). The patient reported that not only had her mood continued to improve, but her outlook on life and her acceptance of herself also improved. Obviously, the same information could have been obtained with detailed interviewing, combined with good clinical acumen, in evaluating this patient on an ongoing basis. But, the author believes that the computerized assessment via the SQ, on a serial basis, allowed us to more quickly assess, than would have otherwise been the case, what was lacking in this patient's initial treatment, rapidly target what was needed (and why), and make an appropriate referral. In these days of intensely managed psychiatric care, it seems obvious how objective data that supports a "costly" referral can be beneficial to the patient.

Case 2

This patient was a 54-year-old white male who had experienced a work injury approximately 2 years before his evaluation, and had since been taken out of work and placed on disability. He had become progressively more depressed over the past 6 months. The initial evaluation indicated a diagnosis of chronic pain syndrome with both psychological and physical factors, and secondary major depression with melancholic features. The initial evaluation clearly indicated against psychotic features. As this patient had failed a trial of an adequate dose of a SSRI, the patient was placed on a tricyclic agent (for which reliable serum level data were available), and titrated to an appropriate serum level. During the first 6 weeks of treatment, this patient responded reasonably well, and his depression symptoms were moving toward remission. However, at the third month of follow-up his depression T score on the SQ had stopped moving down and was holding at a T score of 84. His anger/hostility T score, which had originally been at a T of 60 (within normal limits), had increased to 90 over the past month. More worrisome were his responses to the Medcheck items that measure psychotic thinking. The patient, for the first time since being seen in our offices, affirmed items that indicated that he believed that people were watching him, talking about him, and possibly planning to harm him. This pattern of responses to computer administered items prompted a more detailed interview/discussion than would have likely been the case ordinarily, and his family history and personal history were explored in more detail. The patient, who had initially denied psychotic symptoms, now admitted to a long history of infrequent and widely separated episodes of feeling paranoid about other people. For example, he reported that on two, and possibly three, different occasions since his late 20s, he had developed fears that people on the streets were talking about him and watching him, and that people may be looking in his windows. He denied ever having had hallucinations, and his delusional thoughts were neither systematized nor fixed. But, he did, in fact, have a history of exhibiting, periodically, the same type of paranoid thought processes that he was exhibiting currently. Interestingly, the patient reported that he became more hostile and angry during these paranoid periods in the past. This was clearly the case now as indicated by his elevation on the anger-hostility subscale of the SQ. This pattern was also validated by the patient's wife, who reported being the object of some, but not all, of his anger. Given the possibility that the tricyclic antidepressant pharmacotherapy had stimulated psychotic thought processes, we followed this patient more closely than usual, but decided to treat this psychosis by adding a dopamine-2 receptor blocker (thioridazine, at a low dose of 50 mg QHS for 1 week and then 100 mg QHS). The patient was clearly improved 1 week after initiation of this augmentative therapy, with lessening paranoia and decreased anger and hostility, and his paranoia had essentially cleared after 3 weeks of this therapy. More importantly, the patient's depression T score dropped to 49 1 month after dopamine blockade therapy had been added. His anger-hostility T score had also normalized. The patient reported being much less depressed, with brighter mood, more energy, less anxiety, and essentially no more anger and hostility than he had during his "normal" periods. As was the case with the first case study presented, the astute clinician, spending substantial time in detailed interviewing with the patient, could have obtained the same information that we obtained with the above computerized assessment. However, our team believes that with this case, as in the one previously discussed, computerized assessment allowed for more rapid assessment of therapeutic problems and a more rapid and more effective intervention than might have otherwise been the case.

In a private practice setting where patients are treated primarily with pharmacotherapy with monthly medication check visits, and secondarily with cognitive psychotherapy, computer assisted assessment provides both cost effective and quality enhancing features. Objective measurement of factors that are important to patient outcome (pathology factors and well-being factors) and side effects, allows for more rapid detection of problems that can prolong psychiatric treatment or derail it entirely. Computerized assessment also allows for a comprehensiveness that ensures that details of patient responses can be followed very closely from one follow-up session to another (remember that the computer never forgets to ask any question).

VA Medical Center Psychiatric Medicine Clinic

At the Salem VA Medical Center, which is major residency training site for the University of Virginia School of Medicine's Psychiatric Medicine Residency Program, we have a lab that is very similar to that described above for the private practice setting. At the VA site, we have a computerized psychiatric assessment laboratory that consists of office suites adjacent to a pair of Epson 286 computers, and a Packard Bell 486 computer, each linked to a printer (one is a laser jet printer and the other a 24 pin printer). Residents and attendings orient their own patients to the computerized assessment process, and this is usually done after a brief interview. The patient initially receives a computer administered and scored version of the SQ, the SCL-90, and the Personality Diagnostic Questionnaire-Revised-(C) (computer-assisted) (Hyler, 1988, 1994). The latter represents an increasingly widely used assessment for DSM-IV personality disorders and dysfunctional personality traits.

At the VA site, when patients complete one questionnaire, they generally go on to the next and the next until the computer indicates, with a statement, that they have completed the assessment. At that point patients go to their psychiatrist's office, and the psychiatrist or resident prints out the results of the above assessment. The patient is then taken back to the examination room for the completion of the initial psychiatric assessment.

When patients are followed up, usually in 1 month, and thereafter every 4 to 6 weeks, they complete Medcheck and SQ in a fashion identical to that described for the private practice setting. One exception however is that the patients are not directed by office staff, but are assisted directly by their resident or their psychiatrist. Frequently we have patients who are familiar enough with the system that they simply go to the computer, turn the program on, complete the questionnaire, and then go their psychiatrist's office for their designated appointment, informing the psychiatrist that he/she needs to print out their results (some patients print their own results). The usefulness and cost efficiency of this system at the VA is exemplified by the following cases.

Case 3

This patient is a 46-year-old white male Vietnam veteran with ´a long history of disability due to Post Traumatic Stress Disorder (PTSD) and episodes of major depression. This patient was referred from the medicine clinic due to worsening depression and lack of responsiveness to a low dose SSRI. The patient was initially evaluated and a diagnosis of major depression, recurrent, was made. The patient was placed on a tricyclic antidepressant and titrated to appropriate serum levels, and his SQ *T* scores promptly progressed toward normal. The patient's clinical report was also consistent with the improvements noted on the SQ. However, at a 3 month follow-up visit, the patient's Medcheck report was flagged for extensive sexual side effects. This prompted a detailed clinical interview discussion with the patient about these side effects, and he admitted that he had difficulty talking about this on a face-to-face basis, but that he had no trouble indicating the presence of sexual side effects (in this case ejaculatory dysfunction and decreased libido) "to the computer." The patient stated that he probably would not have told me directly about these side effects had the computer not asked about them, and that he was thinking about stopping his medication and dropping out of treatment because of his sexual frustration. This situation provided an opportunity to educate the patient about aspects of his depression treatment as well as the treatment of this particular set of side effects. We continued the medication, which had been highly efficacious in treating this patient's depression, and added neostigmine 15 mg 30 minutes prior to intercourse. At a 2 week follow-up, the patient reported that he was having no sexual side effects and that he was much better satisfied with his treatment and was now ready to continue. The patient has been in remission for approximately 6 months now and has had no recurrence of sexual side effects (he continues to use neostigmine as directed). It is very clear, in this case, that this patient would have likely dropped out of treatment due to side effects that (by his own admission) he was "ashamed" to convey to his psychiatrist. The computer interface provided a non-judgmental "blank screen" onto which the patient could tell his story, and this likely spared the patient from a recurrence of depression that would have surely taken place had he stopped his medication due to side effects.

Case 4

This patient was a 42-year-old white male who had experienced various psychiatric difficulties since his tour of duty in Vietnam. He carried diagnoses of PTSD, dysthymia, recurrent major depression, and substance abuse. On his initial evaluation, which was conducted by one of our residents, the patient, who had been treated ineffectually with antidepressants on numerous occasions in the past, was found to have subtle but clearly present delusions of persecution and nihilism. When asked about the items that the computer had flagged for psychotic thought processes, the patient indicated that he had never told any of his previous psychiatrists about this and had denied their questions about psychotic thought processes. The patient indicated that he had felt more comfortable admitting to the computer that he believed people were watching and talking about him, and that he felt that the world was going to end soon, all of which worsened his mood dysfunction. The patient was appropriately placed on a combination of antidepressant and dopamine-2 blocker, and obtained remission. The literature in psychotic depression is very clear regarding the lack of efficacy of antidepressant medications alone in this condition. The addition of a dopamine-2 blocker was the pivotal factor that placed this patient in remission. This agent would not have been started had the patient not admitted his psychotic thought processes "to the computer". Furthermore, the patient indicated that he had never admitted these symptoms to his previous psychiatrists and that he probably would have not admitted them to the resident with whom he was working had the computer not asked specifically about these types of thoughts. The value of the computer interface in this situation is obvious. The computer interface made the difference between efficacious treatment of psychotic depression and continued ineffectual attempts to treat PTSD and major depression when psychosis was not detected, attempts that would result in continuous festering of the patient's condition with worsening over time.

Summary

Computerized psychiatric testing, far from being merely conceivable within the next decade, is a viable technology now. Computer-assisted assessment has been in development for many years, primarily by nonphysician mental health providers, and is now in growing use by psychiatrists. Not only does computer-assisted assessment increase the cost effectiveness of outpatient psychiatric services, but it also increases quality by: (a) inserting standardization and increased objectivity into the assessment process; (b) ensuring that the assessment is always comprehensive (i.e., items are never left out by the computer); and (c) allowing for rapid data analysis that can be accessible to the psychiatrist whenever the patient is being seen, thus providing massive information without time costs on the part of the psychiatrist.

The Future

Undoubtedly we will see a wide array of assessment instruments designed for computerized administration and scoring evolve over the next decade. One very interesting development that is only in its infancy involves the use of artificial intelligence or expert systems in the diagnostic and assessment process.

Artificial intelligence is the use of computer technology to replicate human intellectual processes. A subset of this discipline involves expert systems. Expert systems represent computer programs that attempt to mimic the way an expert (in whatever field) analyzes, views, and solves particular problems. In essence, the expert system consists of data acquisition modules and rule structures written into the program, that allow pieces of data to be combined into an overall summary judgment.

Early versions of expert systems in psychiatry involved "therapist programs" such as Eliza, a computer "therapist" who asked questions and responded (based on preprogrammed rule structures) to the "patient's" keyboard input. Although such programs have novelty interest, they have been confined to entertainment uses due to their lack of true sophistication regarding the underlining theories and rules with which psychiatrists operate. However, recently expert systems with substantial power have started to evolve in both general medicine (Berner et al., 1994) and in psychiatry in particular.

Servan–Schreiber (1986) articulated the ways in which computerized expert systems could be used in psychiatric diagnosis. More recently, Stein, Patterson, and Hollander (1994) described workable expert systems for psychiatric pharmacotherapy evaluation. Garfield and Rapp (1994) have developed and described a sophisticated artificial intelligence/expert system for the analysis of psychotic speech processes. Stein and Roose (1994) have developed a commercial artificial intelligence/expert system called Depression Expert, that guides the clinician through complex decision-making processes regarding the diagnosis of various types of depression.

At the University of Virginia School of Medicine Department of Psychiatric Medicine, we are currently developing an artificial intelligence system for the diagnosis of depression subtypes in the primary care environment (Workman, 1994). This system is built upon the ESIE (Expert System Inference Engine) developed by Lightwave Software (1994), and integrates the artificial intelligence system developed by NASA (i.e., CLIPS) for high-level, multifactorial logic processes. The system presents the primary care clinician with a brief series of questions, based on branching logic, and draws conclusions about the subtype of depression for a given patient, based on the pattern of responses given by the primary care physician. If the patient does in fact have a depression spectrum diagnosis, such will be confirmed or disconfirmed, a subtype diagnosis will be made, and the program will make suggestions regarding the type of appropriate pharmacotherapy based on subtype. We are currently in the testing stages of developing this system.

In addition to expert systems for depression, several commercial expert systems are available (Mental Health Connections, 1994) including systems for the diagnosis of obsessive/compulsive disorder, and the evaluation of extrapyramidal symptoms in treatment with dopamine blockade. I anticipate that over the next decade we will see a wide array of such programs come to the market, and we will also likely see many of them integrate highly sophisticated logic circuits such as those that involve "fuzzy logic." Fuzzy logic entails the ability for a program to utilize data that is not in a binary format, but is analog in nature. Instead of processing 0/1, yes/no, or black/white, fuzzy logic systems can acquire and respond to data that reflects gray areas, such as degress of certainty, gradations of quantitative variables, and qualitative differences between data points. Fuzzy logic allows the computer analysis of exactly the types of data with which psychiatrists deal daily.

Conclusions

It seems very clear that computerized psychiatric assessment is a viable technology that will be used more and more widely in the future. We are likely to see development along the lines of a wider array of instruments available for computer administration and scoring, as well as the development of increasingly more sophisticated artificial intelligence/expert systems that will help the clinician make progressively more accurate (i.e., reliable and valid) psychiatric diagnoses. This will likely lead to more targeted treatments, and the ability to more rapidly diagnose and treat serious psychiatric illness. Such technology will not only make us more cost effective in our care of patients, but will also free us from the need to spend time acquiring what may be trivial data, and allow us to focus more on the serious issues that our patients bring to the consulting room. Computerized assessment, thus, may well be a technology that further humanizes the doctor/patient relationship in an era of cost containment and consciousness of, and perhaps obsessiveness with, cost effectiveness.

References

Berner, E., et al. (1994). Performance of four computer based diagnostic systems. *The New England Journal of Medicine, 330*, 1792–1797.

Butcher, J. (1987). The use of computers in psychological assessment: An overview of practices and issues. In J.N. Butcher (Ed.), *Computerized psychological assessment: A practitioner's guide* (pp. 3–14). New York: Basic Books.

Department of Psychiatry, University of Wisconsin. (1993). *Symptom Checklist-90*. Lexington, MA: Mental Health Connections, Inc.

Dunner, D. (1993). Diagnostic assessment. *Psychopharmacology, 16*, 431–438.

Fava, G., et al. (1986). Rating depression in normals and depressives: Observer vs. self-rating scales. Journal of Affective Disorders, *11*, 19–33.

Garfield, D., & Rapp, C. (1994). Application of artificial intelligence principles to the analysis of "crazy" speech. *Journal of Nervous and Mental Disease, 182*, 205–211.

Greaud, V., & Green, B. (1986). Equivalence of conventional and computer presentation of speeded tests. *Applied Psychological Measurement, 10*, 23–34.

Greist, J., Van Cura, L., & Kneppreth, N. (1973). A computer interview for emergency room patients. *Computers and Biomedical Research, 6*, 257.

Harrell, T., & Lombardo, T. (1984). Validation of an automated 16 PF administration procedure. *Journal of Personality Assessment, 48*, 638–642.

Hinkle, J., Sampson, J., & Radonsky, V. (1991). Computer assisted vs. paper and pencil assessment of personal problems in a clinical population. *Computers in Human Behavior, 7*, 237–242.

Hyler, S. (1988). The personality diagnostic questionnaire: Development and preliminary results. Journal of Personality Disorders, *2*, 229–237.

Hyler, S. (1994). PDQ-R (CA) PC Version. NI JO Software/Alpha Logic, Ltd.

Kellner, R. (1987). A symptom questionnaire. *Journal of Clinical Psychiatry, 48*, 268–274.

Lightwave Software. (1994). ESIE—The expert system inference engine. Tampa, FL: Author.

Mental Health Connections, Inc. (1994). [Serial newsletters]. Lexington, MA.

Molnar, G., Fara, G., Zielezny, M., & Spinks, M. (1987). Measurement of subclinical changes during lithium prophylaxis: A longitudinal study. *Psychopathology*, *20*, 155–161.

Othmer, E., & Othmer, S. (1994). *The clinical interview using DSM-IV: Vol. 1, Fundamentals.* Washington, DC: American Psychiatric Press.

Rainwater, G. (1984). *Questmate manual. Indian Harbor Beach*, FL: Psychometric Software, Inc.

Rainwater, G. (1992). *Testmake manual.* Indian Harbor Beach, FL: Psychometric Software, Inc.

Rosenfeld, R., Revren, D., Anderson, D., Kabak, K., & Greist, J. (1992). A computer administered version of the Yale/Brown Obsessive-Compulsive Scale. *Psychological Assessment*, *4*, 329–332.

Servan–Schreiber, D. (1986). Artificial intelligence in psychiatry. *The Journal of Nervous and Mental Disease*, *174*, 191–202.

Stein, D., & Roose, S. (1994) *Depression expert.* Lexington, MA: Mental Health Connections, Inc.

Stein, D., Pattrson, R., & Hollander E. (1994). Expert systems for psychiatric pharmacotherapy. *Psychiatric Annals*, *24*, 37–41.

Tharp, M., & Miller, M. (1992). *Generic questionnaire driver* [Shareware program]. Available on the Testing Station BBS.

Workman, E. (1993). Patient progress assessment in clinical psychopharmacology. *American Society of Clinical Psychopharmacology Progress Notes*, *4*, 1–4.

Workman, E. (1994). *An expert system for assessment of depression subtypes.* NIH Grant proposal, under review.

Workman, E., & Tellian, F. (1994). *A practical handbook of psychopharmacology.* New York: CRC Press.

6
Development, Problem Solving, and Generalized Learning: The Therapeutic Learning Program (TLP)

Roger L. Gould

The Therapeutic Learning Program (TLP) is a computer-assisted therapy program that facilitates the work of the therapist and empowers the patient to do a "unit of work." The computer is a tool that helps clients participate in their care and helps therapists do quality work. It can be used by therapists and counselors of all backgrounds and styles, and by anyone doing assessment, referral, or brief therapy. Personal orientation is not important, and all individual styles work equally well with the program.

The TLP is a mediated therapeutic interaction that helps to establish a new form of communication and therapeutic relationship. The patient becomes a more active, responsible, and informed participant. The TLP simplifies the steps required to successfully change and adapt to a problematic situation. The common sense model underlying the TLP is based on the natural process of development and ongoing adaptation. The TLP program helps the user move forward, going into the past only when it is interfering with the patient's present life. The TLP deals directly with the consequences of childhood by how it distorts how people think today rather than their attempts to remember the often painful past. The focus is the pain in the present.

Over the last 10 years, 14,000 people have been treated by therapists and counselors who have used the TLP. The therapy has proved successful with a wide variety of patients. From incarcerated youths in the California prison system to senior citizens yearning for change, from inpatients to outpatients, people are opening themselves up to the advantage of working with computers. Many people now treat the computer as a useful addition to their own healing process, and believe it is an important aspect of helping them live with less emotional pain. Educating and empowering the patient are crucial aspects of the TLP. The idea is not only to solve a patient's present problem, but to give them useful tools for solving future conflicts. Evidence of generalized learning will be presented in the research results section.

The computer itself is the powerful interactive instrument that teaches the model to the patient, produces the printout, and guides, focuses, and presents options. But the computer may also threaten professionals unless they clearly see it as a tool for themselves and their patients. Viewing the computer program as an adversary or competitor that interferes with the poetry of the relationship between the patient and therapist, is easy because there is now a new mix of cognitive work and relationship: there are two teachers instead of one. The counselor or therapist, in order to use the TLP program, has to resolve this professional adaptational conflict (allow the patient the benefit of the tool) to successfully integrate the program into his or her own practice pattern. Later in this chapter we will demonstrate how the TLP facilitates both the clients' progress and their relationship to the therapist.

The TLP

The TLP is a 10 session interactive computer course that helps participants define a problem, propose an action solution, and resolve the conflict about taking action. The 10 sessions are a sequential unit that must be taken in order. However, each session is comprehensive enough to be a possible ending point of treatment, depending on how much help the client needs. The program represents the condensation of years of therapeutic experience designed into a very explicit model of change and then translated into a computer program.

In each session the patient spends about one-half hour in an interactive program, receives a printout, and talks to a therapist either individually or in a group setting. The printout is the basis for the discussion with the therapist, and focuses the treatment process into a series of decisions that are made by the patient after conversing with the therapist. The patient works with a therapist at the end of each session to accomplish a specific work assignment. A typical decision would be the prioritization of problems at the end of the first session in order to work on one problem at a time, and the prioritization of an action plan at the end of the second session in order to resolve a particular conflict or dilemma. Subsequent sessions provide focus by challenging specific irrational thinking and arriving at cognitive insights about typical obstacles to taking action, such as fear of failure or success, feelings of anger or guilt, and self-doubts. The work of the therapist is to consolidate as well as expand what has been learned.

Adaptational Activity

Although the computer program is novel and the center of attention, a more important feature of the whole program is the therapeutic change model underlying it. In most therapeutic explorations, we find that the patient knows on some level what they need to do to adapt, but that adaptation requires either a hard decision or a requirement to develop some particular ability more fully. They may need to learn to stand up for themselves, become more independent, listen to others more carefully, or concentrate on work rather than engage in office politics, to suggest a few possibilities.

No matter how simple these actions may seem to an outside observer, they represent a significant change for the individual that may trigger a minor identity crisis. Adaptational developmental conflict can occur. In a big way, a small change in behavior opens a whole closet full of fear. The model underlying the TLP leads to the operationalization of a problem statement. A person has a problem when they need to adapt but cannot do so because the new behavior called for is erroneously interpreted as being too dangerous. The "unit of work" to be performed in brief therapy is to resolve this particular urgent developmental problem.

We use the concept of a developmental problem to point to the fact that underneath a problem in living is a problem of development. Some particular ego function that is not completely developed is being challenged. Some way of looking at life or some aspect of the self or self-image is also being challenged. When the patient makes a decision to face a problem in living and consider a new bit of behavior that might resolve that problem in living, they are in the midst of a developmental conflict where two frames of reference collide—the past and the present. That cognitive conflict is not easily available to the patient without doing psychological work. What is available to the patient is the volitional conflict in the form of "I need to do this, but for some reason I am too afraid to try."

The result of adaptational action exploration leads to experimenting with new behavior and getting positive feedback. The patient moves from relative helplessness to empowerment, the ability to find successful adaptational options and act on well thought out decisions. When this happens there is not only symptom reduction and function improvement, but there are also signs of a new vibrancy and zest for life as the patient takes control of a challenge that was previously immobilizing.

The TLP form of short-term therapy based on a developmental problem can be viewed within a life course framework as a form of therapy that helps a person progressively develop through intermittent episodes of treatment rather than traditional long-term continuous treatment. An argument can be made that patients are ready for change during crisis periods and that effective help during crises is a good way of leveraging scarce economic and clinical resources.

Experiencing TLP

In a short period of time, and with great ease, a patient who has never previously used a computer can enter so much data in one half-hour session that trained counselors say it would take them 2 to 3 hours to get the same amount of information in a face-to-face interview.

The extensive research on computerized assessments and questionnaires in almost all settings consistently shows that patients are more honest and open when working on the computer than either with a personal interview or a written questionnaire. They do not have to worry about being judged and they do not have to deal with the limitations of conventional inquiries that cannot make extensive use of branching logic. When the patient sees familiar items on the screen, they recognize that many others have had similar experiences. This "normalizing" facilitates a more honest reporting. The patients perceive the program as a learning experience even though it is called short-term therapy and is given in a mental health setting. The participants in the TLP report that they forget about the program and the computer very quickly because they become so intrigued with their own internal drama. Their emotions are stimulated and they become inward, self-absorbed, and involved in a very intense self-reflective thinking process. In this sense, the person is having a private experience in which the medium is largely obliterated from emotional consciousness. Special programming techniques, particularly the use of patient-favored language patterns, facilitate this self-reflective internal process.

Using TLP

The information that the patient gathers during the course of the interactive program is not used by a therapist for diagnosis; it is self-generated material about the patient's complex life. The facts gathered help the person process the data necessary to complete a unit of adult developmental change within their real life problem situation.

When the patient completes the interactive portion of the session at the end of each module, they receive a printout that documents everything that was explored on the computer, including all of the distinctions between rational and irrational thinking that the person discovered. The format of the printout is straightforward, and the patient's words and choice of language are reflected. The most commonly reported experience from the user is, "That is exactly what I am thinking but I could never have said it more clearly or as exactly." The program and the printout help the patient become more articulate, focused, and clear thinking. In particular, the distinction between current perceptions and past distortions is clearly made. The printout is a very important part of the process. Patients frequently refer to it in between sessions as well as use it as a discussion piece with their therapist. A former inpatient believes, "The computer helped me get to the heart of the problem in much less time then it would take with a therapist alone."

Defining the real problem in a complex life setting is not all that simple. If a person reports anger at his perceived-to-be authoritarian boss, is that the problem? Is the real issue the marital stress at home that puts him on edge before and after work? Or is the accompanying depression that leads to poor performance at work the issue?

These questions are addressed by having the computer program control the structuring of the problem statement to include all the essential elements. We connect the problem context and content to the psychological pain that drives the person to attempt change. We then connect this pain to a deeper problem or source of disappointment. This is usually some important frustrated need that is not being satisfied. We also look at what the patient is currently doing that is not working and how they may have to change to get what they need.

One prototypical problem statement for our sample employee would be "I'm having tension with my boss, Joe, who overpowers me and doesn't listen to me. This makes me feel crushed and depressed. This pain tells me I'm not getting respect, and I have difficulty expressing myself. I may need to be more assertive and persistent."

The sample employee is depressed, his performance is deteriorating, he complains about his authoritarian boss and a stressful home life. He already has several problems to describe, and many different unmet needs. By the time he is finished with the second half of the first computer session, we will have several potential workable problems to choose from. He will have all of them in print to consider, even before starting the first session with the counselor.

If work is really the problem, then the employee with the perceived to be authoritarian boss may truly have a difficult supervisor, or may instead just have a more challenging situation represented by a more focused and demanding manager. The patient will have to consider whether his need for respect and self-expression is being ignored by his boss, or whether his frustration is caused by patterns within himself that he need to change. Maybe it is a combination of both. In either case, he is in the midst of an adaptational challenge.

In the remaining nine sessions of the program, the patient is helped to sort out these kinds of distinctions and get a look at the realities of his life situation in order to explore adaptational options. By the end of the second complete session he will have a "healthy" action step to explore. We then use that intended action step as an experimental probe to help the patient understand and overcome his fears and come to some decision about whether the apprehension he feels about taking appropriate action represents a current realistic concern or just a shadow of the past.

TLP Session Goals

There are unique objectives for each of the 10 TLP sessions. They are as follows:

1. Identifying stress-related problems, conflicts, and symptoms:
   a. to identify sources of stress and ineffective responses;
   b. to sort out stressful issues from developmental stress problems;
   c. to prioritize one clearly stated stress problem that calls for some action.
2. Clarifying goals and focusing on action:
   a. to identify the developmental goal that addresses the adaptational demand;
   b. to clarify and define the action or behavior change that is necessary;
   c. to build an action intention that represents the recovery of the underdeveloped function.
3. Thinking through the consequences of taking action:
   a. to distinguish realistic dangers from exaggerated dangers;
   b. to isolate and expose the fears as predictions confused with memories;
   c. to reach a conscious, cost benefit, positive decision about the intended action.
4. Uncovering hidden motives and fears of failure and success:
   a. to clarify that certain strongly felt fears are not objective dangers;
   b. to weaken the hold of irrational fears;
   c. to learn to identify thinking errors as a useful concept;
   d. to distinguish healthy and unhealthy motives;
   e. to demonstrate that fears of failure and success rarely point to real dangers.
5. Exploring anger and guilt as obstacles to action:
   a. to clarify that certain strong anxiety feelings are not indicative of external dangers;
   b. to demonstrate that angry feelings are controllable by rational considerations;
   c. to demonstrate that the feeling of guilt is information that can be processed to continue to confirm that the intended action is safe and doable.
6. Confronting issues of self-esteem:
   a. to identify and acknowledge self-esteem sensitivities;
   b. to begin to accept the universality and mystery of these sensitivities;
   c. to entertain the thought that this powerful inner voice represents a historical fiction;
   d. to understand that the self-esteem sensitivity is the biggest block to resolving the developmental conflict.

7. Examining old and detrimental patterns of behavior:
   a. to identify the deepest vulnerability that is being challenged by the action intention;
   b. to see how the self-doubt triggers the ineffective protective behavior;
   c. to examine and demonstrate how the self-doubt system feeds itself;
   d. to begin to challenge the automatic response.
8. Understanding the history of the self-doubts:
   a. to expose the illusion of permanent damage;
   b. to see that responses to early events were limited and naturally protective;
   c. to see that these early protective behaviors were automatic responses to feeling inadequate;
   d. to view the self-doubt as an initial response to events by the immature mind.
9. Analyzing a current incident involving the self-doubt:
   a. to demonstrate and diminish self-fulfilling prophecies;
   b. to identify the erroneous thinking that currently feeds the powerful self-doubt;
   c. to understand that feeding the doubt by misinterpretation is a choice, not a necessity;
   d. to recognize that to continue to do this is to avoid growth.
10. Evaluating the changes experienced during the course:
    a. to see that fears are to be overcome and not submitted to;
    b. to see the action intention as part of ongoing recovery of function;
    c. to understand that recovery of function and individuation are necessary;
    d. to consolidate new views of reality.

Generalized Learning

By the time the patient has completed the program they have not only resolved the identified problem, but have also generated their own unique self-help book. This computer generated, individualized self-help book has proved to be a surprisingly valuable part of the after treatment. In fact, in a 3 year follow-up study done by a major client, CIGNA Healthplan, 75% of a sample of 2,000 patients continued to use these self-help books as guides and they claim the books have made a significant difference in the way they approach and resolve problems in living. The TLP is a tool that extends brief therapy into the highly desired realm of generalized learning.

Outcome Studies

Research on the TLP started in 1984, and continues today. The results can be separated into four phases.

Phase I: 1984 to 1987, Early Studies

Through CIGNA Healthplan HMO, 2,000 patients were treated. Five different studies were done representing a total sample of over 500 people in an outpatient program delivered in five, 2 hour group sessions. Fifty therapists were involved in five different cities. Each of the therapists received adequate, but minimal, training and supervision. The population served was a broad spectrum of employed people and their families.

These five studies were:

1. An initial satisfaction study involving therapists and patients with an independent 6 week follow-up corroboration (CIGNA study, 1985, unpublished);
2. A larger sample of patients 2 years later (Talley, 1987);
3. A pre–post pilot psychometric study (Schag, Larsen, & Read, 1985);
4. A 3 year follow-up study done as a Ph.D. thesis (Klein, 1988);
5. A medical cost offset study also done as a Ph.D. thesis (Vosen, 1991).

Satisfaction. The purpose of the initial studies was to establish some baseline information about the program. We established that the TLP was a program well liked by both therapists and patients. The overall satisfaction rate was high: "96% reported they were satisfied with the TLP, while 79% reported the highest levels of satisfaction" (Talley, 1987).

We looked at the various components of satisfaction that are the computer, the group interaction, the learning that took place, and contentment with the therapist along with indirect measures of satisfaction.

Indirect Measures of Satisfaction. 69% felt the TLP was more acceptable to them than a traditional referral to the Department of Psychiatry (CIGNA, 1985).

56% of the participants told other people at their job site about the TLP (CIGNA, 1985).

Another measure of patient overall evaluation of the TLP work was in their interest in TLP services as part of their HMO. Respondents were asked if they would inquire about "TLP-like services if they were confronted with choosing a new HMO plan in another job setting. Two-thirds of the sample reported affirmatively; the overwhelming response was 'very likely'" (Talley, 1987).

A fourth indirect measure of satisfaction was in response to a question comparing TLP group therapy to other group therapy these patients had in the past. Eighty-five percent said that they learned more about themselves and actually changed more in the TLP group therapy even though it was only five sessions long (Talley, 1987).

CIGNA patients were pleased with their group: "Over 90% felt the groups provided plenty of time for them to talk; almost 87% felt the chance to listen to others was also valuable" (Talley, 1987).

Satisfaction with the group:

98%   understood by therapist most of the time,
96%   felt like part of the group most of the time,
74%   easy to speak in group,
94%   helpful to hear others speak (CIGNA, 1985).

Satisfaction With Therapist. CIGNA studies also found patients were generally satisfied with their therapists. Patients rated the therapists "as warm, insightful, competent, and supportive. Although they had a 7-point range for their responses, the overwhelming response on each of these questions was the point of extreme agreement" (Talley, 1987).

The Klein (1988) 3 year follow-up study corroborated Talley's study satisfaction with therapists using this method of treatment. This was an important finding and began to allay the fears of therapists that the computer would interfere with their important relationship with patients.

Satisfaction With Learning. Patients identified the following key concepts of the TLP model as something they understood and found helpful.

Key concepts: 94%   self-doubt emphasis important,
                98%   action step concept clear,
                98%   thinking error concept,
                96%   childhood origin,
                99%   self-doubts interfere with action (CIGNA, 1985).

Satisfaction With Computer. Patients found "the keyboard and mouse generally easy to use (92 and 84%, respectively). The homework was considered valuable (92%) (Talley, 1987).

Even more interesting was their assessment of the more social effects of working with the computer. More than 75% of the patients felt the computer: "helped me think more clearly," "helped me overcome my reluctance to talk," "gave me more to talk about than expected," "was more individual and responsive to my unique concerns than I expected." "The use of the computer clearly contributed not only to the client's work on their own problem, but also to their involvement with group" (Talley, 1987). This evaluation of the computer component has been replicated in all subsequent studies of the TLP, including the most recent Drakeford study (1995, reported in Phase IV) with high school students.

TLP Effectiveness According to Therapists and Patients. The next question to consider is whether or not the program was effective as well as satisfying Talley (1987) and Klein (1988) studied TLP use at CIGNA by 2,000 patients. There was no opportunity to do a formal comparison outcome study against another form of psychotherapy or the waiting list in this first phase, but the five initial studies do give us information about appropriateness, patient improvement, and effectiveness.

Therapists' Report of Appropriateness. Klein found the results of the data analyses indicated that the vast majority of TLP therapists rated the TLP appropriate for patients who were depressed (91% agreed), had work-career stress (100% agreed), medical symptoms stress (82% agreed), and those patients recovering from substance abuse (100% agreed). "In other words, this therapist sample judged the TLP appropriate for a wide range of client problems. Ninety-one percent (91%) of the therapists interviewed, however, disagreed that the TLP was an appropriate treatment for character-personality disorders; but many people believe many therapies are inappropriate for these clients" (Klein, 1988, p. 155).

Exclusion from TLP. The following are categories of patients who should be excluded from the TLP:

1. Acutely psychotic patients or those who have impaired cognitive abilities.
2. Severely learning disabled or retarded, or organically impaired individuals;
3. Patients who are toxic with alcohol or other chemical substances;
4. Patients actively violent or demonstrating out of control behaviors;
5. Patients undergoing ECT;
6. Patients under the age of 12.

Therapists' Report of Patient Improvement. In the CIGNA pilot, therapists were surveyed about patient improvement. Their assessments of their patients' improvement include:

    80%   improved self-esteem,
    79%   improved problem-solving ability,
    83%   improved personal satisfaction,
    69%   improved interpersonal satisfaction,
    73%   decrease in symptoms.

Effectiveness: Comparison of Baseline and 3 Year Follow-Up Study. The following is the summary of the Klein (1988) Ph.D. thesis where he compares his results to the baseline results of the Talley (1987) TLP study.

Client Results: Interpretation of the Findings—The present investigation provided a relatively long-term assessment (1–3 years) of client-reported TLP outcome. Previous researchers investigating the effects of brief, structured, group problem-solving approaches *have noted that most programs have not been investigated for their long-term effectiveness*. This has emanated from the commonly held belief that one must restructure personalities during the course of therapy, resulting in a process that is long term. Thus, long-term therapies received the majority of the long-term effectiveness studies, in the assumption that brief, structured program results do not qualify for such evaluation.

Similarly, the three previous TLP investigations had not studied its long-term effectiveness (initial CIGNA satisfaction studies: Klein, 1988; Talley, 1987; Schag et al., 1985). The current study was intended to be a follow-up to the Organizational Diagnostics' (Talley, 1987) study, and utilized a six item, self-report questionnaire to find that, 1 to 3 years later, *clients reported lower stress levels as compared to pre-TLP stress levels*. They also reported a higher ability to solve problems and were still satisfied with the TLP. In addition, almost *two-thirds of the sample (65%) agreed that the TLP was responsible for their ability to solve problems*. It must be remembered, however, that the meaning of these results is limited by the fact that they are not based on changed scores, only client's estimates of change: They are not based on an actual ability to solve problems, but a perceived ability.

Client Results: Comparison With Organizational Diagnostic's 1987 TLP Study—The results of the present study indicated that 67% of the respondents reported high levels of stress (*much stress* and *great distress*) prior to entering the TLP as compared to 80% of the subjects in the Organizational Diagnostics' 1987 evaluation (Talley, 1987). Seventy-three percent of the current respondents also reported that their stress level was lower 1 to 3 years after completing the TLP than when they began the TLP. In the 1987 study, 78% of its subjects reported that their stress levels had declined between the two points in time.

The present study found that *81% of respondents* surveyed 1 to *3 years after* participating in the TLP reported an *increased ability to problem solve*. The 1987 study only surveyed respondents immediately following their completion of the TLP. Ninety-five percent of those respondents reported an increase in problem-solving skills between the beginning and the end of their TLP experience.

We can conclude from this that the participants' perception is that the effect of the TLP is strong, although this perception appears to diminish over time. It could also be said that with time, one's perception changes, that the problem-solving skills are the same (or better or worse), but their initial perceptions are either retained (as they were in this study) or altered with time.

In addition, *79% of the subjects in the current study reported being satisfied with the TLP 1 to 3 years later*, with 57% reporting high levels of satisfaction. The 1987 post-TLP data reported 96% of the subjects were satisfied with the TLP, with 79% showing high levels of satisfaction.

The earlier study did not ask respondents if they agreed with a statement that their problem-solving ability was due to TLP intervention. The present study asked this question and found that *almost two-thirds (65%) attributed their increased problem-solving ability to the TLP.*

Even though the two samples were not matched, *the current study supports the results reported by the 1987 Organizational Diagnostics investigation* (Organizational Diagnostics, 1987). The Organizational Diagnostics sample included only those clients who had completed the TLP between February 1986 and April 1987. The current study surveyed those subjects, yet added clients who completed the TLP between April 1985 and February 1986, before the 1987 survey went into operation.

Effectiveness: Psychometric Study. Researchers from the California School of Professional Psychology (Schag, et al., 1985) did a small pre–post test with a 6 month postpsychometric study on 6 patients undergoing group therapy at CIGNA Healthplan in Los Angeles. The number was small but the psychometrics were interesting inasmuch as significant changes were made in hard to change scales on the Tennessee Self Concept Scale and the Profile of Mood States (POMS), with a marked positive improvement in the self-concept scale over the period of the study. Participants had an increase in their activity level and a decrease in anxiety, depression, anger, and confusion. Their comments on their results are as follows (p. 9):

> The results are encouraging for several reasons. First, they hang together and seem to be entirely consistent with the goals and objectives of the TLP. There were no surprises, i.e., statistically meaningful findings that ran counter to expectation. Second, the changes on the Tennessee and the POMS are impressive given that only a handful of previous studies have been able to record any significant effects with these measures. And finally, the size of the sample always plays a big part in determining statistical significance. Had the recorded changes occurred with a larger sample, the increased number of significant effects would have made the TLP look even more impressive. Moreover, the group means suggest considerable individual improvement since the averages must take into account regression to the mean as well as individual "backsliding."
>
> *Six Week Follow-Up* Six weeks after the last session all participants were interviewed. Most individuals felt the TLP was a more helpful program than they had anticipated before they began. Many of the group members believed they already knew what the problem was in their lives but they were also surprised to see and feel the emotional connection to their childhood perceptions. Some people were able to feel "understanding" as to why they act the way they do now; while others felt awareness but were

unable to move beyond. Most felt a sense of "putting it all together" for themselves and feel more in control of themselves and their lives. While most saw their previous therapy as positive, they felt the TLP was a definite growth experience. They reported that they were able to make changes in their lives, enabling them to be happier persons.

Participants felt a sense of relief in talking about their self-doubts with others who were experiencing the same kinds of feelings. The examination of thinking patterns made it easier for the individuals to sort out what areas of their cognitions were trapping them. It is as if a tool was given with which to understand one's own process and this was further clarified by the working through of the individualized homework assignments. Two individuals felt some heightened awareness of their problem but qualified it by stating more of the program would be needed for the awareness to result in action.

All felt the program was beneficial and would recommend it highly. The therapists as well as the group interaction were perceived as critical in supporting and contributing to the individual's experience.

Six Month Follow-Up. Schag and group (1985, p. 10) did a 6 month follow-up and readministered the psychological battery and reinterviewed the patients. They summarized their follow up interviews,

> In the follow-up interview subjects offered their phenomenological impressions of the TLP. All felt that the group experience had been worthwhile and would recommend it to others. There was a general feeling that the basic idea of the program—identifying a problem and resolving to take action on it—had been helpful. One participant summed up the program's impact on her by saying that she is now less passive and more active. She said that she is "now thinking more and looking for solutions instead of not acting." Another person described the program as "not structured for hand-holding but for opening doors so one can move through on one's own steam." A third member concluded that the TLP had produced a change in her coping style toward "a cognitive approach that has helped me to "put it all together."
>
> While the participants felt clear and comfortable with the skills acquired from the TLP, some also expressed the need to have the kind of reinforcing experience with new problems and situations that they had during the five week TLP. Consequently, most indicated they would "like to take the program again or receive additional instruction."

In addition, Schag et al.'s findings of an increased vigor-activity change is consistent with patient's statements that they became much more active in confronting problems and finding solutions. This is also corroborated by the Klein (1988) 3 year follow-up study and our own Gould Center follow-up studies.

Effectiveness: Medical Cost Offset Study. A Ph.D. study of 357 patients was done by Barbara F. Vosen to determine the effect of the TLP on health care costs. She used a multifactorial model and regression analysis against patient utilization data. "Participation in the TLP was associated with a post-TLP reduction in medical costs for inpatient and outpatient services at a 0.0001 level of significance. Post-TLP medical services costs decreased an estimated $13.89 per month for each additional TLP session attended, reflecting a dose–response effect. Although inconclusive in the absence of comparison groups, this result suggests that completion of the TLP may be important for optimal cost savings. The study findings are consistent with the literature, that reports that brief psychotherapy of 1 to 10 sessions is frequently associated with a reduction in medical costs" (Vosen, 1991, chap. V, p. 1).

Phase II: 1988 to 1992, Hospital Studies

During this phase, the TLP program was enlarged and modified from a 5-session group program to 10 individual sessions that were used primarily with individual therapy, but also used in a group format. During this period of time we began to use the TLP on inpatient wards in private and community psychiatric hospitals around the country. Over 8,000 patients were treated during this period of time. These studies continued to demonstrate that the TLP was safe, effective, and satisfying, using both the therapist and patient assessments of effectiveness as our measures. Surprisingly, the TLP was found to be as useful in the hospital as in the outpatient setting. The effectiveness seemed to cross diagnostic categories. We believe that one of the reasons for the effectiveness in the hospital setting is because it allows patients, therapists, and ancillary hospital personnel to work together on the unsolved problems of living that put the patient into the hospital in the first place. This takes place while the patient's psychopharmacological care is directed toward symptom relief and management of the diagnosed psychopathology.

One outcome study, done with 637 inpatients from five different hospitals, is reported here. In this study we took a global "mass action" approach in probing two important questions: What did the patient population learn? and What magnitude of symptom improvement occurred in this entire hospitalized population as a result of 10 TLP sessions?

1. Did the patient learn something that is useful? The average patient endorsed 4.6 positive statements. The top 4 statements endorsed are: "Yes, I am . . ."
   a. "less likely to give other people too much power to influence my feelings and stop me from doing what I need to do.";
   b. "more likely to remember that I have rights to do what I need to do for myself.";
   c. "more likely to experiment with new actions because I now realize that I can take just one step and then see what happens. I no longer feel committed to go through with something if along the way I find it's wrong for me.";

   d. "less afraid of my anger because I am more able now to sort out my angry feelings and where they're coming from.";
2. Was there symptom improvement? We use three scales to compose our psychological pain index. We use physical symptoms, function change such as sleeping and appetite, and bodily pain sensations such as crushed, torn apart, and crying inside. Before TLP patients endorsed 10.3 symptoms. Following treatment, patients felt that they needed no further help on 8.9 of those initial items.

On a population basis, these results could be interpreted as an 85% effectiveness rate for a hospitalized population.

The other findings of this study are consistent with the finding reported in Phase I. This is supported by the following quote from Tom Woolf, LCSW, the Director of Adult Services at the University of Utah Neuropsychiatric Institute (personal communication, November 1994). His view on the TLP is as follows:

> We have very actively utilized the TLP as a key therapeutic tool in both our adult and adolescent recovery programs over the last three years. In fact, the TLP has been so well received by our adult recovery patients that we have structured an evening, intense outpatient program that embraces TLP work as one of its central (and most popular) components.

Phase III: 1992 to 1995, Gould Center Experiences

It was during this period of time that the TLP was used primarily in an outpatient managed care setting where both length of stay and quality of care were carefully assessed and monitored. Over 3,000 patients were treated during this period of time, primarily in Los Angeles.

Using the TLP in our own outpatient clinics we have found that the therapists take to the model quickly and find it an invaluable tool to do brief therapy; they are encouraged because they see the clients' improvement in such a short period of time. The typical case is completed within 6 to 8 sessions (an average of 7.2 sessions). Clients leave with clarity, hope, and direction. Ninety-five percent say they would recommend the Gould Centers to others.

Report Card. The primary managed care company that we work with has recently issued a "report card" comparing our services to other providers on the panel using the Global Assessment of Functioning (GAF) that is axis 5 of the Diagnostic and Statistic Manual of Mental Disorders (DSM-IV) diagnostic schedule. Two hundred and thirty-six of our clients pre- and postmeasures were compared to 13,233 of other therapists in the network. The results show 53% of the Gould Center patients improved versus 32% improvement in the rest of the network; 41% were maintained versus only 58% maintained in the network; and only 6% of the Gould Center clients regressed while 10% of those in the network regressed.

Keep in mind that these results of increased functioning were attained in 7.2 sessions (with our model and tool) versus 11 sessions average for other therapists in this panel.

Generalized Learning. We sent out a follow-up survey to 118 clients in three groups: Group 1, 3 to 5 months posttreatment; Group 2, 6 to 8 months; and Group 3, 9 to 11 months. We found the same kind of small decrease in clients' perception of TLP's impact over time as reported in the Klein 3 year follow-up study. The self-reported ability to sort out problems increased over time from 43% in Group 1, to 53% in Group 2, and 67% in Group 3. This 67% figure is close to the 81% plateau reported in the 3 year follow-up.

This increased ability is illustrated by a quote from one of the outpatient follow-up surveys.

> The single most helpful benefit I got was the "action step." I use it all the time. It has become like a mantra—"How do I feel, do I want to feel like this, can I change it, what are the consequences, can I live with them, yes; take the action.' It gave me a concrete usable tool for my everyday life.

Phase IV: 1993 to 1995

During this current phase of research activity we created an adolescent version of the TLP that was used by high school students in both California and New York, and expanded the usage of the TLP into nonmedical settings. The most striking new findings just reported requires a corroborative study because of its obvious importance. In the Fresno continuation high school (the at-risk population), the annual drop-out rate is 25 to 30%. The TLP group was 50 students selected as most likely to drop out. Ten months later the drop-out rate for these 50 students was only 6%.

A more formal study is a just published Ph.D. thesis by Cynthia Drakeford (1995). The study was designed to investigate the use of the TLP for the mainstream high school population in New York. There were 20 randomly assigned participants in the control group and 20 participants in the experimental group. The students were between the 9th and 12th grade. Two counselors did both the control and experimental groups.

The research findings suggest that the TLP is a superior and effective method of providing counseling services in schools. There was a marked decrease in the anxiety/stress level in the experimental group and there was a marked increase in the activity and participation level in the experimental group. A hundred percent of the experimental counseling group was satisfied with their counseling program at the end of the study compared to 60% of the control group. The students were surprised that the TLP was so highly individualized, made good use of their printouts, and used their printouts at home and during the counseling sessions to be able to pinpoint and work with the problems that were bothering them. Students not only felt the printout helped them clarify their feelings, but they actually felt understood by someone even though that someone, they knew, was a computer program.

The counselors did not see the computer process as inhibiting the relationship between them and their students. They felt the students were better equipped to participate, were more active, and presented more real problems requiring more follow-up and contact with a therapist than the control group. Counselors felt the computer-assisted therapy supported the development of a caring and collaborative relationship with a more knowledgeable student who was equipped to take a more proactive role in the development of a course of action for themselves.

Not only did the results favor the TLP in this study, but the results were obtained with minimal training and only half the amount of counselor time. That is, the control group had two face to face group meetings per week with the counselor while the experimental group only had one face to face meeting (the other weekly session was taking the TLP in the computer laboratory).

Kaiser-Permanente and UCLA Studies. The Kaiser Permanente Garfield Foundation funded two studies, the first at Kaiser Permanente Los Angeles Department of Psychiatry (Belar, 1991; Dolezal, Snibbe, & Belar, 1993; Dolezal, Snibbe, & Belar, 1995), followed by a joint UCLA-Kaiser study conducted at UCLA. The Kaiser study compared 54 patients treated by TLP group therapy with 55 patients treated by cognitive behavioral group therapy. The findings replicated the results on CIGNA TLP group therapy a decade earlier as reported in Phase I. This included the same high degree of satisfaction, effectiveness, and therapist rating of effectiveness. This study added new weight to the evidence for the TLP as a treatment tool. It was a well-conducted, random assignment, comparison study using standard pre–post measurement tools for depression, anxiety, and severity, and sophisticated data analysis techniques. At the end of 10 group sessions and at the 6 month follow-up, both the experimental and control group were significantly and equally improved. When the Kaiser study group compared TLP group effectiveness ratings to the literature on brief therapy, they found the TLP group to be rated quite a bit higher at the end of 10 sessions (82 vs. 50%) and much quicker in achieving equal effectiveness (10 vs. 26 sessions).

The UCLA-Kaiser study (Jacobs, Christiensen, Snibbe, Dolezal, Huber, & Polterock, 1995) studied individual treatment rather than group treatment. They used essentially the same measurement tools on 100 outpatients divided into control and experimental groups. By the end of the treatment and at the 6 month follow-up, both groups had improved significantly, with no significant differences between groups.

This study adds new information about potential use of the TLP as a self-help tool as well as evidence for its effectiveness and efficiency as a therapeutic tool. The TLP was used in a unique way. The experimental group received 10 TLP sessions but only about 15 minutes with a therapist focused on the TLP printout from that session. The comparison group was given 10 full therapeutic hours without the TLP.

Ending up with no statistically significant difference in expenditure of therapist time opens the door to the possible use of the TLP as a self-help tool, as a follow-up to brief therapy (many of the brief therapy control patients requested the use of the computer program during their follow-up interviews), or as an efficient way of utilizing therapist time.

Summary to Date and Future Research

All the reports over a decade corroborate the initial studies that the TLP is a safe and effective program with broad applications in outpatient managed care, inpatient hospitals, schools, adults and youths in non-medical settings, and self-help programs.

Future research will include comparison outcome studies with other short-term therapies, and the following research questions:

1. How does the program actually work? We will study the correspondence between the model behind the program and what the patient learns at each session.
2. We will link the step by step process to outcomes in order to improve the program by understanding which parts and which concepts are the most effective.
3. We will subtype the problem areas to try to determine which processes are more effective for which subtypes of patient populations.
4. We will study the combinations of short-term therapy and medication for the treatment of depression.
5. We will study the efficacy of the TLP as a short-term class for individuals in self-help programs and in stress related medical programs.

Conclusion

Whether it is the TLP, or some other form of therapy yet to be created with the ever-changing technology all around us, it is crucial that all caregivers stay open to new ways to better serve their patients. In this day of the ever-shrinking medical dollar, the need to have affordable care is more important than ever.

While the pressure is on to provide both brief therapy and quality care at the same time, the TLP or other computer-assisted therapy programs can help the therapist provide, with dignity, the kind of quality help that the patients can also take with them after the treatment episode is over.

References

Belar, C. (1991, Jan.). *Computer-assisted psychotherapy*. Invited Colloquium, Department of Psychology, University of Central Florida, Orlando, FL.

Dolezal, S., Snibbe, J., & Belar, C. (1993). *Innovations in short-term psychotherapy: Computer-assisted psychotherapy vs. standard cognitive behavioral group therapy*. Presented at the Kaiser-Permanente Medical Center Annual Research Symposium, Los Angeles, CA.

Dolezal, S., Snibbe, J., & Belar, C. (1995). *Computer-assisted psychotherapy vs. standard cognitive-behavioral group therapy: Do computers have a future?* Presented at the Annual Symposium of the Western Psychological Association, Los Angeles, CA.

Drakeford, C.A. (1995). *High school guidance counseling by computers: A study of the Therapeutic Learning Program (TLP)*. Unpublished doctoral dissertation Columbia University, New York.

Jacobs, M., Christensen, A., Snibbe, J., Dolezal, S., Huber, A., & Polterock, A. (1995). *Computer-assisted individual therapy vs. standard, brief individual therapy*. Presented at the Annual Symposium of the Western Psychological Association, Los Angeles, CA.

Klein, Ronald (1988). *The effects of implementation on program outcome: An evaluation of the Therapeutic Learning Program (TLP) at CIGNA Healthplan*. Unpublished doctoral dissertation, University of Southern California.

Schag, D.S., Larsen, T., & Read, L. (1985). *Evaluation of the Therapeutic Learning Program Ross–Loos Clinic, Torrance, California*. Los Angeles, CA: California School of Professional Psychology.

Talley, J.L. (1987). *TLP Evaluation Study*. Palo Alto, CA: Organizational Diagnostics.

Vosen, B.F. (1991). *The effect of the Therapeutic Learning Program on health care costs and member retention in an HMO*. Unpublished doctoral dissertation, University of Southern California.

TLP Bibliography

Gould, R.L. (1979). Psychoanalytic theory of adulthood consciousness. In S.I. Greenspan & G.H. Pollack (Eds.), *The course of life/III: Adulthood and the aging process* (pp. 55–89). Adelphi, MD: National Institute of Mental-Health.

Gould, R.L. (1989). Adulthood. In H.I. Kaplan & B.J. Sadock (Eds.), *Comprehensive textbook of psychiatry/V* (pp. 1998–2012). Baltimore, MD: Williams & Wilkins.

Gould, R.L. (1990). The therapeutic Learning Program (TLP): Computer-assisted short-term therapy. In G. Gumpert & S. Fish (Eds.), *Talking to strangers: Mediated therapeutic communication* (pp. 184–199). Norwood, NJ: Ablex Publishing Corporation.

Gould, R.L. (1992). Adult development and brief computer-assisted therapy in mental health and managed care. In J.L. Feldman & R.J. Fitzpatrick (Eds.), *Managed mental health care: Administrative & clinical issues* (pp. 347–358). Washington, DC: American Psychiatric Press, Inc.

Gould, R.L. (1994). Computer-assisted therapy. *Employee assistance: Solutions to Problems*, 7, 22–26.

7
Voice Interactive Computers for Attitudinal Interviewing

Stuart Gitlow and David R. Gastfriend

Computers released prior to the mid-1980s had a variety of interfaces; each application's programmer would determine and write an interface that was believed to be the "best." The end user would then be challenged by a continually changing face of computing in which each application had a different command set, appearance, and response methodology. In this early context, applications each had their own command set to be memorized by the operator.

In the early 1980s, the Macintosh development team at Apple Computer was determined that their computer would be easy to use. At the start, they borrowed heavily from one of Xerox's advanced research groups to achieve the final outcome—an operating system interface that was intuitive. More importantly, however, the Macintosh's developers realized that for their new prodigy to be successful, it would have to stand out via ease of use. They gradually wrote what would eventually be called the Human Interface Guidelines (HIG) (Apple, 1987). These guidelines specified items we now take for granted in both the Macintosh and Microsoft Windows domains: a mouse-driven command structure, a menu bar, scroll bars at the side and bottom of windows, and a single title bar for each window on the screen.

After the introduction of the Macintosh in 1984, nearly all applications that did not closely follow the HIG failed in the marketplace. Users reportedly enjoyed the improving learning curve—once they had learned how to react to and give information to a single application, they could do the same for most other applications. With the advent of color in the Macintosh in 1987, an additional factor was added. In adding color to the mix, Apple's goal was to "add meaning, not just to color things so they 'look good'" (Withey & Wagner, 1987). Application developers learned that programs should be designed in black and white, with color used only as a supplementation to the overall scheme (Schneiderman, 1987). Since that time, animation presentation techniques have been perfected.

Sound input and output have also been added to computers, with many new monitors containing built-in stereo speakers. Several monitors incorporate sensitive microphones as well.

Interface Techniques

Since the personal computer first became an economic and commercial reality with the Radio Shack TRS-80 and the Apple II, computer interfaces have advanced considerably. In the 1970s, an individual operator would communicate with the computer by entering information on a keyboard. The user could, for example, press "Y" for a Yes answer or enter a number in response to a multiple-choice question. Movement on the screen, entries of information, and graphic design all required keyboard commands.

In the early 1980s, the mouse was added to personal computers as an alternative input technique. The mouse would give instructions to a cursor on the screen, allowing the operator to "point and click" on potential answers presented on the computer's monitor. The mouse assisted those unwilling or unable to use the keyboard and allowed graphic design to be accomplished in a more intuitive manner, with the user using the mouse as a pen. Touch screens provide a similar capability wherein the user points to and touches the monitor screen at a desired location to indicate a response to the computer. Touch screens remain a more expensive interface than other available devices.

Speech Interface

More recent advances in multimedia computing allow for a voice interface to be used inexpensively. Early voice interfaces required the computer to be "trained" for each user's voice. Training is no longer necessary with current technology. Voice interfaces permit the computer to "speak" questions to the user, using either digitized wide-spectrum recordings or a voice created with the assistance of a digital signal processor, and permits the user to answer directly into a microphone. A voice created with the assistance of the computer requires reasonable processing speed, enough random access memory (RAM) to contain each spoken phrase, and a compatible operating system but no storage requirements beyond that of the system software itself. In this instance, the computer can be programmed to read directly from a text file that itself would take minimal hard drive storage. Currently available 80486, 68040, or PPC-based computers are all able to accomplish this task. Unfortunately, the state of the art for desktop computers still results in speech that is clearly computer generated. It may be difficult to understand for some users, especially those for whom the language used is not their primary language.

Recorded, digitized speech represents the use of recorded human voice, replayed by the computer for the user. The reproduced voice can be of audio compact disc quality; further, multiple languages can be recorded such that the user can choose their preferred language for playback. Processing speed of the computer is less important for this situation, but large amounts of storage space are necessary for an extensive application. Depending on the recording technique, a 10 second sound file will require roughly 200 kilobytes of storage space. This storage method is preferable, however, to that of computer generated speech, and the storage requirement is easily overcome by using a CD-ROM as an application interface. Hiring a professional voice expert for the recording session is advisable if it fits into the budget. The production of a CD-ROM after appropriate testing of the application and recording has been complete is easily available and has become inexpensive. Over 600 megabytes of information can be stored on a single CD-ROM. The application should be programmed to access updates, if any exist, from a local hard drive, thereby allowing updates to be made without the need for mastering a new CD. As of this writing, the cost of a recordable CD-ROM drive that is SCSI compatible (and therefore useful for both Macintosh and IBM PC compatible systems) is under $2000.

Speech Recognition

Early in the computerized use of sound, audio was used in two general ways. The first was to integrate sound throughout the standard interface to help make the user aware of the state of the computer or application. The second was to alert the user when something happens unexpectedly in the background (Withey & Wagner, 1987). As speech recognition technologies improved, three axes were postulated (Negroponte, 1990). The first axis is user-dependent versus user-independent speech; the goal is for the computer not to have to be trained for each word spoken by the user. The second axis is that of small versus large vocabularies. Here, one might also recognize that a variety of languages can be recognized by the computer such that the user's language of choice becomes less germane to their interaction with the computer. The last axis is discrete versus connected speech. Until very recently, most computer speech recognition routines required the user to pause between each word. Within speech recognition applications, four response types must generally be expected (Schmandt, 1990). The user might be silent, indicating that the computer should continue speaking; the user might acknowledge understanding; the user might indicate a lack of understanding; the user might indicate a desire that the computer change the speed of its presentation. Clearly, in the case of a direct query, the computer should expect a specific response set in addition to the possible utterances just mentioned.

Within the most recent release of the Macintosh Operating System (MOS), version 7.5, 51 phonemes are recognizable by the computer (Heid, 1994). When a spoken command is presented to the computer, the MOS analyzes the data to determine the volume of various frequencies; it then compares the results to its data base of phonemes. Once a word has been recognized, the MOS generates an event message that is sent to the active program. The program then responds accordingly. This process can take up to several seconds, depending on processor speed. Additional functionality is also present wherein the computer can read text that is present within an appropriately programmed presentation. Numbers, proper names, and nonstandard languages are acceptable. For example, "Dr. White" is pronounced "Doctor White" whereas "disk dr." is pronounced as "disk drive." Text to speech allows the computer to be programmed to allow telephone-controlled data access or manipulation (Poole, 1994). It also allows working with visually impaired users or to serve as a voice for those who have difficulty with speech themselves. Computers can now produce verbal information in any language, in a male or female voice, and at any speed desired. Frequency and amplitude may both be adjusted to the needs of the listener. Computer applications utilizing this interface are programmed to expect certain potential responses and can request verification of responses that do not appear to fit the programmed possibilities. More advanced programs can allow the computer to respond to potential questions posed by the individual at the workstation.

Patient Acceptance of Computer Interface

Shortly after the introduction of personal computers, computers were shown to be acceptable to the general public for purposes of health-related instruction (Chen, Houston, & Burson, undated; Ellis & Raines, 1981). Computerized instruction allows dialogue to be individualized. Self-pacing and self-testing within a private environment is easily achieved. The use of a computer facilitates standardization of an interview, permitting a higher degree of uniformity in the interview situation, and controlling for diverse sources of variability in the patient–interviewer interaction such as language difficulties and countertransference reactions. Computer reports also reduce the likelihood of subjective bias in reporting of results (Butcher, 1994).

Automated interviewing provides improved logistical feasibility. Software has consistency and constant availability. On-line documentation is available when programmed. Any language or speed consistent with any single patient's needs can be used. The combination of visual and oral cues improves the chance that users are exposed to the medium that works best for them (Brown, Wright, & Christensen, 1987).

Data collection from patients by computers presents several potential drawbacks. First among them is the expense of the workstation, although this can be offset by the degree to which the computer is used for other purposes. The computer misses certain inputs that would be taken for granted by a clinical observer, such as body language, pitch and intensity of verbal input, and latency of response. As programming techniques improve, several of these variables could indeed be measured. Finally, while new technologies have greatly enhanced the potential for useful computerized interfaces, typical computer programs for patient use are didactic and fail to tailor information to an individual's specific needs (Skinner, Siegfried, Kegler, & Strecher, 1993).

Patients found computers not to be demeaning or threatening; they reported feeling more comfortable reporting sensitive information to a nonjudgmental computer than to a physician (Ghosh & Greist, 1988; Servan–Schreiber, 1986). When women were given either computerized, verbal, written, or no instructions for collection of a clean urine specimen, those receiving computerized instruction produced urine specimens with the fewest bacterial contaminants (Fisher, Johnson, Porter, Bleich, & Slack, 1977). Computers have been successfully enlisted as interview aides in psychiatry (Carr & Ghosh, 1983; Greist, 1984; Slack & Slack, 1977) as well as in chemical dependence, specifically (Duffy & Waterton, 1977; Lucas, Mullin, Luna, & McInroy, 1977) for at least 15 years.

Patients describe deviant behavior or stigmatized symptoms more easily to a computer than to human interviewers. Those patients with alcohol-based diagnoses will admit greater quantities and frequencies of alcohol use to a computer than to a psychiatrist presenting the same questions (Duffy & Waterton, 1977; Lucas et al., 1977). Studies of alcoholic and schizophrenic patients indicate computer interactive programs to be at least as effective for educational purposes as videotape (Alterman & Baughman, 1991) and printed word (Gitlow, 1991) methods of pre-sentation. These findings suggest that computer technology might offer significant advantages in administering a questionnaire about patients' attitudes regarding chemical dependence treatment and recovery. The majority of computerized versus paper-and-pencil presentations in the past have concluded that the two types of testing are equivalent (Flowers' Booraem, & Schwartz, 1993). These studies did not generally include voice interactive methods of interfacing the patient with the computer.

Computerizing RAATE Questionnaire

One method of assessing resistance and obstacles to chemical dependence treatment is the Recovery Attitude and Treatment Evaluator (RAATE) Questionnaire. The RAATE assesses the patient at a single cross section in time and is suitable for serial administration. It is a comprehensive, standardized, and quantitative means of assessing resistance and obstacles to recovery (Mee–Lee, 1988). Developed to help clinicians improve clinical assessments, the computerized version of the RAATE has a standard report capability that is thorough and based upon a uniform method of data gathering (Mee–Lee, 1985).

The RAATE Questionnaire has 94 true/false items comprising five subscales: Resistance to Treatment, Resistance to Continuing Care, Acuity of Biomedical Problems, Acuity of Psychiatric/Psychological Problems, and Social/Systems/Family Problems Unsupportive to Recovery. Content of the RAATE is clearly sensitive; the population of interest has variable levels of cognition and varying degrees of denial that present a challenging test of feasibility and performance for voice-based computer interviews.

Gastfriend, in 1992, constructed a computer program to offer the RAATE by high-fidelity digitally recorded human voice. The computer recognizes patient responses spoken into the computer's microphone. An Apple Macintosh IIsi computer was adapted with Voice Navigator voice recognition hardware (Articulate Systems, Inc., Woburn, MA) and a custom HyperCard software application (Apple Computer, Inc., Cupertino, CA). This specific hardware would no longer be necessary with many contemporary computers containing internal microphones and speech recognition capabilities.

Computerized RAATE Research Protocol

Each patient was presented with one of four RAATE questionnaires: conventional paper and pencil, computerized text output to the screen/mouse-selected patient input, voice output/mouse input, and voice output/patient voice input. Patients using the computer received brief instructions and supervision. All computer formats were timed by the computer; other forms of RAATE administrations were timed by the Intake Coordinator. Patients were asked to rate their confidence in their answers, their satisfaction with the questionnaire, and their perception of the usefulness of the questions in planning their treatment. Because this study was conducted using a prototype system, patients who were randomized to the voice/voice version underwent a brief process to "train" the computer to recognize their voice. This process would no longer be necessary with current operating systems. Sixty-eight patients participated in this study, 78% of whom were men, with half having alcohol as their drug of choice.

The mean duration of test administration across all four versions was 15.5 minutes, with a standard deviation of 4.4 minutes. There were no significant differences among the groups. There was, however, a trend for differences in uniformity, in which the voice/voice version produced the least variance among subjects' durations of response ($p = 0.062$). Thus, the Voice–Voice format yielded the best combination of brevity and uniformity of test administration.

All patients agreed to complete the instrument, regardless of format. The patients' mean confidence ratings regarding the accuracy of their answers revealed the mean confidence rating to be greatest in the voice/voice group. However, the differences among the four groups were not significant. Again, there was a trend in which the voice/voice version yielded the most homogeneous distribution of responses ($p = 0.091$). Patients showed more intersubject uniformity in their confidence of their responses using the voice/voice format. No differences were observed between the four formats in terms of patient satisfaction ratings or perceived usefulness of the questions in their treatment planning. The computerized voice interactive presentation is a highly efficient process that produces high levels of satisfaction reported by patients. These results are consistent with studies of paper-and-pencil vs. computerized interviews in general.

Summary

Desktop computers have capabilities that represent a marked improvement over that available only 1 to 2 years ago. The recent combination of audio and video technology with that of the personal computer allows the use of movie footage from laser disc or videotape to be combined with compact disc quality sound in the creation of an application that is understandable by even the computer-phobic population. Several new systems have RCA-type and S-video input jacks identical to those used on stereo components for the input of audio and video information. Combining these abilities with a high-level programming language and modern operating system can lead to the rapid development of a fully interactive application.

Computerized voice interactive interviewing is not only feasible, but efficient and effective. The use of computers shortens test durations and increases uniformity of administration. The use of a voice interface increases access for vision-impaired or foreign language speakers and increases data entry efficiency and accuracy. Interviews assessing stigmatized syndromes through the use of potentially provocative questions may particularly benefit from the use of a computerized interface. A consistent, controlled, and nonjudgmental interview interaction may now be provided by the interested clinician.

References

Alterman, A.I., & Baughman, T.G. (1991). Videotape versus computer interactive education in alcoholic and nonalcoholic controls. *Alcoholism, Clinical and Experimental Research, 15,* 39–44.

Apple Computer Inc. (1987). *Human interface guidelines: The Apple desktop interface*. Reading, MA: Addison–Wesley Publishing Co.

Brown, C.S., Wright, R.G., & Christensen, D.B. (1987). Association between type of medication instruction and patients' knowledge, side effects, and compliance. *Hospital & Community Psychiatry, 38*, 55–60.

Butcher, J.N. (1994). Psychological assessment by computer: Potential gains and problems to avoid. *Psychiatric Annals, 24*, 20–24.

Carr, A.C., & Ghosh, A. (1983). Can a computer take a psychiatric history? *Psychological Medicine, 13*, 151–158.

Chen, M.S., Houston, T.P., & Burson, J.L. (undated). *Microcomputer-based health education in the waiting room: A feasibility study*. Ph.D. Thesis, Ohio State University.

Duffy, J.C., & Waterton, J.J. (1977). Under-reporting of alcohol consumption in sample surveys: The effect of computer interviewing in fieldwork. *British Journal of Addiction, 79*, 303–308.

Ellis, L.B.M., & Raines, J.R. (1981). Health education using microcomputers: Initial acceptability. *Preventive Medicine, 10*, 77–84.

Fisher, L.A., Johnson, T.S., Porter, D., Bleich, H.L., & Slack, W.V. (1977). Collection of a clean voided urine specimen: A comparison among spoken, written, and computer-based instructions. *American Journal of Public Health, 67*, 640–644.

Flowers, J.V., Booraem, C.D., & Schwartz, B. (1993). Impact of computerized rapid assessment instruments on counselors and client outcome. *Computers in Human Services, 10*, 9–15.

Ghosh, A., & Greist, J.H. (1988). Computer treatment in psychiatry. *Psychiatric Annals, 18*, 246–250.

Gitlow, S. (1991). *Medication: educating the psychiatric patient*. Master's thesis, University of Pittsburgh School of Public Health, Pittsburgh, PA.

Greist, J.H. (1984). Conservative radicalism: An approach to computers in mental health. In M.D. Schwartz (Ed.), *Using computers in clinical practice*. New York: Haworth Press.

Heid, J. (1994). *Macworld complete Mac handbook*. San Mateo, CA: IDG Books.

Lucas, R., Mullin, P., Luna, C., & McInroy, D. (1977). Psychiatrists and a computer as interrogators of patients with alcohol-related ilnesses: A comparison. *British Journal of Psychiatry, 131*, 160–167.

McLellan, A., Luborsky, L., & Woody, G. (1980). An improved diagnostic evaluation instrument for substance abuse patients: The Addiction Severity Index. *Journal of Nervous and Mental Disorders, 168*, 26–33.

Mee–Lee, D. (1985). The Recovery Attitude and Treatment Evaluator (RAATE): An instrument for patient progress and treatment assignment. *Proding of the 34th Internation Congress on Alcoholism and Drug Dependency*, pp. 424–426.

Mee–Lee, D. (1988). An instrument for treatment progress and matching: The Recovery Attitude and Treatment Evaluator (RAATE). *Journal of Substance Abuse and Treatment, 5*, 183–186.

Negroponte, N. (1990). Hospital corners. In B. Laurel (Ed.), *The art of human–computer interface design*. Reading, MA: Addison–Wesley.

Poole, L. (1994). *Macworld system 7.5 bible*. San Mateo, CA: IDG Books.

Schmandt C. (1990). Illusion in the interface. In B. Laurel (Ed.), *The art of human–computer interface design*. Reading, MA: Addison – Wesley Publishing Co.

Schneiderman, B. (1987). *Designing the user interface: Strategies for effective human–computer interaction*. Reading, MA: Addison–Wesley Publishing Co.

Servan–Schreiber, S.D. (1986). Artificial intelligence and psychiatry. *Journal of Nervous and Menal Disease, 174*, 191–202.

Skinner, C.S., Siegfried, J.C., Kegler, M.C., & Strecher, V.J. (1993). *The potential of computers in patient education. Patient Education and Counseling, 22*, 27–34.

Slack, W.V., & Slack, C.W. (1977). Talking to a computer about emotional problems: A comparative study. *Psychotherapy Theory Res Practice, 14*, 156–163.

Withey, K., & Wagner, A. (1987). *Human interface technical note*. Apple Computer, Inc.

8
How to Create Your Own Computerized Questionnaires
Marvin J. Miller and Morgan Tharp

We now have a 25 year history of using computerized interviews for the testing of psychiatric patients (Maultsby & Slack, 1971). The real and the potential benefits of computerized testing have been documented in various studies. Computerized interviews are very inexpensive and are very systematic in remembering to present all the questions needed to make a thorough evaluation (Slack, Hicks, Reed, & Van Cura, 1966; Downing, Francis, & Brockington, 1980). The systematic approach of the computerized interview often elicits symptoms missed in routine clinical interviews.

Patients are able to focus on material more carefully because one question at a time is presented to the screen. The patient directs the speed of the interview at his/her own comfort level and the computer is generally seen as less threatening than a human interviewer. In one studies, the interview itself reduces the level of stress and anxiety (Greist, Gustafson, & Strauss, 1973). This program was also able to predict the potential for suicide attempts and the persons interviewed reported a good level of comfort in giving information to a computer. Depression is a symptom area that can be evaluated well by computer (Ancill, Rogers, & Carr, 1985).

Topics that would traditionally be threatening or embarrassing are more easily handled by the computer. Patients' self-report of alcohol consumption is often twice as high when reported to the computer as compared with reporting to other interviewers (Lucas, Mullin, Luna, & McInroy, 1977).

There is generally less fear and resistance from patients than is found in clinicians. Computers are present in so many areas of life today that patients report being very comfortable in giving their information to a computer (Lucas, Card, Knill-Jones, Watkinson, & Crean, 1976; Carr, Ghosh, & Ancill, 1983). Some even perceive a clinic as more up to date when computerized assessment tools are present.

Clinicians benefit from computerized interviews in several ways. They have a comprehensive set of screening information with which to conduct their own specialized, in-depth evaluation. The thoroughness of the computerized interview often raises pieces of information that might have escaped attention otherwise. The printed summary of the computerized interview is much more legible and more likely to be read and utilized in the treatment program than handwritten material.

Difficulties in Computerized Testing

While it is not very difficult to program a questionnaire for computer administration, it does require skills that are not present in every psychiatric clinic or private office. There are many "questionnaire drivers" available that provide a short cut to this process. The text of a proposed questionnaire is developed on a word processor with embedded codes that tell the driver what to do. The driver then administers the questionnaire to the patient. The answers are saved and can be summarized in a formatted summary of the test. The same questionnaire driver can administer many different questionnaires if they are properly configured and available on the same computer as the driver. This driver is available as shareware on various BBS and FTP sites. The following is a set of instructions about composing and administering a questionnaire using this generic driver.

The Questionnaire Driver

This questionnaire driver is a program in the Basic language designed to use a separate text file to administer a set of questions and appropriate responses stored in the text file. The text file must be appropriately coded with a format to be used by the questionnaire driver. An explanation and a sample text file are discussed here so that the reader can construct and use a questionnaire.

The Driver allows administration of the test that is in the text file. The results are then stored on disk. These results may be retrieved from the disk by the Driver, and the results printed out for use by the test administrator.

Setting Up a Text File Questionnaire

The text file has codes that tells the Driver program what to do with each line from the text file. The Driver reads each line from the text file separately, then looks at the leftmost character to see if it is a code symbol shown below. If the leftmost character is a code symbol, the Driver uses that line as directed by the code symbol. If the leftmost character is not one of these symbols, then the line is treated as a continuation of the previous line. (The # and % signs require an additional character or two to the right of them of further direct the Driver. This will be explained later.)

The following are the symbols and a brief summary of what they mean. A more detailed explanation is given later in this document.

−: A remark line in the program (will be ignored by the Driver)
+: A title or general category that the question is in
*: A brief summary of the question
$: End of the question, time for the response to be entered.
&: An on-screen note to the test taker (information note)
#: The beginning of a multiple-choice response
%: The beginning of a multiple-choice response that will be printed on-screen more than once (stored for later use).
Sx or Rx: Store or retrieve a set of frequently used set of multiple choice responses.
Any numeral: marks the beginning of a yes-no or multiple-choice type question.
Space: If at the beginning of a question, marks it as a text answer type question; otherwise, the line is treated as a continuation of the previous line.
Blank lines are ignored (except in on-screen notes); all other lines (not marked by an action modifier above) are treated as the previous line was treated.
Note: The symbols above are treated as special symbols, only when located in the very leftmost position of the line.

Sample Program

This section explains the sample text file at the end of this document so that one can better understand how to set up text files for the questionnaire Driver.

The next section is a note; it begins with the ampersand (&). Each line until the next symbol ($) is treated as a part of the note. In notes, blank lines in the text file are not ignored. This first note is the introduction to the questionnaire to be administered. The dollar sign ($) at the end of this note tells the Driver to hold. The reader must press the Return key to continue.

Following this is another on-screen note, explaining the text. This gives one a chance to explain any terms the patient will need to know or to give directions. Notes may be displayed before or between questions anywhere in the questionnaire.

The first question begins with the numeral "1." Any numeral in the leftmost position at the beginning of a question sets up the question as a yes-no or multiple-choice type question. The next symbol is the pound sign (#). This tells the computer two things. First, this is a multiple-choice type question. Second, this marks the beginning of a choice. The computer now looks at the second leftmost character (a 0 here); this number represents the response the patient must give if this fits him.

The next symbol is again the #. This tells the computer the first multiple-choice response possibility is over, and marks the beginning of the second. The second leftmost character is a "1"; this is the appropriate response for the choice: "I occasionally avoid them for this reason."

The third choice is marked by a # followed by a 2. The computer next sees the $, and it marks the end of this question. The Driver now prompts the patient for his response. The response must be either a 0, 1, or 2 in this example, as suggested by the symbols. If it is not, the computer reminds the patient that these are the only acceptable responses.

The next symbol is an asterisk (*), and it marks a brief summary of the question. This brief summary may be used on the final printout to remind the administrator of the question content without printing the whole question. These should be kept as brief as possible.

The next symbol is again a number (2). Thus, this is either a yes-no or multiple-choice question. The computer prints this question on the screen until it comes to the next symbol, the #, suggesting the beginning of multiple choices. The character immediately following the # is a 1, so the appropriate response for this choice is a 1. Similarly, each of the next choices are 2, 3, and 4. Thus, the patient must respond with a 1, 2, 3, or 4 or the computer will not accept the answer and prompts to enter one of these characters. Following this is the $, end of question, and the summary (*) of the question. The next symbol is again a numeral, 3. Thus, this again is a yes-no or multiple-choice question. The next symbol is a $, showing the end of the question. Because there is no # to suggest multiple choice (or % as we shall see later), this is presented as a yes-no question to the patient. After this is the * indicating question summary. Next comes the + sign. This is the category or title of the preceding questions. The category can be listed for *each* question, or on the *last* question of the category only. The category Contamination Obsessions could have been listed at the end of questions 1, 2, and 3, or as done here. Because it occurs at the end of question 3, questions 1, 2, and 3 are all assumed to be in this category of questions.

The next question again begins with a numeral, indicating yes-no or multiple-choice format. Following the question we note the % symbol. This shows a group of multiple choices that will be repeated several times throughout the text. The Driver next looks at the symbol to the right of the %, which must be an R or an S. This means "Repeat a previously stored group" or "Store this group of choices after printing it on-screen."

The symbol is an S, so this set of multiple choice responses will be stored. The third symbol is next looked at; it must be either a 1, 2, or 3. This indicates which set of repeated choices will be stored. Thus, 3 different sets of repetitive choices can be stored and repeated on the screen at any time.

The following line again has the % symbol, suggesting a set of choices to be repeated. Because the Driver has been set in the mode to store this set of choices, it looks for the # sign next to tell it this is a new multiple-choice possibility. Following the # symbol is the appropriate response for the answer. Following this possible choice, the next set of symbols is the %#2, indicating a choice to be stored, with the appropriate response being 2. After this choice comes %#3, indicating to store this possible response with the proper response being 3. Next comes a $, showing the end of the question. The previous multiple choices are now stored as multiple-choice set 1, and can be repeated following later questions, as we shall see. The question summary then follows (*).

Question 5, denoted by the numeral 5, will next be printed on-screen. Following the question, the Driver will see the symbol %, again suggesting a repetitive set of multiple choices. Following the %, on the same line, the Driver looks for an R or an S. Here, the symbol is R, which will repeat a previously stored set of responses. The DRIVER next looks at the character following the R to see which set of responses, 1, 2, or 3, to print (set #1 here).

The Driver now repeats multiple-choices set 1 on the screen. The $ is the next symbol, showing the end of the question. The computer now prompts for the patient to give an appropriate response. Following this is the question summary (*), and then the general category (+). Again, the category is placed on the *last* question to which it applies, so the Driver places the prior unclassified questions in this category; in this case questions 4 and 5 are stored in the category Aggressive Obsessions. (Note that the repetitive multiple choice sets can be stored as set 1, 2, and/or 3. Thus, three different sets of repetitive choices can be stored and reused when needed. Also, any set can be changed later in the questionnaire. For example, set 1 in this sample was stored in question 4. If later in the questionnaire it is desired to have a different repetitive set 1, the same format for storing set 1 is followed as is shown in question 4.).

The next question in the example text program begins with a space. Thus, the Driver treats this question as a text answer type question. The $ symbol is seen following the question, prompting the Driver to ask the patient for a response. The patient may now type in one line of text before pressing enter. Following this is the question symmary (*), and the category (+).

The next question starts with a numeral (7), suggesting yes-no or multiple choice. Note that the number counts the text answer question previously as number 6, as this is the way the Driver treats the text

question. Following this question is the $ (end of question) and the *
(summary) followed by the + (the title).

The Driver next sees that this is the end of the text file, and displays a
note on the screen that the questionnaire is over.

Hints for Writing Text File

Use the repetitive multiple-choice format as much as possible; this makes
the text file simpler and greatly speeds the administration of the questionnaire. Keep the multiple-choice response concise. Keep question
summaries as brief as possible (two or three words if possible). Title
headings should be capitalized. Put ample on-screen notes in the questionnaire to explain the test and its terminology.

Administering the Questionnaire

After loading Basic, the Driver program is loaded from the disk by typing
load "driver." When the OK prompt is again displayed, type Run to
begin the test. After the initial screen, press Enter to continue. The
Driver can also be compiled with one of many Basic compilers so that the
above steps are simplified.

The first aspect of the program to appear is the main menu. Press 1
then Enter to administer the questionnaire. Next, the Driver will ask for
the name of the text file in which the questionnaire is stored. At this
prompt, type in the proper file name (filename.ext), then press Enter. If
the file is not found an error message will be displayed.

The Driver will next ask for the patient's ID number. Enter a number
that uniquely represents this patient. This ID number will be the file
name under which the results of this questionnaire will be stored. (Con-
sequently, if the same patient will be taking more than one questionnaire,
the results must be stored on different disks, or in different subdirectories,
or the results of the previous questionnaire will be erased.) After pressing
Enter, the program asks for the patient's name. Once this has been
entered, the questionnaire is presented on the screen.

While taking the test, the patient will be given yes-no, multiple-choice,
or text answer type questions as stored in the text file. The patient must
press Enter after each response to enter it in the computer. The patient
may backup any time simply by typing the word back when the prompt is
given to respond to a question. The option also exists to halt the test by
typing stop at this prompt. The program stores results of the completed
questions and a note is made in the file that the test was stopped
prematurely.

After the test is completed, a message is displayed on-screen that the test is over, and to notify the test administrator. The Driver now waits for the proper disk (for storing the patient's responses to the questionnaire) to be placed in the drive; when this is the case, the administrator is to press Enter. The test is now complete, and the screen returns to the main menu. The Driver program is in the public domain and can be obtained from various BBSs and FTP sites as DRIVER.ZIP.

Obtaining Results on a Printout

From the Main Menu, press 2 then Enter to reach the Print Menu. At this point, there are two options for printing. One option is to obtain a listing of all questions to which the patient gave a specified response. A printout is obtained by pressing 1 then Enter from the Print Menu. The Driver will ask which specific answers are being requested. That is, one may want a list of all questions to which the patient responded with a 1, a listing of all questions to which the response was 4, etc. At this point, press the number of each specific answer for which a listing is desired, followed by pressing Enter. After entering the number for each list that wanted, type Stop followed by Enter. After checking the printer for readiness to print, press Enter and the printout will be generated.

The second option for printouts is to obtain a listing of each question and the response that the patient gave. To do so, press 2 at the Print Menu, then press Enter. Verify that the printer is ready, press Enter, and the printout will be generated. After either option has been completed, one is returned to the Print Menu. The third option at this point is to press 3 then Enter, which will return one to the main menu. The program is ready to offer any of the options discussed earlier.

References

Ancill, R.J., Rogers, D., & Carr, A.C. (1985). Comparison of computerized self-rating scales for depression with conventional observer ratings. *Acta Psychiatrica Scandinavica, 71*, 315–317.

Carr, A.C., Ghosh, A., & Ancill, R.J. (1983). Can a computer take a psychiatric history? *Psycholical Medicine, 13*, 151–158.

Downing, A.R., Francis, A.F., & Brockington, I.F. (1980). A comparison of information sources in the study of psychotic illness. *British Journal of Psychiatry, 137*, 38–44.

Greist, J.H., Gustafson, D.H., & Stauss, F.F. (1973). A computer interview for suicide risk prediction. *American Journal of Psychiatry, 130*, 1327–1332.

Lucas, R.W., Card, W.I., Knill–Jones, R.P., Wakinson, G., & Grean, G.P. (1976). Computer interrogation of patients. *British Medical Journal, 2*, 623–625.

Lucas, R.W., Mullin P.J., Luna C.B.X., & McInroy D.C. (1977). Psychiatrists and a computer as interrogators of patients with alcohol related illnesses: A comparison. *British Journal of Psychiatry, 131*, 160–167.

Maultsby, M.C., & Slack, W.V. (1971). A computer based psychiatric history system. *Archives of General Psychiatry, 25*, 570–572.

Slack, W.V., Hicks, G.P., Reed, C.E., & Van Cura, L.J. (1966). A computer-based medical-history system. *New England Journal of Medicine, 274*, 194–198.

Appendix I: Text File of Sample Program

& SAMPLE PROGRAM
written by
John Q. Doctor, M.D.

$
& This questionnaire is a set of multiple-choice, yes-no, and text-answer type questions. The question will appear on the screen, and you will then be shown a set of responses from which you must choose the one that best fits you.
$
1. Have you ever avoided using cabs/taxis because they might be dirty or have germs, even though you actually knew it didn't make sense?

#00 = This has never happened
#11 = I occasionally avoid them for this reason
#22 = I frequently avoid using them for this reason
$
* Avoids cabs/taxis because of germs

2. Have you ever worried excessively about getting germs if you touch a public telephone (even if you wash your hands afterward)?

#11 = I have never been worried by this
#22 = I seldom worry about germs from telephones
#33 = I frequently worry about germs from telephones
#44 = I avoid telephones because of germs
$
*Excessive concern with contamination from telephones

3. Have you ever been bothered by the thought that your hands are dirty after touching doorknobs?

$

* Excessive concern with contamination from doorknobs
+ CONTAMINATION OBSESSIONS

4. Have you been frightened or upset by thoughts or ideas that you might start a fire even though you know you don't want to?
%S1
%#1 1 = Never
%#2 2 = Occasionally
%#3 3 = Frequently
$
* Fear might start a fire

5. Are you constantly bothered by the thought that you may have done something that will harm another person even though you didn't intend this?
%R1
$
* Fear might harm others
+ AGGRESSIVE OBSESSIONS

Do you have any other obsessions that we did not ask you about?
$
*Other obsessions
+ OPEN-ANSWER QUESTION

7. Do you often make two or more trips through your house or apart-ment before leaving just to make sure that everything is OK?
%R1
$

* Multiple checks before leaving house
+ CHECKING COMPULSIONS

Appendix II: Printout of Sample Test Results

Name: John Doe   ID Number: 123
Questionnaire: Test1   Date: 3/14/94

Heading	Question	Answer
Contamination obsession		
	1. * Avoids cabs/taxis because of germs	1
	2. * Excessive concern with contamination from telephones	2
	3. * Excessive concern with contamination from door knobs	y
Aggressive obsessions		
	4. * Fear might start fire	2
	5. * Fear might harm others	3
Checking obsessions		
	7. * Multiple checks before leaving house	3

Test-answer questions:
* Other obsessions
The person responded as
   follows:
I don't want to talk
   about them.

9
Clinical Experience With a Prescription Writer Program
T. Bradley Tanner and Mary P. Metcalf

Writing prescriptions for patients can be tedious and prone to error. Particular care must be taken with psychiatric medications. A single mistake in a routine reorder of these medicine can have catastrophic consequences: too little medication can lead to a relapse; too much can cause to arrhythmia's dystonias, or unstable gait. Further, psychiatric illness is frequently chronic and multifaceted, with the result that patients may be using several medications simultaneously, as well as having been prescribed a high number of different medications over the course of their treatment. Patients with suicidality or cognitive impairment require particularly close follow-up and monitoring of their use of medication. Writing prescriptions for more than 1 week's supply, or with many refills, may not be appropriate for these patients.

In these (as in all patient) situations, the process of prescription writing involves more than filling out the appropriate form. Choice of the number and frequency of refills, dosing regime, and tracking the patient's other medications is essential. Several problems confront the doctor and mental health professional in regard to these issues. For example, frequent writing of refill prescriptions is time consuming, and in a busy outpatient treatment setting where patients are being seen for 15 minute medication checks, time is precious. The need to hurry can detract from accuracy of prescription writing and from the quality of patient care.

A related task is the time consuming, yet useful, one of maintaining a record of a patient's past and present medications. A well-maintained record can be critical to determining the best course of treatment. This task must compete with other functions such as documentation of clinical status and patient education. Often, there simply may not be time for everything, and the medication record is overlooked.

Patients, their families, and caregivers often request a listing of the current medications. These lists help patients remember what medications they are taking and when they should take them. A complete list of active medications is an excellent way to bring patients and their nonprofessional providers into the treatment process. Nonetheless, time constraints often limit providers to hastily handwritten lists of medication names. The benefit of a fresh typewritten listing is easily outweighed by the time expense.

All of these tasks are perfectly suited for computerization. With appropriate software, a computer can flawlessly prepare prescription after prescription, each one exactly like the previous one and correctly dated. A computer can keep track of thousands of medications over many years. It can compile a medication history including medication name, dose, start date, stop date, dosing instruction, typical refills, and prescriber. On command, a computer can create a useful listing of medications for the patient; no additional work is required. A few programs exist to perform these functions. This chapter will briefly discuss currently available prescription writing programs and then will discuss one, Prescription Writer™), in depth. This will allow the reader to determine how a prescription writing program could be of benefit, and then to familiarize him with one such program for a more complete understanding.

Commercially Available Software

S-O-A-P Drug Interaction and Prescription Writing Program™, AskRx™ Plus, RxWriter™, HNPRX™, and Prescription Writer™ are all commercially available programs with prescription writing capabilities. Availability is noted at the end of the chapter. Costs typically range from $100 to $200 for the initial version of the software. Thus, such programs are within the cost range of the solo practitioner and group practice. Features include simple prescription printing, refill functions, and demographic/medical information storage for patients.

All of these products can perform the basic function of printing a prescription based on data entered into the computer. The features of interest to the particular user vary. For example, some programs include a list of frequently prescribed medications; others allow the physician to custom build a list. Such a "customizable" list of medication may be of most use to the psychiatrist. The computer hardware environment of all of these programs is the IBM PC or compatible. Some run under Windows; others only require DOS. Some can function over a network; others are designed for single user situations.

The ability to indicate drug interaction problems is an important component of both AskRx and the S-O-A-P programs. These programs combine prescription writing features with reference material. Whether the individual physician sees this as an advantage or disadvantage is personal. The advantage would be the ready availability of information on a medication one is about to prescribe. However, such information is currently available in common reference books. Further, each of these programs would require updating, just as do standard (paper-based) reference materials. This increases the cost of the programs, and requires continued maintenance. Because it is unlikely that paper-based reference manuals will be eliminated from the medical setting, a practitioner might not be interested in this ability.

RxWriter, HNPRX, and Prescription Writer all focus primarily on simplifying the task of writing the script. Each allows the physician user to log medication information, and create a custom list of medications. A brief description of the five programs follows.

S-O-A-P Drug Interaction and Prescription Writing Program

S-O-A-P is a DOS program that is intended for use in a variety of settings (i.e., physician office, nursing home). Records of patient drug use and medical summaries can be maintained using S-O-A-P. In addition, the program has built-in data on the interactions and possible side effects of more than 2,500 medications. S-O-A-P automatically checks for problem drug interactions when a medication is added to a patient's list, and indicates such problems. Two-hundred-fifty prescriptions are built-in to the program, and an additional 250 more may be added by the user. In order to "write" a prescription, the user may choose one of three approaches: enter new data, alter an existing prescription (such as the built-ins) or simply choose a built-in script. Some report generating features (such as a patient chart) are available.

An enhanced version of this program is the S-O-A-P Patient Medical Records System 2, which includes all of the features of the Drug Interaction and Prescription Writer program. It includes additional text capabilities for patient records, can link to common billing programs, and is networkable. The cost is substantially higher than the simpler version. Update versions are offered twice yearly. The program is also DOS based.

AskRx Plus

AskRx Plus is a Windows program available on CD-ROM. It allows storage of patient data, and also notes problem drug interactions. Based on the USP DI of the U.S. Pharmacopial convention, AskRx includes a great deal of reference material. Detailed information on medications, including the information typically associated with the "insert" (i.e., indications, contraindications, even bibliographic references), is available. In addition, the program can suggest medications for specific problems, such as high blood pressure, and note medications to avoid in patients with specific conditions. Report generating functions exist to create listings of patients, medications, and combinations of these. A network version is available, as are annual updates of the drug information.

RxWriter

RxWriter runs under DOS. RxWriter concentrates on automating the process of writing prescriptions and tracking that data for patients. Using RxWriter the physician can link personal notes to specific medications. When that medication is prescribed the computer sounds a "warble" to remind the physician of his note. In addition, scripts written with RxWriter can be as simple or complex prescriptions as desired. A refill feature has recently been added.

HNPRX

HNPRX runs using DOS, Windows, and Pen Windows. HNPRX also focuses on the automation of prescription writing and tracking patient data. HNPRX produces prescriptions and logs all medicine and dosing changes. The product is advertised as simple and easy to learn.

Prescription Writer

Prescription Writer is a Windows program with a graphical interface. Prescription Writer is a data base program developed by the author to address the needs of an outpatient physician in a very busy treatment environment. It can be used singly or as part of a network. The software was designed on the assumption that a computer, software, and printer would be present during the patient's evaluation. It was first used in an outpatient clinic providing outpatient treatment to patients with psychotic and mood disorders, especially schizophrenia and schizoaffective disorders.

Schizophrenia treatment requires close attention to medication benefits and side effects. Patients often require one or more medications for symptom relief and a medication for side effects. The clinic fully tested the ability of the software to track multiple patients given a variety of ongoing medications. The software successfully assisted in the task of generating prescriptions, reviewing medications, and generating medication listings.

Description of Prescription Writer

Overview

Prescription Writer computerizes the essentials of outpatient treatment, especially the prescribing of medications. Each user (physician or clinician) chooses from a list of only those patients assigned to him or her.

From that list, users access medication, demographic, or other treatment information. Prescription Writer automates prescription writing, generates medication histories, and creates medication lists for patients. The software also helps organize patient medical history and diagnoses; this information can be used to generate typed progress notes. Finally, the user can print a report of his or her caseload including patient's names, addresses, and medications. The software is primarily intended for physicians; however, it has functions useful for other clinicians, such as the storage of demographic information and medication lists.

Different levels of access to the data base information exist. For example, one clinician might be allowed to view patient data, but not to change any of the information. An "administer" level user is able to enter, delete, and change data, as well as to view the log of other users' activities. Additional security features are discussed below.

Environment

Prescription Writer is a Microsoft Access™ client application. The software incorporates a fully graphical user interface that should be comfortable for any Windows user. Prescription Writer can run on a stand-alone PC or in a networked environment. A 486/50 PC with 8 MB of RAM and Windows™ 3.11 or NT 3.5 Workstation is the minimal configuration for acceptable performance. The software includes the full security including password protection and logging of all usage.

Data Base Structure

Patient Data. The software records basic patient demographic data including birth date, sex, race, marital status, address, phone number, social security number, medical assistance number, and catchment area. Primary diagnosis, pharmacy, and pharmacy telephone number are also stored. The software allows the user to note if the patient requires a special prescription that must be handwritten.

Staff Data. The software collects basic demographic data on all staff, including phone and room numbers, educational degree, position, typical role (e.g., treating psychiatrist, clinician), professional license number, social security number, and Drug Enforcement Agency (DEA) number. The data base administrator can limit access to the demographic screen; some users can be denied access to staff information such as the Drug Enforcement Agency number.

Medication/Prescription Data. For each prescription, the physician chooses the medication name from a formulary, a list of acceptable medications. This list is created by the physician users, who can also add to this list at any time. Each prescription includes the medication name, dose, dosing instructions, days supply, refills, prescriber, and need for a name brand. In addition, the data base keeps track of the start date, stop date, and the staff member who originally entered the medication. The software calculates total pills per prescription and anticipated date for renewal based on the data in the prescription.

Progress Note Ability. The data base also keeps track of basic treatment information. A free form field can include a brief history, diagnostic formulation, assessment, and plan. This data plus medication and demographic information is used to print a progress note. The user can easily determine the last assessment for a patient because the software notes the last time a progress note was printed.

Tracking Use/Security Features. The process of admitting a patient to a clinic (i.e., adding a patient to the data base) captures who the admitting staff member was. Similarly, requesting access to a patient's records allows the data base to record who has requested access. If a patient's confidentiality has been breached, the software can determine who has requested access to the patient's information and what role they envisioned for themselves. A clinician can allay the fears of a patient who is concerned that "Anyone can read my record and you'll never know." By recording any and all requests to retrieve information from patients chart, the data base is more secure than a paper record. In addition, access to this log of "who requested information" is also restricted to higher level users.

Use of Software

A user first signs onto the system by entering his or her ID, clinic name, and password. The process insures that patients are added only once to the data base, clinic, and user caseload.

Adding a Patient to Data Base and Clinic. If the patient has never been entered into the system, he or she is first added to the data base by entering the patient's identification number. If the patient already exists, the full demographic information will be presented for possible correction. Upon the user's request, the patient will be admitted to the same clinic that the user chose when he or she signed on. Once a patient has been admitted to a clinic, the user can request that the patient be added to his or her caseload.

Adding a Patient to Your Caseload. The user chooses from the list of patient's admitted to the clinic, chooses an expected role (e.g., consulting psychiatrist), and requests that the patient be added to his or her caseload. This process captures all requests for access to a patients records.

Viewing a List of Your Patients. The user works with a list of all patients assigned to him or her in a certain clinic. From that list the user chooses to view or edit some aspect of the patient's care. Figure 1 depicts a user who has chosen to examine the medication information for a patient. Users can also examine historical or diagnostic data, demographic information, or a list of other staff working with the patient.

Working With Medication Information. If the user chooses to view medication information, the screen displays a list of current medications. From this window, the user can print prescriptions or a list of medications, add or stop a medication, or review a history of medications.

Printing Prescriptions or a Medication Listing. Printing a prescription is a simple matter. Prior to printing a prescription, the user can adjust the total days supply and number of refills. The user prints prescriptions on 5 by 8 inch paper using a nearby laser or inkjet printer; just one prescription or all can be printed. Paper with a color logo is recommended to insure prescriptions are not easily copied. If the medicine is a controlled substance, the physician's DEA number prints on the prescription (the laser-printer generated prescription is not valid for schedule II substances). The user can also print a listing of current medications to give to the patient, family member, or caregiver.

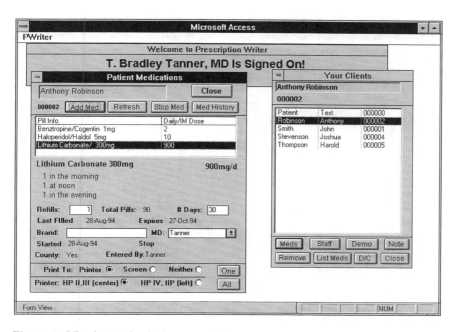

Figure 1. Viewing and printing prescriptions.

Adding a New Prescription to a Patient Record. Any change in dose or dosing requires the user to stop the old medication and then to generate a new prescription (Fig. 2). Thus to change the prescription from 2 mg at night to 3 mg at night, the user must first stop the medication and reenter the new dosing information. This process insures that medication histories include all dosage and dosing changes.

Adding a new medication requires the user to choose the medication name from a list of acceptable medications; the list can be added to by any physician user. Dosing instructions are entered as the number of pills to take in the morning, at noon, in the evening and at bedtime rather than the usual qd, BID, TID, qhs notations. This system allows more complicated regimes (e.g., one in the morning and two in the evening) and more clearly defines when a medication should be taken. Finally, the user chooses a number of days, number of refills, and (if necessary) brand name. The software calculates the total number of pills required given the dosing instructions and number of days requested.

Reviewing Present and Past Medications. If the user chooses to review old medications, a medication history is generated (Fig. 3). This list includes medication name, dose, dosing instructions, total daily dose, total days supply, and refills. The data base notes who started a medication and the last prescribing physician. Users can review the date a medication was

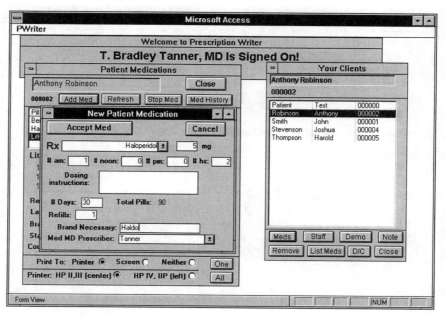

Figure 2. Adding a new prescription.

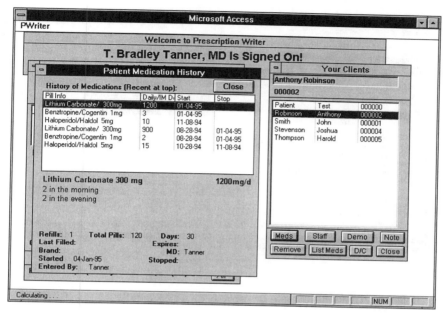

Figure 3. Reviewing present and past medications.

started, last prescribed, and (if applicable) stopped. The list allows the user to rapidly assess past medication treatment for proper dosing and adequate trial length. It can be especially helpful if one must gradually increase or taper a medication (e.g., tapering alprazolam slowly to minimize the risk of seizures).

Creating and Printing a Progress Note. Users can use a free-form text area to note the historical data, diagnostic impression, assessment, and treatment plan. The computer can combine this information with demographic data and the current medications to generate a progress note (Fig. 4). In keeping with the software's focus on prescription writing, the data base does not save past progress notes. It is assumed that a paper chart will remain the true medical record.

Printing Caseload Reports. The software prints out several useful reports. It can generate a listing of one's assigned patients including their address, phone number, primary diagnosis, who else in involved in their treatment, and what each person's role is. Another list includes demographic information and current medication information. The lists are convenient aids for covering clinicians or physicians.

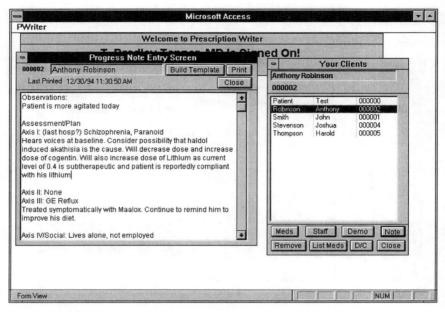

Figure 4. Creating a progress note.

Benefit of the Software

Time spent confirming the patient's ongoing medications and writing a new prescription was decreased substantially. Because the computer and printer was located at the treatment site, the time spent locating a patient's medications in the data base or waiting for the printer to print could be put to good use. The author would typically use this time to answer questions about the medication or side effects.

Occasionally patients have difficulty taking medications as prescribed. A very anxious patient occasionally took two pills instead of one; she would often use a 30 day supply in 21 days, then request a refill. A week without medications might have led to a relapse; thus she would be given a new prescription, and the cycle would begin again. The patient's treatment plan was changed so that a new prescription was given every week. The treatment plan could be easily implemented because the software made weekly prescriptions easy to generate. The patient continued to occasionally take extra pills, but the prescription was never refilled more than once per week. She eventually became more responsible in managing her medications. Regular prescriptions, combined with pill bottle checks, can best insure a patient does not take too many pills (and thus run out early) or too few.

The software's ability to generate a medication history was used daily to determine if the current medication regiment could be improved. The medication history made it possible to review the length and dose of past medication trials and assess if another trial was warranted. Also, the information could be passed on to patients requesting a change in medication or dose. For one patient, it was very helpful to point out that we were increasing the medication dose every 3 months, and next month would be the next time to assess improvement and make a decision.

The computer's ability to provide a listing of medications was praised repeatedly by patient, families, and caregivers. Patients also appreciated that the computer generated prescriptions were legible. As a result, it appeared that patients and their caregivers were more involved in the medical management of their illness. Additionally, pharmacists preferred the legible and mathematically correct prescriptions generated by the software.

Conclusion

Several commercially available software programs to aid prescription writing exist. These programs can produce substantial benefits for the clinician user. Accurate and up-to-date recording of medication is one of the primary advantages of these programs. In addition, prescription writing programs can save substantial amounts of time when frequent refills are required, as is common with psychiatric medications. The software can accurately calculate the number of pills required and produce a clear, easily read prescription for the patient and pharmacist. Drug interaction information is included with some programs. One program, Prescription Writer, was described in detail. This program allows the printing of medication lists for physician use and for patients and other caregivers. In addition, progress notes may be generated. Security features track all users of the program to assure confidentiality and prevent inappropriate use of the software. The Prescription Writer software was piloted in a busy, outpatient mental health clinic. Physicians, clinicians, patients, patient families, and pharmacists reported positive reactions to the prescriptions and other lists generated using Prescription Writer.

The prescription writing programs can be of substantial assistance to the mental health care medical professional.

Program Sources

S-O-A-P Drug interaction Program, Richard M. Hope, M.D., Patient Medical Records, Inc., available from Alpha Media, Marina Del Ray, CA.

AskRx Plus, Patient Diagnostic Solutions, available from Continuing
   Medical Education Associates, Inc., Chicago, IL.
S-O-A-P Patient Medical Records System, Patient Medical Records, Inc.,
   HNPRX, Health Care Data, and RxWriter, Hall Design, all available
   from Medical Software Products, Campbell, CA.
Prescription Writer, Clinical Tools, Inc., available from Clinical Tools,
   Inc., Pittsburgh, PA.

Part II
Quality and Cost Control Issues

10
Planning for Large-Scale Integrated Clinical Information Systems
Virginia S. Price and Robert M. Kolodner

Since the 1960s, clinicians have been looking forward to the time when computers would be used routinely in the day-to-day delivery of mental health care (APA, 1969). Since then, a significant body of work has been published on the use of general clinical computer applications in the mental health field (Glueck, 1974; Sidowski, Johnson, & Williams, 1980; Hedlund et al., 1981; Schwartz, 1984; Lieff, 1987; Kolodner, 1990). However, except for psychological testing and patient interviewing, most mental health treatment environments are not routinely using clinical computer applications as an integral part of the health care delivery process (Glueck, 1974; Laska, 1976; Kolodner, 1986). Several reasons have been suggested for this, such as clinician (specifically physician) resistance, lack of clinician involvement in system design, and lack of managerial or financial support from within the health care institution (Hedlund et al., 1981).

In contrast, the Department of Veterans Affairs (VA) has been able to provide mental health professionals with clinical information systems that play an integral role in the delivery of care. Although several areas remain that can be significantly improved, on the whole the VA experience demonstrates that large-scale, integrated clinical information systems can provide a level of support that can significantly improve the delivery of quality care in the mental health care environment.

Automated Support for a Total Health Care Environment

In 1982, the VA made the commitment to develop and implement a Decentralized Hospital Computer Program (DHCP). The vision was to develop modules of software designed to satisfy the needs of end users at VA medical centers. After certain core software was installed, each medical center was able to implement those modules that best suited the needs of that health care environment. All these modules worked together in an integrated fashion as a complete hospital information system.

The plan involved capitalizing on work already in progress, and developing software in a decentralized fashion at the medical centers themselves. This was accomplished through a coordinated, "grass roots" effort at selected facilities, linking programmers with end users (clinicians and managers) as a team to develop the necessary software using a method of rapid prototyping of new software applications.

By 1986, the core applications of patient registration, admission/discharge/transfer, outpatient scheduling, outpatient pharmacy, and clinical laboratory had been developed and implemented throughout the VA. Other service-oriented applications, such as Mental Health (including psychological testing), Surgery, Nursing, Radiology, Medicine, and Oncology followed, providing the medical centers with a rich data base of patient information.

VA's Mental Health System (MHS)

The cornerstone of automated support for the VA mental health professional is the MHS. The MHS shares the standard DHCP user interface, which uses menus and prompts, and has a two-level password security system. Within the MHS itself, information access is controlled by assigning security keys and by limiting available menu choices. This prevents unauthorized users from modifying, or even accessing, patient information. For some applications, such as progress notes, a third password is required to affix an electronic signature to the note before it becomes a part of the patient's record. This electronic signature meets all Federal requirements and is regarded as the equivalent of a written signature.

The MHS was intended to be used by front-line clinicians in the course of daily activities. The designers of the software recognized that when information is useful to the individual who is recording it, and when that information can be easily retrieved, that individual's commitment to accuracy is increased. Therefore, the MHS was designed to help clinicians to easily obtain information about patients they are treating and to quickly and efficiently record clinical observations, examinations, assessments, and treatment plans. MHS menus minimize the number of keystrokes needed to select menu options and patients, and an even faster method of navigating the system is provided for advanced users.

Components of MHS

The MHS provides computer support for both clinical and administrative patient care activities. Psychiatrists and psychologists have directed its design, with active input from all affected health care disciplines. The guiding principle has always been to produce software that makes the clinician's job easier and leads to better patient care.

A by-product of this approach has been the creation of a clinical data base that is useful to mental health program managers in many ways. Using features of the MHS, clinical managers are able to evaluate clinical productivity, monitor and improve the quality of care, and follow trends involving various patient care events.

The MHS is comprehensive, high quality, and accessible from terminals throughout medical centers and clinics. The MHS has three components: the clinical record, the inpatient features, and the patient testing module.

Clinical Record

In effect, the MHS software provides a mini clinical record. A patient profile includes demographic information and a brief index to other clinically relevant information, including physical examinations, psychological tests, clinical interviews, problem list, and diagnoses. Clinicians can enter patient diagnoses using a complete listing of Diagnostic and Statistical Manual of Mental Disorders (DSM-IV) and International Classification of Diseases (ICD-9) diagnoses. Because the DHCP system is tightly integrated, any piece of information available in the local facility's system (such as laboratory results, medications dispensed by the pharmacy, and health summaries) can be added to the menu to supplement mental health information with further clinical data.

The problem list and diagnosis options provide a way to record diagnoses and patient difficulties in 29 nondiagnostic problem areas relevant to the care of patients with mental health problems. Items that might warrant special attention of the caregiver, such as assessments of the patient's suicidal and violence risks and the presence or absence of such key symptoms as psychosis and drug or alcohol abuse, are displayed on a critical item screen. Clinicians can enter or retrieve information regarding the patient's diagnoses, recorded in DSM-IV and ICD-9 nomenclature.

The diagnosis option of the MHS has received an enthusiastic reception from clinicians and is widely used. By contrast, the problem list option has not been widely used because of clinician difficulty with data entry methods and limited clinical utility. VA is addressing these concerns by developing a generalized problem list application with a broader spectrum, interdisiplinary view, and by making new input methodologies available to front-line clinicians.

The History and Physical option allows the clinician to enter basic results of a patient's physical examination and to print the results for inclusion in the patient's chart. The MHS steps through each organ system, and prompts the clinician to indicate whether that portion of the exam was normal, omitted, or abnormal. If abnormalities are found, the clinician can type in a brief description of them. After information on the physical examination has been entered using this rapid method, a complete physical examination report can be printed for inclusion in the chart. Organ systems that were normal are described in a paragraph of pre-defined, "canned" text indicating the details of a normal exam.

Progress notes may be entered and printed for inclusion in the patient's chart. A standardized note can be created, and then copied to a new individual and edited to tailor the note for that patient. The MHS does allow progress notes to be corrected; however, in keeping with legal requirements, no progress note is ever destroyed or altered after being signed electronically. Instead a comment is attached, indicating that information was entered in error. The progress note option has gained extensive use at a number of VA sites, despite the predictions that clinicians would not type notes into the computer.

Additional options are available on the MHS Clinical Record menu for retrieving patient reports of their past medical history, social history, review of systems, and other tests and interviews. This feature gives clinicians a way to enter and retrieve a history of present illness, crisis notes, and patient messages corresponding to notes on the outside of the patient's chart.

Inpatient Features

This portion of the MHS capitalizes on the availability of information entered into DHCP by medical administration, and supports the clustering of patients by treatment teams. Users can rapidly review the census on mental health inpatient units and on individual teams on those units to determine available beds and team work loads. The census report also calculates occupancy rate, indicates any scheduled admissions that are due in the near future, and indicates the next team designated to receive an admission.

Clinicians can print a list of patients on each team in one of several formats. A short list provides a patient's name, social security number, age, admission date, and the number of days the patient has been on the unit. A work sheet form with this information can be printed, so that the clinicians can make notes or record observations as they are conducting their rounds and daily activities. Information regarding specific patient-related data for the entire team can be retrieved either on-line or in a printed report, providing clinicians with an easy way to obtain information for all of their inpatients.

These treatment team management features enable front-line clinicians to enter and retrieve patient information in a way consistent with the organization of most inpatient psychiatry units. A summary can be generated of tests administered to all patients assigned to a certain team, and treatment plan tracking is available on request. The system can also provide "alerts" that treatment plans are due shortly or are overdue.

Management information is generated as a by-product of this system. For example, a length of unit stay report can be printed that summarizes the average length of stay for patients on that ward and for each of the individual teams. A number of reports regarding admissions and/or discharges by ward and team can be produced. As an example, one report indicates whether the care delivered by each team results in a positive or negative status, using VA-specific DRG weightings.

Patient Testing

One of the oldest components of the MHS is psychological testing and interviews. Patients are able to take most of these tests and interviews at a terminal, saving considerable clinician time.

The MHS currently contains 35 structured tests. Additional tests are added as contracts are signed with the copyright holders. Thirty-three interviews are also available, covering such areas as medical history, review of systems, alcohol history, legal and marital problems, and sexual history and functioning. Tests and interviews can be clustered so that a group of tests can be easily administered on a regular basis.

One question at a time is presented on the screen to the patient, who then indicates his or her answer by pressing the appropriate key on a standard keyboard. Patients may stop a test and resume later if they are unable to complete the entire testing in one session. After completing the test instrument(s), patients are automatically exited from the system so that system security is not compromised by unauthorized access.

The software permits clinicians to enter data, review, and append comments to tests and interviews. Some tests, such as the Minnesota Multiphasic Personality Inventory (MMPI), print an interpretive report based upon the test results. Because these are generated in an automated fashion, they must be reviewed by a trained clinician before the results are released. This utility allows the clinician's comments to be available on-line whenever the report is reviewed by authorized users.

Additional features of the MHS include the ability to create, update, and search a job bank; to manage limited clinical resources by maintaining waiting lists; to support clerk entry of tests and interview data; and to record information on patients who are in seclusion and restraint.

Moving Toward the Computer-Based Patient Record

It became apparent that the DHCP MHS features such as crisis and progress notes, history and physical, problem list, patient profile, electronic signature, and patient lists should be generalized for use by the larger clinical community. In 1987, a user group was formed to guide the transition to the automated clinical record. The Clinical Record Special Interest User Group was an interdisciplinary group of clinicians, administrators, and allied health professionals. This group was able to build on the experience of the original MHS and other clinical modules, and broaden the functional specifications.

The experience of clinicians using these MHS applications has provided important first steps in the continued evolution and development of these functions throughout the VA. One application fielded by this group was a flexible way of retrieving information on groups of patients seen in either inpatient or outpatient treatment settings. These health summaries are made up of building blocks of patient information. A health segment is built for each DHCP application that produces clinically relevant information, for example, demographic information, laboratory, pharmacy, or radiology data. Different "filters" can be applied to the information to limit the number of occurrences or the time frame within which data will be displayed.

A health summary is then constructed by combining different health segments to construct a report that facilitates the delivery of health care in a specific clinical setting. In this way, the report generated for patients seen in an endocrinology clinic can be different than the report for patients being treated in cardiology or mental hygiene.

Care providers found that having access to a wide range of clinically relevant data from other DHCP applications (such as medication profiles, test results from laboratory, EEG, EKG, radiology, etc., nutritive analyses, and social work reports) gave them a more complete clinical picture. They also found that presenting the information at different levels enabled the same information to serve the various needs of all involved in providing care, including psychiatrists, psychologists, nurses, nursing assistants, social workers, physician assistants, students, psychology technicians, administrators, and clerks.

DHCP: VA's Large-Scale Integrated Clinical Information System

Today, DHCP is a highly successful hospital information system that provides administrative, management, financial, quality management, and clinical functionality. This comprehensive system has now been installed throughout the VA medical care network of over 160 medical centers, 350 outpatient clinics, 131 nursing homes, and 35 domiciliaries. The VA health care delivery system provides care for a large patient population, comprised of 2.6 million veterans (out of a total veteran population of approximately 27 million). Its activity level is of major proportions: in fiscal year 1993, DHCP systems supported 1.1 million inpatient episodes of care and 24 million outpatient visits, 1.3 million dental services, 50 million prescriptions, and 250 million laboratory tests.

DHCP is also used widely by government and private sector institutions both in this country and abroad, including university health services, Indian health service and military facilities, and state and county hospitals. Two factors that have contributed to the successful implementation of DHCP in such a wide variety of health care settings are the public domain availability of all DHCP programs, and the availability of the language environment in which it functions, M (previously known as MUMPS), from commercial vendors under several operating systems. DHCP currently runs on a variety of scaleable hardware platforms.

Each VA medical center can choose from over 60 integrated DHCP applications from which to build a flexible information system to support its individual health care delivery environment and mix of services.

DHCP applications span a broad range of clinical and administrative functionalities, and an ongoing development program addresses the critical clinical and administrative information needs of the medical centers (see Table 1). All DHCP modules are integrated through use of a common data base, with the result that data need only be entered once to be immediately available to users throughout the hospital. Standard approaches to application development have resulted in a uniform and consistent user interface, and software that can run on many kinds of computer hardware and under many operating systems.

DHCP development was organized around several principles that were intended to yield software products that would offer the benefits of standard corporate options across the VA hospital network, and yet maintain a great deal of flexibility and autonomy at the local level. These organizing principles and the actions that VA took to bring DHCP into reality have been summarized in Table 2.

Integrating Commercial Off-the-Shelf Products

The DHCP M-based applications are the base information system for every VA medical center. For the most part, they continue to meet the basic needs of the VA health care network in a cost-effective manner. VA has developed a strategy to allow VA medical centers to supplement these applications with some of the excellent commercial off-the-shelf (COTS) technologies available on the market in areas where medical centers are seeking automated support (e.g., ICU, EKG, reference retrieval systems, office automation). Through the Hybrid Open System Technology (HOST) initiative, VA is developing standards-based approaches to allow VA medical centers to take advantage of commercial clinical applications in cases where there is no DHCP module or where

Table 1. DHCP Evolving Clinical Record Functionality

Available in 1995	To be added
Admissions, discharge, transfer	A variety of different methods for entering data (ranging from pen-based to voice)
Allergies and adverse reactions	Clinical decision support
Billing	Data presentation for clinicians (e.g., cover sheets displaying the information clinicians most desire to see on their patients)
Clinic scheduling	Event linkages
Consults	Full range of clinical modules
Data exchange and transport utility	Health reminders
Dentistry	Medication administration
Dietetics	Order checking
Digital medical imaging	Order sets
Discharge summary	Patient histories (past medical, psychosocial, etc.)
Encounter forms	Physical examination findings
Funds control and accounting	Patient provider linkages
Health summaries	Query tool
Immunology case registry	Specifying and tracking clinical privileges
Links to on-line reference literature	Tailoring of reports
Medicine	Tools to identify and track cohorts
Mental health (includes psychological testing)	Windows-type user interface
Notifications and alerts	Workstation technology
Nursing	
Oncology	
Order entry/results reporting	
Pharmacy	
Problem list	
Progress notes	
Quality management	
Radiology	
Records tracking	
Social work	
Surgery	
Time and attendance	
Vitals/measurements	

commercial packages offer additional capabilities and are more cost-effective. This will enable VA medical centers to take advantage of commercial software while retaining standardization in areas where this is important to effective management of the nationwide VA system.

Table 2. DHCP Design Principles and Implementation Strategies

Principle	Implementation Strategy
Serve the needs of the user community effectively	Maximize "grass roots" user involvement in developing functional specifications; decentralize hardware and systems support to the medical centers; conduct national training programs; appoint application coordinators to assist with on-site implementation and user training
Achieve maximum portability and vendor independence	Use existing industry standards to the greatest extent practicable (ANSI standard language, standard file management utilities, and data dictionaries, etc.); develop internal standards and programming conventions; build software on a data base management system; develop common device handling, access, and security measures
Provide a common user interface	Provide a common "look and feel" across applications through internal standards and programming conventions
Develop cost-effective solutions	Engineer central equipment buys to achieve economies of scale; develop "common-denominator" software applications that run on many hardware platforms; decentralize equipment location and system support
Allow each site to tailor the implementation to local needs	Develop standard data dictionaries and site parameter files to facilitate local changes without programmer intervention
Satisfy privacy and confidentiality requirements	Design system to control user access; control central system access and security on a need-to-know basis

Computerized Patient Records (CPR): Meeting Clinical and Administrative Goals

VA's experience shows that computers are valuable clinical tools that can be instrumental in improving the quality of patient care and the efficiency and effectiveness of administrative and billing functions. Within the computer, all clinical information can be gathered in one place, and analysis can be more easily performed. This offers the opportunity to reduce conflicting or redundant information, reordering of tests due to missing results or illegible notes, and time-consuming searches for the patient's chart. In a system in which patients are often treated by a variety of providers over time, DHCP can increase continuity of care by improving communication among providers. In addition, today's health care delivery environment is undergoing many changes that are making data-driven management practices extremely attractive and generating demands for a free exchange of information with other VA and local community health care providers.

In this new environment, the clinical and administrative goal is the same: to provide immediate access to the medical record information needed to perform the task at hand. To achieve this goal, health care providers must have the information to make well-informed, medically sound judgments; preventive medical measures must be identified and implemented; and patients must not be subjected to visits and procedures that can be avoided. All of these considerations entered into VA's decision to embark on development of a full CPR.

Keeping Pace With the Changing Health Care Environment

The basic goal of the CPR is to derive information from complete and accurate clinical data entered at the point of patient care, and to use that information set to serve the multiple needs of clinical, administrative, financial, quality management, research, and education activities. The patient record will be expected to organize all relevant data on a patient (demographic data, medical history and conditions, problems and diagnoses, risk factors, diagnostic studies, and therapeutic procedures and interventions) in a way that directly supports clinical activity and indirectly feeds management and administrative systems. Intelligent decision support (for example, drug–drug interactions, clinical practice guidelines, and preventive health reminders) and the capability to share data with other VA and non-VA facilities will be integral attributes of the patient record.

The CPR provides users with an accurate longitudinal account of care along with the ability to retrieve and display the information in formats tailored to their specific needs. The CPR will provide new dimensions of functionality through links to other systems, decision support tools, and the reliable transmission of detailed information across substantial distances.

The CPR will assist the VA in meeting the ongoing challenges of a medical information explosion. The CPR will provide our health care professionals with tools they need to continue to provide our veterans with quality care while working to reduce the rising cost of health care.

Moving Forward

Further progress toward a complete CPR will require VA to meet a number of major challenges. These involve migrating from a department-centered architecture to one that adequately supports both departmental and patient-centered functionality, and providing the flexibility to respond to major changes in the VA environment such as primary care initiatives and health care reform. These changes must take place while maintaining the integrity of day-to-day operations.

Other challenges include: (1) implementing a user interface that is intuitive, easy to use, and responsive to clinician needs; (2) achieving integration of commercial and VA-developed applications; (3) improving access to data in various formats (text, images, and multimedia); (4) establishing a repository for clinical data that can be accessed throughout the system; and (5) providing the ability for data to be exchanged among VA medical centers and between VA and non-VA sites of care.

VA is now moving toward implementing a standards-based, flexible telecommunications technology capable of rapidly transmitting patient information, including electronic data and digital images, at all medical centers and outpatient clinics. When this is in place system-wide, veterans will be able to move freely throughout the system and receive coordinated treatment at multiple facilities. Although veterans will most likely continue to be treated primarily at one medical center, they will be patients of the entire VA system with established referral patterns and access to any facility where treatment is required.

VA Experience: Lessons Learned and Keys to Success

Involving Top Management

The factors most closely correlating with a successful implementation seem to be: gaining the support of top management, finding or generating a climate where users are enthusiastic, and being willing to take risks. One clinical coordinator expressed it this way:

> My first implementation was on the most difficult ward in the medical center. Everyone said it was a mistake, but I had top management support and a gung-ho surgeon and Administrative Assistant who made it work. The theory was if we could make it work there, we could make it work anywhere and it proved to be a great way to work out all the "bugs." I am currently implementing [it] on a unit that is not so supportive and I am encountering a lot of resistance. What I have learned from this is that it is not the pace of the unit that makes the difference, it's the level of support you get from the key physician players. Physician order entry is a huge paradigm shift for the docs, some love it, some aren't sure and some hate it . . . The fact is that it does take them longer to enter orders into the computer than writing it on paper and it is difficult to see the end benefits up front (e.g., faster action on orders; less chance for transcription errors; a more complete patient data base that is readily accessed by clinicians vs. digging through endless reams of paper). My advice is to assess who is most enthusiastic among the physicians and start there.

Achieving Clinician Acceptance

In addition to the benefits previously discussed, offering functionality that provides clinical relevance has proved a powerful inducement for clinicians to enter data and orders directly into the information system. Clinicians have been especially interested in the clinical benefits of progress notes, discharge summary, and patient lists, and have shown a willingness to enter data to reap these benefits. This has yielded other benefits for the clinician, such as concurrent monitoring; immediate clinician feedback; hand-off to billing/cost recovery operations; and exchange with other community health care providers for referral and follow-up.

Appointing a Clinical Coordinator

The most successful clinical DHCP systems have been those where a dedicated clinical coordinator handles the entire implementation. The responsibilities of the clinical coordinator include designing the implementation (order of implementation varies tremendously with the individual facility); preimplementation interviews and public relations with the potential user community; and one-on-one training for clinicians.

Freely Exchanging Information

The VA has an electronic messaging facility that provides for the exchange of ideas among all professionals in the VA system involved in implementing clinical systems. It is hard to overstate the benefits of having an ongoing dialogue available where implementors, systems people, and professional trainers are able to answer questions before, during, and after implementation in a specific clinical setting.

Recognizing Pitfalls

Our clinical coordinators have identified several factors to be considered when choosing a pilot site for beginning an implementation. These factors include: (1) user mix and staff turnover; (2) order type, frequency, and complexity; (3) work flow and pace; (4) stability of the environment; (5) amount of disruption to normal routine; (6) identification of key staff; and (7) the acceptance level of potential users.

Most recommend establishing a base pilot implementation that can be modified for the specialty areas. But contrast this with the testimony of one of our most successful implementors:

> We started on the busiest medical unit and "lived in" for a while. The group basically figured if we could get it running in a "hostile," untested environment and work out all the bugs, we'd be better off in the long run. We started on one unit, even with docs on other units rotating call (very

interesting scenario) and then spread throughout, bringing up one ward from each bed service, specifically so we could deal with the issues of cross-coverage training. . . .

All of this proves that each individual implementation is as individual as the individuals on staff, and can only benefit from getting buy-in from the user community and the implementation committee.

Summary

In any large-scale system implementation, good planning is a key to success. However, today the standards are not fully developed, and technology is changing so fast that it is extremely difficult to adequately address all aspects of a system or an implementation. It is important to avoid the trap of "analysis paralysis," where the standards are never mature enough, or the technology is never robust enough to handle the task. In implementing DHCP, VA has attempted to strike a balance by defining sound development and implementation principles, providing a growth path for the future, and moving with dispatch to provide automated support throughout the VA medical center network.

References

American Psychiatric Association. (1969). Computers in psychiatry. *American Journal of Psychiatry, 125*, Suppl.

Glueck, B.D. (1974). Computers at the Institute of Living. In J.L. Crawford, D.W. Morgan, & D.T. Gianturco (Eds.), *Progress in mental health information systems: Computer applications*. Cambridge, MA: Balliger.

Hedlund, J.L., Vieweg, B.W., Wood, J.B., Cho, D.W., Evenson, R.C., Hickman, C.V., & Holland, R.A. (1981). Computers in mental health: A review and annotated bibliography (DHHS Publication No. ADM 81-1090). Washington, DC: U.S. Government Printing Office.

Kolodner, R.M. (1986). Clinical computer applications for mental health treatment in the Veterans Administration system. In J.E. Mezzich (Ed.), *Clinical care and information systems*. Washington, DC: American Psychiatric Press, Inc.

Kolodner, R.M. (1990). Mental health clinical computer applications that succeed: The VA experience. In M. Miller (Ed.), *Computer applications in mental health*. New York: Haworth Press.

Laska, E.M. (1976). The Multi-State Information System for psychiatric patients. *Medical Care, 14* (Suppl.), 223–229.

Lieff, J.L. (1987). *Computer applications in psychiatry*. Washington, DC: American Psychiatric Press.

Schwartz, M.D. (Ed.). (1984). *Using computers in clinical practice*. New York: Haworth Press.

Sidowski, J.B., Johnson, J.H., & Williams, T.A. (1980). *Technology in mental health care delivery systems*. Norwood, NJ: Ablex Publishing Co.

11
Shifting the Paradigm in Outcome Quality Management
Murray P. Naditch

Outcome Measurement Rooted in Old Assumptions

A robust interest in outcome measurement is being fueled by potential health care reform, the need to do more with less, and a growing demand for accountability from payers and patient advocates.

Researchers at Strategic Advantage, Inc. (SAI) have had the opportunity to implement continuous outcome monitoring systems in more than 300 adult, adolescent, and children's psychiatric, dual diagnostic, and chemical dependency treatment programs during the last 5 years.

Although most of these systems have been successful in collecting, analyzing, and reporting outcome information (Naditch, 1993), this experience has made us aware of some significant inherent problematic issues in the methods being used to collect and analyze outcome information. These issues are discussed in this chapter and an alternative data collection paradigm that addresses these problems is presented.

Efforts to measure outcomes in clinical settings usually involve the capture of information about patients using paper-and-pencil questionnaires. Questionnaires are filled out by patients or clinicians, sometimes supplemented with information from clinical records.

We have encountered a number of problematic issues using this type of system. These include:

1. High cost;
2. Problems in data accuracy;
3. Difficulty in maintaining adequate staff motivation and compliance;
4. Difficulty in getting patient compliance;
5. Reporting limitations; and
6. Problems associated with integration of outcome data with other clinical information and processes.

152

High Cost

Information in most outcome systems is collected at intake, treatment termination, and at some follow-up period (usually 6 months) after treatment termination and may include questionnaires and one or more psychological tests at each of these points, as well as information transferred from medical records. In a paper-based system, it is not uncommon to batch and coordinate seven or more separate questionnaires to complete one patient outcome record.

Production, inventory, distribution, and tracking of all of these forms is enormously complicated and expensive. Lost, inadequately filled out forms, or single forms with missing or inadequate patient identification can negate the value of all of the other information collected about that patient. Compensating for these incomplete forms can sharply increase costs because it means that information has to be collected from a larger sample of patients to ensure the necessary number of complete records and because of the expense involved in attempting to find missing information for incomplete forms. Staff training, quality control, and staff time required to track, distribute, administer, and return these forms for data entry and analysis also involves significant expense.

The expense involved in treatment staff training, retraining, and communications to be certain that forms are available, that proper forms and versions of each form are given to an appropriate sample of patients, and that these forms are correctly completed is also significant.

Once forms are complete the next step in the process, data entry, whether through scanning or key entry, involves significant costs and staff time. And, with key entry, there are additional problems concerning accuracy, time, and logistics, which in turn increase project costs.

The final step in the process—development, printing, and distribution of paper reports—also adds to the financial burden of pencil-and-paper outcome systems.

Data Accuracy Problems

SAI does an extensive amount of work with participating treatment programs through mail, telephone, and direct contact to ensure that patients fill out questionnaires accurately. In addition, there is a program coordinator at every treatment site whose task it is to focus on this issue. Even with these quality control efforts, we consistently find a significant number of forms that have been inadequately filled out. Forms most commonly have missing identification information, skipped items, or blank sides.

Patients have usually terminated treatment by the time forms are processed. In some cases accuracy problems can be corrected by retrospectively reviewing clinical records—a staff-intensive, expensive task.

Missing information, such as an identification number or before and after measures for important outcome variables, results in deletion of the patient from the analysis or limitation of questions that can be addressed. These problems add cost as well as limit the usefulness of information collected.

Difficulty in Maintaining Adequate Staff Motivation and Compliance

The press for more cost-effective health care, which leads to tougher entry requirements, and the press of utilization review, which leads to more frequent turnover because of decreasing length of stay, have resulted in clinics having sicker patients. In most clinics, staff have little time or inclination to embrace the added paper work that is part of an outcome monitoring system. Staff cooperation and support in performing the extra tasks that may be introduced with an outcome system—such as selecting patients, giving them forms to fill out, filling out forms about patients, keeping track of forms, and getting forms to whoever is in charge of processing them—may be one of the most seriously problematic aspects of achieving acceptable functionality in an outcome system. In our experience, this is true even in situations where almost every form is patient self-administered and where clinical staff are not required to fill out any forms about patients.

Staff compliance issues can be addressed with staff training and with an enthusiastic and persuasive local coordinator whose job it is to motivate staff to participate. Nevertheless, inadequate staff motivation, or the disjuncture in program functioning that may occur with staff or administrative turnover, can result in outcome information slowing or totally drying up in a site, an increase in sampling problems, and an increase in expense and data inaccuracy because of the failure to adequately review and track forms.

Difficulty in Getting Patient Compliance

Incoming patients may be faced with a near overwhelming number of forms when entering treatment: multiple, uncoordinated forms that require a patient to provide the same information over and over at a time of acute emotional difficulty. Coupling this with a perfunctory staff attitude about completing outcome forms can result in low levels of participation and poor quality data.

In addition, as clinics are dealing with sicker patients at intake, a larger portion of these patients are unable to complete self-administered, paper forms.

Reporting Limitations

It is not uncommon for delivery of an initial outcome report to take more than a year and a half from the time the site begins collecting outcome data. When reports are generated their potential utility is often not realized. This occurs for two reasons: managers do not know how to effectively use the information to affect clinical and strategic decision making and the timing or content of the reports does not facilitate this kind of decision making. Conventional paper-and-pencil outcome reporting does not provide the information people need, when they need it.

Problems Integrating Outcome Data With Other Clinical Information and Processes

Paper-and-pencil outcome monitoring is most often an adjunctive system tacked onto existing clinical systems. The lack of integration with existing clinical systems leads to redundant data collection, problems in compliance and sampling, and an inability to use the same information that is collected for outcomes to do clinical assessment and treatment planning.

Blueprint for a Solution Addressing Limitations in Conventional Methods

The research group at SAI has developed an electronic system to address problems inherent in paper-and-pencil systems. The principal components of this system, RES-Q (Reliable Electronic Survey Questionnaire), include:

1. An electronic questionnaire;
2. A multimedia instructional motivator;
3. A link to a national data base;
4. On-line, real-time reporting capability; and
5. Links to other patient information systems.

Electronic Questionnaire

The RES-Q electronic questionnaire displays questionnaire items on a computer screen. The patient enters responses via a touch screen.

Electronic delivery facilitates branching logic within the questionnaire so that patients are only asked to respond to items relevant to them. This shortens the questionnaire, eliminates response errors related to inability to follow branching instructions in a paper-and-pencil questionnaire, and eliminates the need to have multiple versions of paper questionnaires for different types of patients and programs.

Errors related to incomplete identification numbers, needed to connect various instruments, are eliminated. The system also has the capability to check the validity of patient responses in real time while a patient is filling in responses. This is done by screening for incomplete and illogical responses. The patient is asked to rethink and reenter unacceptable answers. When a patient does not answer within a 1 minute time interval or continues to enter invalid responses, a staff person is called to assist and the data entry into the computer proceeds via an interview format.

This process substantially improves data quality as well as extends use of the system to sicker patients. Electronic data entry system essentially eliminates all paper in the system, thus eliminating the costs associated with printing, inventory, sorting, distribution, shipping, processing, data entry, and the staff and management time and training associated with these processes.

Multimedia Instructional Motivator

The RES-Q System is designed to decrease patient resistance by utilizing recent advances in computer technology.

Patients are greeted by the video image of a woman who acts as a narrator for the interview process. She reads all interview questions, following whatever branching logic applies for a particular patient. The narrator can be changed to accommodate languages other than English.

Voice and video accompaniment of the questions extends the instrument further toward less literate, more confused, and sicker patients. Patients have the option of eliminating the voice accompaniment at any time during the interview. This enables patients to move through the interview at a faster pace if they so desire.

The consistent voice and video orientation to the system reduces the staff time it takes to introduce patients an outcome system, and should increase reliability because of the consistency of the orientation message.

The narrator also interacts with an animated character. This character, a scruffy bear named RES-Q, raises the points of resistance the patient may be experiencing such as: "How long is this going to take? What are you going to do with the information? Why do I have to do this when this is such a difficult time for me?" The intention is to decrease patient resistance and increase compliance by raising and responding to patient objections and by presenting information in a novel manner, one that is more interesting than filling out a conventional paper-and-pencil questionnaire.

RES-Q also uses patient incentives at the end of each section including maps that show patients how far they have come, positive feedback, and other reinforcing devices.

The SAI research group is empirically testing the value and application of the multimedia approach by testing multimedia and nonmultimedia versions of RES-Q in different clinical programs with varying types of patients.

Link to National Data base

Data collected at each terminal is transmitted on a regular basis to a central data base via modem. A complete client–server network architecture and communications protocol (known within SAI as Res-Q Net) has been developed to provide this communications infrastructure. Reports are calculated at a central location and completed reports are downloaded to the originating terminal.

Information from all clients is compiled in a national data base. The data base has more than 30,000 patient records at the time of this writing. The national data is used to calculate national as well as risk-adjusted norms, both of which are optionally available via the electronic reporting process, whenever they are needed. (The method for calculation of risk-adjusted norms is illustrated in a later section.)

The RES-Q architecture also facilitates increased flexibility in making instrument changes. Changing an item in a paper-and-pencil system involves a new printing, writing off all old form inventory, and working with sites to abandon use of the old forms and institute new forms. This is a laborious, expensive, and error prone process. The electronic system can modify, add, or delete items throughout the system with a few keystrokes. The electronic files to supersede or optionally customize the survey instrument may be updated on-line from the SAI National Support Center (NSC). The SAI NSC and the Res-Q application provide the ability to update the files from the NSC, with little or no computer expertise at the client treatment site.

Real-Time Reporting

Aggregated outcome reports are available to appropriate staff on demand. Staff review a menu of standardized reporting options and can select whatever reporting is appropriate. Reports can be printed on site using the same terminal and printer that collected client data. Outcome reports can include normative outcome information that has been empirically risk rated for each treatment program. These reports include patient psychosocial histories, diagnostics reporting, and reports that match patients to the treatments most appropriate for them.

Links to Other Patient Information Systems

Admission to treatment from a patient's perspective may involve filling out a number of forms containing redundant information. The RES-Q System can be modified at a treatment site to avoid redundancy with information being collected in other data collection efforts at the treatment site.

Most paper-and-pencil systems collect information from a sample of patients rather than all patients coming into treatment. Because outcome conclusions can be drawn about the entire population from an appropriately drawn sample, this avoids the forms and testing costs associated with collecting information from all patients. An outcome system relying on less than a 100% patient sample cannot be used as a segment of a treatment facility's clinical information system because information will not have been collected on some patients. Using an electronic system, the marginal cost of collecting data from all patients is small, making a 100% patient sample feasible, thus facilitating use of these data for case management and other clinical purposes.

Electronic storage and retrieval of patient outcome data also facilitates integration of outcome information with other clinical information systems. Combining outcome and treatment exposure information enables researchers to address more complex questions such as matching patients to the treatments that will be most effective for them.

Using Outcome Information to Affect Clinical and Strategic Decisions

The availability of real-time outcome information creates expanded possibilities for utilization of outcome information to make clinical and strategic decisions. Researchers at SAI have been conducting interviews with treatment center staff who are using the RES-Q System in order to evolve reports that will be more likely to drive real-time decisions.

A survey of 51 medical directors and chief executive officers at free standing psychiatric treatment facilities in the United States conducted in December 1994, indicated that risk-adjusted, normative outcome comparisons would be very important in interpreting their outcome information. It is not clear to a medical director or CEO, for example, whether a 9 point change in depression from intake to follow-up, represents either outstanding or below average performance relative to other providers.

Normative comparisons are complicated by the fact that providers may not be treating patients of comparable difficulty. If one provider is treating severely disturbed chronic patients and another provider is treating patients with situational stress disorders, comparing the two populations to a normative standard can make the provider with more difficult patients appear to be achieving worse results.

This problem can be avoided by using normative outcome information that is empirically risk adjusted for patient difficulty. Risk-adjusted norms can be used by providers to compare their outcomes to appropriate norms, compare therapists, or compare treatment programs. Risk-adjusted normative outcome information can also be used by payers to establish normative standards and to manage and evaluate the performance of provider networks. Risk-adjusted norms can further be used by providers or payers to risk rate potential populations to determine expected outcomes and expected resources utilized to achieve these outcomes.

Normative Risk Rating Methodology

The methodology used by researchers at SAI to empirically risk rated outcome measures is explained in this section using an illustrative example. Approximately 300 behavioral health treatment programs are currently using SAI's outcome measure instruments and procedures. Each of these treatment programs collects approximately 240 patient psychosocial characteristic variables. Psychosocial characteristic measures are variables that have been found to relate to differential outcomes for psychiatric or chemical dependency treatment for adults or adolescents in the published clinical literature. They include measures of psychosocial history, current life situation, and symptomology at intake.

Outcomes, measured as difference scores from intake to treatment termination and/or follow-up 6 months after treatment, include measures of mental health status, work and other role functionality, medical resource utilization, quality of life, chemical dependency, and satisfaction with program services.

A separate risk-adjusted norm is calculated for each outcome dimension such as psychiatric status, medical offset, work adjustment, quality of life, or patient satisfaction. Risk rating for one area of psychiatric status, change in paranoid ideation from intake to discharge, is used here as an illustrative example.

An initial risk rating calculation was performed by drawing a sample of 2,961 inpatient psychiatric patients who had completed the Brief Symptom Inventory (BSI) (Derogotis, 1975) at intake and discharge and who had a length of stay (LOS) greater than 8 days (average LOS = 15.3 days). This represented a sample of 131 treatment programs who had collected this information between January 1992 and December 1994.

Each of the 240 psychosocial characteristics was correlated with change in paranoid ideation from intake to follow-up. A statistical cutoff point of $p < 0.0005$ was used to eliminate false positives. This univariate procedure resulted in approximately 30 psychosocial characteristics significantly associated with the change in paranoid ideation between intake and treatment termination.

A stepwise multiple regression equation was calculated using these psychosocial characteristics as independent variables and change in paranoid ideation from intake to treatment termination as the dependent variable. This procedure resulted in four psychosocial characteristics predicting change in paranoid ideation. The results of this regression equation are shown in Table 1.

This association between psychosocial characteristics and change in paranoid ideation is a method for determining patient difficulty.

Table 1. Change in paranoid ideation: Risk Adjustment

Variable	Response Range	b^a	T	P Value	Standardized b^b	% of Variance
BSI Intake Paranoid Ideation	20–80	0.51	23.08	0.0000	0.50	21.64
BSI Intake Phobic Anxiety	20–80	−0.09	−4.03	0.0001	−0.09	0.72
Previous hospitalization for mental health	0 = No 1 = Yes	−1.57	−3.71	0.0002	−0.07	0.50
Patient wanted treatment	0 = No 1 = Yes	1.57	2.68	0.0074	0.05	0.26

Note: $R^2 = 0.23$; $n = 2.125$; Range of Paranoid Ideation = −38 to 47. Sample comes from adult MH inpatients. Difference between BSI Paranoid Ideation T-score form intake to discharge.

[a] b: One unit change in BSI Phobic Anxiety means −0.09 change in Paranoid Ideation.

[b] Standardized b: regression coefficients when all variables are expressed in standardized (Z-score) form. This makes the coefficient more comparable.

It indicates which types of patients are more or less difficult to treat (achieved change in the paranoid ideation outcome variable from intake to treatment termination) and how important each of these patient psychosocial characteristics are in affecting treatment outcomes.

If two treatment sites are being compared, these data can be used to adjust expected outcomes based on patient difficulty. This is illustrated for one treatment site in Table 2. The mean score on each of the psychosocial predictors for patients at the sample treatment site are shown in the first column. The national means on these psychosocial predictors, taken from SAI's national data base, are shown in the second column. The differences between the site mean and the national mean (the third column) is multiplied by the relative importance of each psychosocial characteristic in determining change in paranoid ideation from intake to treatment termination (the b coefficient in the regression equation). This difference, shown in the fourth column, is the adjustment factor for the sample treatment program. The adjustment factor for each relevant patient psychosocial characteristics is added, providing a total adjusted score. This whole procedure is represented by the formula:

$$\text{adjusted score} = \sum ((\text{site norm} - \text{national norm}) * \text{weight}).$$

This adjusted score is added to the national norm to provide a risk-adjusted norm for the sample treatment program. In this example, this program site has an adjusted norm of 0.85 more than the national norm, indicating that this site had patients who were less difficult to treat, for example, more likely to respond to treatment with a decrease in paranoid ideation.

Figure 1 shows the actual comparison between this site and a second site drawn at random from SAI's national data base. This figure shows

Table 2. How Risk-Adjusted Norms Are Calculated

Variable	Site Norm	National Norm	Difference[a]	Weight[b]	Adjustment[c]
BSI Intake Paranoid	69.91	67.84	2.07	0.51	1.06
BSI Intake Phobic Anxiety	67.28	65.50	1.78	-0.09	-0.16
Previous hospitalization for mental health	0.35	0.34	0.01	-1.57	-0.02
Patient wanted treatment	0.84	0.86	-0.02	1.57	-0.03

Total adjusted score is 0.85 and is the sum of values in the adjustement column.
[a] (site norm) − (national norm).
[b] b Regression weight found in Table 1.
[c] (difference) * (weight).

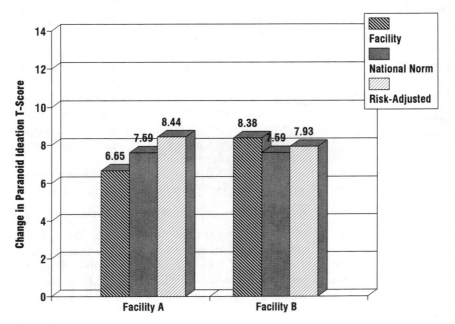

Change In Paranoid Ideation From Intake To Treatment Termination Compared To National And Risk-Adjusted Norms For Two Facilities

Figure 1.

the actual change in paranoid ideation scores for each of these two treatment programs from intake to treatment termination. Treatment Program A had a 6.83 point change in paranoid ideation from intake to treatment termination while Treatment Program B was able to achieve a 8.98 point change. The national normative average in the SAI data base for change in paranoid ideation from intake to treatment termination (shown in the second bar in the chart) is 7.8 points. The risk-adjusted mean for these two sites is shown in the third bar. Even though Treatment Program A had patients who were less difficult to treat and Treatment Program B had patients who were more difficult to treat than the national norm, Treatment Program B has better results in reducing paranoid ideation.

This method is used to risk rate each area of outcomes to determine which treatment sites have patients more or less difficult to treat on each measure of outcomes and to compare their results to these risk-adjusted norms.

A variation of this method can be used to determine the amount of treatment resources required to achieve acceptable outcomes in a given population. This could be accomplished, using the paranoid ideation risk adjustment example described, by pursuing the following additional steps:

1. Select those patients whose change in paranoid ideation from intake to follow-up is equal to or exceeds the norm. This defines a population with acceptable outcomes.
2. Create a measure of treatment costs or treatment resources utilized. This can be a total cost of treatment measure if it is available, a surrogate treatment exposure measure such as number of outpatient sessions, or length of stay in an inpatient setting.
3. For the acceptable outcome portion of the population, regress the psychosocial characteristics variables on the treatment cost or treatment resources utilized variable. This equation provides information about the relative importance of specific patient psychosocial characteristics related to the costs of producing acceptable outcomes in a population.
4. For a potential population being considered for treatment, measure or estimate the normative scores on the psychosocial characteristics in the regression equation predicting resources using patient psychosocial characteristics for the population who achieved successful outcomes. This calculation estimates costs or resources required to produce acceptable outcomes in the population being considered.
5. By repeating the above steps with populations selected who have achieved a somewhat lesser, or a somewhat greater change in paranoid ideation, the user can estimate ranges of treatment effectiveness that can be achieved at varying costs with a population under consideration.

Moving Forward

Emergence of the type of technology applications described here offer providers and payers a new paradigm through which to measure and apply outcome management. The application described addresses serious problems encountered using conventional approaches to outcome measurement, improves data quality, provides outcome information in real time, and provides outcome information less expensively and with less staff involvement.

The immediate challenge we face at SAI involves evolution of methods to implement the system beyond the initial beta test sites and to empirically test key parameters within it. We are using quasiexperimental design to test the efficacy of each facet of the multimedia application such as voice, video, and the animated character to determine how these elements affect compliance and data quality for different patient groups.

We are also testing integration of this system with other electronic clinical information systems. This involves integration of the RES-Q

Outcome System with a practice management information system in two pilot sites that are exploring effective ways to combine clinical, financial, and outcome information. These applications have particular relevance for the evolution of advanced patient treatment matching rules that depend on the interaction of patient psychosocial characteristics, clinical exposure, and outcome information.

This system also offers the potential of more rapid psychological test development. Item analysis associated with tests of convergent validity or internal consistency, for example, can be facilitated and accelerated by testing associations, adding or deleting new items throughout the system from a central location, and retesting with large numbers.

The most profound, and the most potentially problematic, opportunity presented by the emergence of these new technologies has to do with the potential effect real-time outcome information may have on clinical and strategic decision making. Clinicians have not typically had access to these kinds of data, and it is not uncommon for an outcome report to be presented, passed around, and perhaps used in a marketing application before being consigned to the file drawer. Real-time patient treatment matching information and on-demand menus of outcome reports provide opportunities for staff to make clinical decisions on a patient by patient basis, making clinical management and outcome systems seamless, rather than two independently functioning systems. The same information used to measure baselines for outcomes will be used for treatment planning.

The research group at SAI is involved in a continuous evolutionary process with system users to modify report content to create report information most likely to affect clinical decisions. This process causes us to continually revise the ways we report data, and causes users to reconsider how they make clinical decisions.

New paradigms can lead the way to unexpected opportunities and offer potentials that may or may not be realized. Change in practice patterns does not come easily because it threatens established procedures. However, each of us will have the burden and the opportunity of exploring how to use this kind of new tool as a way to reexamine what we do and to potentially offer more efficient and more effective health care services.

References

Deregotis, L.R. (1975). *Brief Symptom Inventory*. Baltimore, MD. Clinical Psychometric Research.

Naditch, M.P. (1993). Get the most value from treatment programs. *Journal of Health Care Benefits*, March/April, 20–25.

12
Using Information Systems to Improve Quality of Care
Kenric W. Hammond

The benefit gained from applying information systems to quality assurance and quality improvement depends on the capabilities of the information system and the leadership of the health care organization. Understanding the strengths and limitations of information systems in managing health care quality is critical. The sophistication and content of the information infrastructure matters, but the vital ingredient of success is an explicit vision of quality priorities shared by as many employees as possible. Once such direction is established, examination of data flow within the organization will identify opportunities to reach quality goals. Not infrequently, such analysis leads to improvements in the information system as well.

When the guiding vision is *ethically* grounded in sound science and economics, valid information, amplified and integrated by competent technology, can properly focus a quality strategy. It can drive a self-reinforcing cycle of process improvement, cost-effectiveness, and favorable clinical outcomes. When vision is lacking, not even excellent information systems are immune from misuse in the name of quality improvement. If, for example, a powerful information system focuses on any one key factor—for example, process, cost, or outcome—at the expense of the other two, the quality initiative will be weak. Impressive statistical reports, outstanding results on accreditation surveys, or even academic prestige may conceal that a quality management program has lost its way and lulled leadership into complacency. The quality activist who observes leaders, caregivers, and patients pursuing separate and discordant agendas should suspect a "vision problem" that needs correcting before attempting to find a fix in information technology.

Health care quality management programs in the 1970s and 1980s were hindered by faulty methodology and severe limitations in collecting and analyzing enough data to meaningfully analyze, let alone improve quality. The retrospective reviews and medical audits common in that era made counting mistakes and fixing blame easy, but provided few insights to eliminate problems. Performance feedback was given, but usually too late to help. Reviews measured the "measurable," rather than the relevant issues. The chief outcomes of quality management then, as possibly now, were passing inspections and steady reimbursement streams, *not* convincingly improved care. Since 1990, distress over rampant cost growth, expensive but unproven treatment, and unequal access within the United States health care industry has exploded, accentuating concerns about the quality of health care services.

Despite many incantations, a definition of quality has been elusive at best. Recently health services researchers and quality experts have begun to borrow a perspective from manufacturing industries that presents a clearer concept of what patients and health care purchasers want and need (Berwick, Godfrey, Blanton, & Roessner, 1990). If the national system of health care delivery ever actually evolves into a freely competitive market, it, like other free markets, will be driven by public perceptions of product quality. Savvy purchasers and consumers will want valid measures to compare the value of services they buy. Service providers competing to deliver higher quality at lower cost will demand intimate knowledge of their production processes. Both will focus on four cardinal characteristics of quality health care:

1. Consistency,
2. Timeliness,
3. Availability, and
4. Acceptability.

Consistency implies that services are the same every time they are performed. This could apply equally well to laboratory testing, cardiac surgery, or psychiatric assessment. Identifying and reducing *variation* in the delivery of health care is an excellent place to begin a quality improvement strategy. Organizations lacking a program to reduce variation should accord high priority to implementing one, especially if a superior practice pattern is known, such as one outlined in the AHCPR Guidelines for the Treatment of Depression (Agency for Health Care Policy Research, 1993). Reduction in practice variation has repeatedly been shown to reduce risk and costs and promote more uniform health care outcomes (Lohr, 1994).

Timeliness means that services are performed at the *right* time. Delay in necessary care produces adverse outcomes, but delivering a service prematurely may increase costs without producing commensurate benefit.

Availability correlates powerfully with patients perceptions of quality. Availability reinforces timeliness, because available practitioners work with patients to identify the "right" time for service. Hard to reach caregivers may end up seeing too many patients who have delayed seeking care too long. Unavailability can make clinician–patient communication less collaborative and mutual, promoting extreme strategies on the part of patients and "defensive" practice on the part of therapists. In settings where access is difficult, patients may exaggerate symptoms to obtain specific services they perceive they need, whether or not acceptable alternatives exist.

Acceptability involves furnishing products that people want and need. For the health care organization, this means market making, and involves both analysis and promotion. Health care providers must understand the services patients like *as well as* deliver the outcomes they expect. Education is an excellent and cost-effective way to encourage patients to be better health care consumers and more effective partners in maintaining good health.

If the above discussion sounded a lot like a business pep talk, that was intentional. Do *business* systems available to mental health care organizations offer much to support continuous quality improvement along the dimensions listed? Probably not, if their billing and financial capability is isolated from the processes and people that produce care. The closer the information system is to the delivery of care, the more opportunites will exist to use data resources to promote consistency, timeliness, availability, and acceptability. Characteristics of information systems that are well-equipped to assist quality management include:

1. Integrated management and production data bases,
2. Mechanisms to feed information back to the care process, and
3. Flexible query capabilities to meet changing information needs.

Applications of Information Systems in Quality Improvement

Reports of computer usage in quality management break into three categories. The first concerns usage of information technology to assist the work of the quality manager. Infection control and risk management data bases are representative examples. These are compiled and maintained by quality personnel and permit retrospective analyses that can be fed back to organizational policy. Graphical and analytic techniques afforded by computers improve the productivity and effectiveness of the quality analysts who manage these systems.

A second category is characterized by descriptions of using computer applications to implement quality management programs. More narrowly focused, these reports describe how computer systems have supported a quality management initiative, but may not convincingly demonstrate achievement of tangible health care, or economic or behavioral outcomes.

A third, increasingly seen, approach, concerns production information systems that prospectively intervene in processes of care. Their appeal is an ability to influence practice decisions during care delivery, eliminating feedback delays associated with retrospective review. Computer usage in quality improvement is multifaceted, and effective systems blend elements of all three approaches. This discussion will emphasize the second and third categories. These have the greatest potential to alter outcomes, and depend most heavily on the design and implementation of patient information systems. Many of the examples to follow are based on experience in Department of Veterans Affairs (VA) medical centers. VA facilities differ from many delivery settings, but the completeness of the clinical and production data bases in VA's Decentralized Hospital Computing Program (DHCP) make VA a good environment for exploring the limits of computer-facilitated quality management (Andrews & Beauchamp, 1989).

In a signficant review of the field, Haynes and Walker (1987) reviewed 135 studies of computer applications to medical quality assurance. Fourteen of the studies involved controlled clinical trials. More recently Aronow and Coltin (1993a, 1993b) reviewed 120 systems. Haynes concluded that computer systems were capable of inducing targeted behavior changes among health care providers, but found that actual changes in clinical outcome were difficult to demonstrate. Aronow and Coltin similarly concluded that computer-assisted quality management has promise, but is presently hampered by limited penetration of information systems into routine clinical practice, especially in the area of computer-based patient record systems.

Surveillance Systems and Joint Commission

One cannot discuss health care quality management without acknowledging the transcendent role of the Joint Commission on Accreditation of Health Care Organizations (JCAHO). Despite criticisms of its older methodological flaws, no force in United States health care has had a greater influence on advancing the practical art of health care quality management. Representing an alliance of management and provider interests, JCAHO earns credit for prominent and persistent attention to health care quality, willingness to admit new knowledge into its sphere, and its delicate balancing of political forces. Institutions accredited by the JCAHO must periodically monitor aspects of care that occur frequently or entail risk, and many of the projects described below were inspired by JCAHO standards. JCAHO compliance is, however, only a start. The definitive transition from reactive to proactive quality management occurs when institutions discover that their integrity and survival depend on managing quality in every aspect of their functioning. Below we will describe how information systems facilitate the transition from inspection complicance to continuous quality management.

Data-Based Quality Management

Drug Utilization Evaluation

Drug Utilization Evaluation (DUE), required by JCAHO, is readily implemented if a pharmacy data base is available. Stored information can identify a cohort of patients receiving a drug for further review. The following examples of DUE are from a setting where virtually all patient prescriptions are represented in the data base. DUE based on partial samples may provide useful hints about drug safety and effectiveness in a setting, but claims about overall organizational performance based on incomplete or nonrepresentative samples must be qualified. Currently, JCAHO does not make such a fine distinction, and accepts an otherwise well-justified DUE based on available in-house pharmacy data.

At the American Lake VA Medical Center, DUE of lithium therapy was conducted for several years, using pharmacy and laboratory data bases to track doctors' compliance with obtaining periodic lithium renal and thyroid tests among lithium recipients. Over the DUE life cycle, compliance with a standard of annual thyroid and kidney testing and biannual lithium levels rose from 70% to above 95%. The monitor was judged a success because it covered all lithium patients, and because all needed data could be retrieved from the computer, minimizing the data collection effort. The practitioners who drafted the review criteria accepted the computer-generated feedback letters reminding them of overdue tests.

A similar DUE for carbamazepine (Tegretol) therapy was more difficult to implement. Identifying patients and checking the laboratory data base for liver tests and drug levels was easy, but a requirement to document informed consent or patient education forced time-consuming chart review. The single manual procedure eclipsed other efficiencies gained from using a data base. Manual review forced partial sampling, and feedback came slowly and late. Not surprisingly, the level of informed consent documentation has remained about 50%. Until the required documentation becomes part of the computer data base, further improvement is doubtful.

A follow-up lithium monitor based on a different VA software tool was useful once compliance reached 95%, allowing the formal lithium DUE to be retired. Ability to integrate pharmacy and laboratory data in DHCP's data base permitted configuring the Action Profile, a prescription reorder form produced prior to each outpatient clinic appointment, to print for specified drugs predefined sets of laboratory results adjacent to the reorder segment. In the case of lithium, showing the most recent lithium level was sufficient to encourage ongoing adherence to the monitoring standard. The procedure worked well, because the reminder appeared at a convenient time to order the test.

Action Profile software also permits triggering the printing of a questionnaire, a message, or even a consultation request as a trailer to the reorder form when a target drug is present. Appended questionnaires can gather data for DUE studies and messages can provide warnings or furnish advice. In one example, after psychiatric staff concluded that one serotonin reuptake inhibitor (SRI) was just as effective as another SRI costing twice as much, use of the Action Profile's ability to issue a low-key reminder to consider switching drugs resulted in significant savings and avoided more intrusive measures. The notification influenced initial choice of therapy as well. Automatic drug-specific questionnaires appended to turnaround forms reduce manual chart reviews and allow a quality management project to involve greater numbers of patients at lower cost than retrospective reviews. Data captured directly from prescribers was more valid than that gathered by medical records technicians and eliminated many secondary reviews by clinical staff.

DUE programs work better when integrated with care processes. Success depends on the information system's capacity to *detect* events such as outpatient visits, and to use events to trigger checking patient data against predetermined criteria. Tirelessly vigilant computers, driven by work events and accessing complete and valid data bases, *amplify* professional judgment, benefiting patients while skirting incursion on clinical autonomy. Quality improvement tactics are sometimes unpopular with clinicians, but these experiences suggest that methods complementing clincans' strengths and agreeing with their aims are welcome. Event-driven reminders maximize opportunities to make the right decisions at the right time. Increased frequency of "correct" provider actions theoretically results in improved health outcomes for target populations.

VA's adoption of the antipsychotic drug clozapine provides another example of a quality assurance mechanism driven by information in a production system. Clozapine therapy can dramatically benefit patients who do not respond to other drugs, but carries high risk of depressing blood cell production in bone marrow. Long barred from the United States market, clozapine was finally granted Food and Drug Administration approval in 1988 when an administrative procedure that bundled dispensing a week's supply of the drug with a mandatory weekly blood count was devised. The annual retail cost of this program, performed by a commercial laboratory chain, approached $8,000, about $4,000 each for drug and testing. VA, potentially a large clozapine market, balked at the expense, but ultimately received a waiver from the drug manufacturer when it delivered assurance that it could provide equivalent surveillance by programming its pharmacy system to block prescriptions until the laboratory system indicated a blood test had been drawn. VA reduced its costs, and payed for the drug alone. In a further refinement, the program detected early trends of marrow failure, blocking refills pending a clinician review. Imaginative integration of data from two different production data bases improved safety while affording an effective treatment option at lower cost. Clozapine therapy has freed up 15 to 20% of American Lake's psychiatry beds.

Clinical Reminder Systems

Almost without exception, Haynes found that computer systems with the greatest demonstrable impact on care were clinical *reminder* systems. Pioneered by Barnett and McDonald (Barnett, 1984; Wilson, McDonald, & McCabe, 1982), these systems issue warnings or advice when caregivers see patients. Reminders, triggered by predefined data base conditions, typically urge performance of neglected preventive care, for example ordering influenza vaccine for the elderly, periodic retinal exams for diabetic patients, or mammograms. Reminders can be issued on-line, via printouts available at appointments, or via office mail. Reminders are effective motivators of behavior change, but when they stop, target behavior reverts to baseline. Most physicians, realistic about the limits of human memory, value reminders that prompt them to take actions they endorse.

Reminder systems are limited more by the contents of production data bases than by the imaginations of their designers. Most systems reported to date involve analysis of data typically found in hospital information systems: appointments, drug therapy, laboratory values, diagnoses, and demographics. Imagination comes into play when figuring out how to use combinations of available data to promote desired quality outcomes. Integrated, patient-centered data bases make the task somewhat easier.

One such reminder developed at the American Lake VA Medical Center helped solve an otherwise intractable quality management problem: inadequate surveillance for tardive dyskinesia among recipients of antipsychotic drugs (Hammond, Snowden, Risse, Adkins, & O'Brien, 1995). The topic was chosen because the prevalence of this irreversible syndrome among patients on chronic neuroleptic therapy can approach 30%. Before the reminder system was begun, the fraction of records documenting examinations rarely exceeded 50% in a population of over 600 at-risk patients, despite extensive urgings and physician willingness to do examinations. Following a process analysis, the decision was made to require a standard examination, the Abnormal Involuntary Movement Scale (AIMS) (Guy, 1976). An automated reminder driven by pharmacy and appointment data was devised, and a registry of antipsychotic recipients storing AIMS scores and dates was created. Searches of pharmacy data periodically identifed new names for the registry, and the software that produced clinic appointment lists was modified to flag patients who needed exams. Once an exam was conducted, the score was entered in the registry, and a timer, triggering another reminder in 6 months, was reset. In 15 months following implementation, compliance with examinations rose from 53 to

85%, and compliance with documentation of informed consent rose from 38 to 74%. Subsequently, adherence to standards continued to rise, approaching 100%. Integrated data base design permitted the necessary links between pharmacy, appointment, and AIMS registry data, promoting marked and sustained change in documentation patterns. Figure 1 displays the result.

So far we have described reminders driven by data bases for support services, such as pharmacy, laboratory, and scheduling systems. In defined-enrollment health care systems, such data sets are likely to be complete, because the information systems perform key operational functions. Basing reminders on incomplete data sets is more problematic. Discharge diagnoses are usually available in hospital systems, but may not apply to outpatients. Also, diagnoses of record may be misleading, especially if a reimbursement policy rewards complex diagnoses. This can happen when a Diagnosis Related Group (DRG) "grouper" program is available to the medical records department. Even so, useful reminders driven by a combination of diagnostic and production data are possible. Examples applicable to psychiatric populations include issuance of alerts when patients with a history of epilepsy are prescribed seizure threshold-lowering drugs, and provider notification when a disease, such as hypertension, appears to be untreated.

Recognition of the utility of better outpatient diagnosis and problem data bases has driven recent developments in VA's DHCP system. Precisely targeted reminders require current, complete clinical data. When support for *patient* information systems becomes routine, the ability of

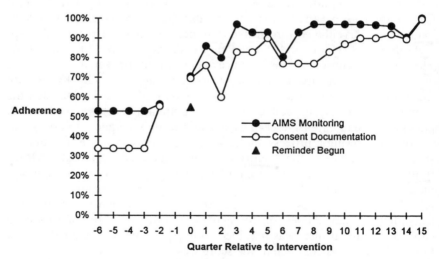

Figure 1. Impact of automated reminders on monitoring antipsychotic drug therapy.

production data bases to assure quality will increase. Effective reminder systems will promote better health outcomes, and in turn reduce costs of care. Financial and competitive advantages will reward those who practice data-based quality management, and encourage development of more capable computer-based patient record systems.

"Epidemiological" Management

Case Study: Using a Reminder System to Reduce Risk in a Defined Population. When data for a target group are *uniformly* present, valid inferences may be drawn about populations. Achieving the goal of reliable dyskinesia monitoring, for example, has set the stage for meaningful intervention. Despite its success in encouraging monitoring, the chief outcome of the reminder system described was protection against liability for negligence or failure to obtain consent. When the project began, intervention options for tardive dyskinesia were limited to lowering antipsychotic drug dosages and hoping that dyskinesia would improve without worsening the psychotic symptoms. Since then, promising new treatments have been identified, including use of vitamin E for newly detected dyskinesia and clozapine therapy for ongoing psychotic symptoms. Because the patient registry accumulated reasonably reliable outcome data in the form of AIMS dyskinesia ratings, it became straightforward to identify patients who might benefit from new interventions.

Figure 2 illustrates the registry's value in case finding. It shows representative samples of trended AIMS scores selected from cases where at least one of the serial ratings was 5 or more, the low threshold for recognition of dyskinesia. The upper graph shows a case with a single elevated score, commonly seen, that indicates no need for action. The smaller graphs show other patterns, mostly static, or with reduced severity over time. Two cases, highlighted in boxes, show rising trends, indicating risk, and opportunity for intervention. Among the 648 active patients in the American Lake registry, 83 (13%) had at least one AIMS score of 5 or above, indicating significant tardive dyskinesia at some point in treatment. Of these, nine (1.4%) exhibited a rising trend. Ability to identify these cases and document treatment attempts presented an important opportunity to manage risk and direct treatment efforts toward patients who would benefit most. In a larger context, the data present a picture of institutional risk exposure and allow comparison with other populations.

Consistently applied reproducible measurements permit strong conclusions about quality. They support more cost-effective, targeted interventions and may improve financial performance. Consistent accurate feedback can lessen anxieties that foster superstitious practices excused as "defensive medicine." The above data moderated pressure to utilize expensive "atypical" antipsychotic agents as first-line therapy because of a reputed lower potential for tardive dyskinesia and "liability." The

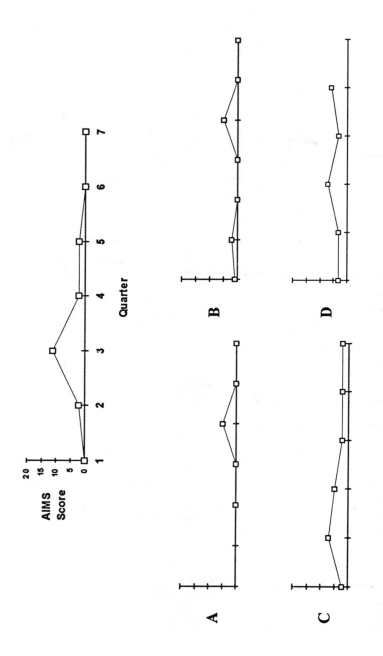

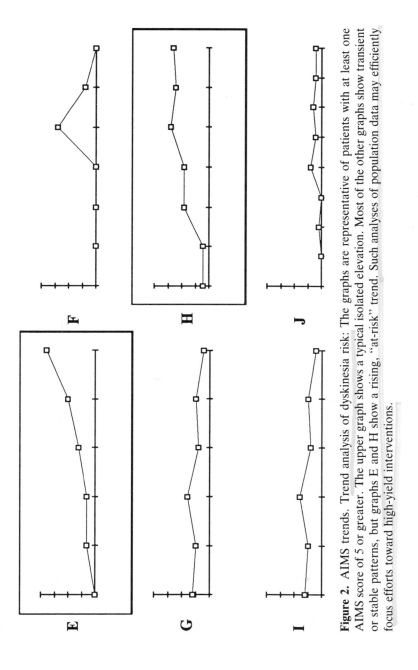

Figure 2. AIMS trends. Trend analysis of dyskinesia risk: The graphs are representative of patients with at least one AIMS score of 5 or greater. The upper graph shows a typical isolated elevation. Most of the other graphs show transient or stable patterns, but graphs E and H show a rising, "at-risk" trend. Such analyses of population data may efficiently focus efforts toward high-yield interventions.

steady stream of monitoring data permitted us to worry less about dyskinesia and focus attention on more pressing risks.

Using Outcome Instruments to Analyze the Health Status of Patient Populations

Applied *regularly*, clinical data sets assist managing the health of populations. From time to time, use of screening laboratory tests (HIV tests of inpatients, urine tests for drugs of abuse, multiple blood chemistries) have been proposed for this purpose, but except for a few tests targeted at newborns, high costs and low yields have forced abandoning this approach. We expect a different fate for prospective gathering of questionnaire-based health status data. Recently developed well-validated instruments such as the royalty-free Short Form (SF)-36 questionnaire used in the RAND Corporation Medical Outcome Study (Stewart, Hayes, & Ware, 1988) have been shown to be sensitive and accurate predictors of health status and service utilization, precisely the information needed by health care organizations to plan resource needs. Instruments can be used for screening and surveillance. For example, the depression and anxiety subscales of the SF-36 can identify individuals who may benefit from mental health intervention. A validated health status measurement can track health outcomes, monitor practitioners and program effectiveness, and provide valuable *objective* data for management decisions. Integrated clinical information systems can assure consistent and reliable administration of these measuring tools. Many of the instruments are brief and lend themselves to administration directly at a computer screen. We anticipate that many of these tests will be administered in waiting and examination rooms. Automated scoring and direct storage of results in electronic patient records will allow prompt notification of results. The data can be linked to other facts in the clinical data base, permitting correlative analyses, as well as automated interaction with appointment scheduling systems to facilitate periodic follow-up interviews. The greatest benefit of surveillance occurs when an entire population is monitored regularly and integrated information environments can assure this.

A relevant mental health care application might be periodic monitoring of mood disorder and substance abuse risk among general medical patients or employee populations using computer administered self-report instruments such as the SF-36 subscales and the CAGE (Cut down, Annoyed, Guilty Feelings, Eye-opener) alcoholism screener (Jones, Lindsey, Yount, Soltys, & Farani–Enayat, 1993). Identification and early treatment of these conditions is quite cost effective. It is well-established that untreated depressed patients utilize more medical services than nondepressed patients (Callahan, Hui, Nienaber, Musick, & Tierney, 1994) and early treatment can reduce the need for psychiatric hospitalizations. Surveillance offers dual advantages of promoting better health status *and* better patterns of resource utilization. It should figure importantly in any risk-reduction program. Anticipating this in the design specifications for information systems will support gathering this valuable information at minimal additional cost, and steer caregivers toward productive interventions via reminders.

Despite extensive use of psychometric instruments in diagnosis and research, no consensus exists about the best instrument for monitoring a general psychiatric population. The SF-36 is standardized and addresses physical illness dimensions often underrecognized in specialized mental health settings. The Diagnostic and Statistical Manual of Mental Disorders' (DSM-IV) Axis 5, the Global Assessment of Functioning, lacks standardization and anchoring of its scores and may have limited reliability and value for this purpose. The Brief Psychiatric Rating Scale (Overall & Gorham, 1962) and the Hamilton Depression and Anxiety Scales (Hamilton, 1959, 1960) are well established, but require a trained rater and are limited to clinical subsets. The self-report Beck Depression Inventory can tracks change in patients with depressive disorders (Beck, Ward, Mendelson, Mock, & Erbaugh, 1961). Because it includes questions about suicidal ideation, its administration must be carefully structured to assure prompt clinical review of patient responses. The Symptoms Checklist-90 (SCL-90) and the Beck Hopelessness Scale address generic clinical concerns and appear suitable for surveillance of psychiatric populations (Derogatis, 1977; Beck & Steer, 1988).

Utilization of Service by Populations

Although useful to characterize health status, most rating scales have not been extensively correlated with service utilization, the crucial determinant of financial risk under capitated reimbursement. Diagnoses and DRGs are of limited value in "epidemiological" quality management, certainly so in outpatient settings and in mental health inpatient settings as well (Taub, Lee, & Forthofer, 1984). Despite improved reliability, DSM-III+ diagnoses per se explain less of the variance in utilization than associated factors such as comorbid substance use, housing and socioeconomic status, and general psychological characteristics. The best predictor is a patient's historical pattern. Information systems tracking resource consumption can identify heavy utilizers. Figure 3 profiles annual utilization of inpatient, outpatient, and pharmacy resources among 4,000 patients receiving psychiatric care in our VA Medical center. It dramatically illustrates the impact of a few very ill patients on a global budget. Utilization data derived from systems that support service delivery can identify the sources of greatest financial risk. Correlating utilization data with demographic and clinical outcome information creates a powerful opportunity to establish priorities for managing costs while maintaining an ethical commitment to patient welfare. More often than not, as occurred with clozapine

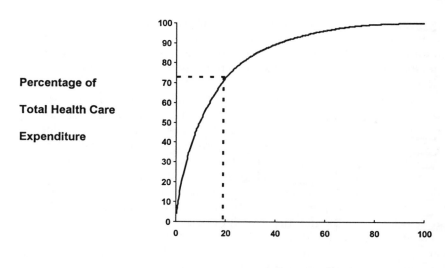

Percentage of Population

Figure 3. Utilization profile of a psychiatric population. This Pareto diagram plots cumulative percentage of total resource utilization against the cumulative number of patients in a VA mental health population sorted by unit annual health services cost from greatest to least. The intersection shows that the most expensive 20% of patients account for over 70% of the total cost of treating the entire population.

treatment for treatment-refractory schizophrenics and a carefully studied geriatric population, approaches that produced better patient outcomes also reduced overall costs of care (Meltzer et al., 1993; Reid, Mason, & Toprac, 1994; Hammond, Prather, Date, & King, 1990).

Tracking Quality Across Institutions

The 1994 derailment of national health care reform interrupted ambitious efforts to promote quality and reduce variations in practice on a national basis. Nevertheless, the increasing costs and persistent maldistribution of health care will keep the topic alive in a changing political climate. The AHCPR, charged with developing effectiveness-based care standards of care, recently published practice guidelines for the diagnosis and treatment of depressive disorders (Agency for Health Care Policy Research, 1993), the first in a series for several major mental disorders that eventually will include standards for treatment of schizophrenia, bipolar, substance use, and anxiety disorders. The American Psychiatric Association has also released guidelines for treatment of major depressive and bipolar disorders. These benchmarks offer health care purchasers an important basis for comparing one delivery package to another.

Responding to similar concerns, the VA instituted in 1992 a case-based external peer review program (EPRP) performed by a private contractor applying identical standards at all of VA's 160-odd medical centers. Using remote data-extraction methods pioneered with the earlier Quality Improvement Checklist project (Barbour, 1994), the DHCP system was used extensively to reduce the labor costs of the review. Cases with target discharge diagnoses are automatically and randomly sampled at each medical center. Pertinent laboratory, appointment, length of stay, and pharmacy data are abstracted and transmitted to reviewers along with copies of a discharge summary. EPRP has promoted increased uniformity of prescribing pneumonia vaccine, and has focused attention on documenting severity of illness among patients hospitalized with major depressive disorder.

Still new, EPRP reveals the strengths and shortcomings of relying on production data bases to effect quality reviews. Random case sampling, automated screening of lab and pharmacy summaries, and the application of uniform review standards across the care network work well when quality questions can be unambiguously answered from the data base; but in the major depression study a complex criteria set required extensive manual review and involvement of physician secondary reviewers. Clear conclusions about quality were not easily drawn. Despite innovative use of data resources, the major depression review pushed the limits of fully automated reviews. EPRP can pinpoint interfacility variations in care practices, mortality, length of stay, and readmissions, but is insensitive to differences in treatment outcome. Routine use of outcome measurement tools will improve the utility of automated review and permit valid comparative judgements.

Putting the Pieces Together

The examples above are a series of "snapshots" of what happens when information systems are harnessed to a quality improvement strategy. Most intriguing has been the discovery that prospecitive tracking of "live" information in a production system brings unexpected vitality and adaptability to quality management strategies. Projects begun to meet external monitoring requirements regularly take on a life of their own, sometimes blending into the background of routine clinical activity and sometimes leading to new avenues. Synergies regularly emerge when clinical and outcome data link over time, projecting quality management over entire populations. One obvious benefit has been to relieve quality management and clinical staff from low-yield chart reviews. Concrete benefits in patient care and utilization have helped garner support for ongoing quality management projects. Experience gained in implementing reminder systems has been fed back to the designers of appointment scheduling, order entry, and clinical record systems, strengthening the utility and relevance of computer-assisted methods.

Organizations that blend strategic vision and data-based comprehensive quality management will outperform competitors that fail to do so. The information systems of such organizations must integrate supporting subsystems such as laboratory, pharmacy, appointment scheduling, and patient records. This permits utilization profiling and embedding of event detectors to trigger reminders at the point of care. Ability to administer, score, and store questionnaires will be desirable, as will be flexibility to add new instruments when they are needed. Questionnaire systems must be coordinated with appointment systems to assure regular testing and extra time for administration. Ad hoc data query tools usable by quality management and administrative staff will be needed to run correlative studies and generate outcome feedback to clinical staff and program managers.

Mental health care delivery organizations are well positioned to profit from data-based comprehensive quality management for a number of reasons. The systems theory perspective of comprehensive quality management is compatible with the intellectual background of most mental health practitioners. Mental health practitioners are comfortable with psychometric instruments. Providers who sell managed behavioral health services to organizations may find it advantageous to screen employee and HMO populations for depressive and substance use disorders to encourage early interventions. And finally, because mental health care is reimbursed less freely than general medical care, mental health providers may have greater incentive to mobilize the favorable fiscal dynamics of outcome-based quality improvement. To thrive in today's health care environment, mental health organizations should plan to acquire or build information systems with sufficient power and flexibility to handle the evolving requirements of comprehensive data-based quality management. If they match this with effective strategic vision, they should be amply rewarded.

References

Agency for Health Care Policy Research (1993). *Depression in Primary Care* (2 vol.), AHCPR Publication 93-0550/1). Rockville, Md., U.S. Dept of Health and Human Services.

Andrews, R.D., & Beauchamp, C. (1989). A clinical database management system for improved integration of the Veterans Affairs hospital information system. *Journal of Medical Systems*, *13*, 309–320.

Aronow, D.B., & Coltin, K.L. (1993a). Information technology applications in quality assurance and quality improvement, Part I. *Joint Commission Journal on Quality Improvement*, *19*, 403–415.

Aronow, D.B., & Coltin, K.L. (1993b). Information technology applications in quality assurance and quality improvement, Part II. *Joint Commission Journal on Quality Improvement, 19*, 465–478.

Barbour, G.L. (1994). Development of a quality improvement checklist for the Department of Veterans Affairs. *Joint Commission Journal on Quality Improvement, 20*, 127–139.

Barnett, G.O. (1984). The application of computer-based medical records in ambulatory practice. *New England Journal of Medical, 310*, 1643–1650.

Beck, A.T., & Steer, R.A. (1988). *Manual for the Beck Hopelessness Scale.* San Antonio, TX: Psychological Corporation.

Beck, A.T., Ward, C.H., Mendelson, M., Mock, J., & Erbaugh, J. (1961). An inventory for measuring depression. *Archives of General Psychiatry, 4*, 561–571.

Berwick, D.M., Godfrey, A., Blanton, A., & Roessner, J. (1990). Curing health care: New strategies for quality improvement. San Francisco: Jossey–Bass.

Callahan, C.M., Hui, S.L., Nienaber, N.A., Musick, B.S., & Tierney, W.M. (1994). Longitudinal study of depression and health services use among elderly primary care patients. *Journal of the American Geriatric Society, 42*, 833–838.

Derogatis, L.R. (1977). *SCL-90-R administration, scoring and procedure manual II.* Towson, MD: Clinical Psychometric Research.

Guy, W. (Ed.). (1976). *ECDEU Assessment Manual for Psychopharmacology* (Publication ADM 76-338, pp. 534–537). Washington, DC: U.S. Department of Health Education and Welfare.

Hamilton, M. (1959). The assessment of anxiety states by rating. *British Journal of Medical Psychology, 32*, 50–55.

Hamilton, M. (1960). A rating scale for depression. *Journal of Neurology, Neurosurgery, and Psychiatry, 23*, 56–62.

Hammond, K.W., Prather, R.J., Date, V.V., & King, C.A. (1990). A provider-interactive medical record system can favorably influence costs and quality of medical care. *Computers in Biology and Medicine, 20*, 267–279.

Hammond, K.W., Snowden, M., Risse, S.C., Adkins, T.G., & O'Brien, J.S. (1995). An effective computer-based tardive dyskinesia monitoring system. *American Journal of Medical Quality, 10*, 133–137.

Haynes, R.B., & Walker, C.J. (1987). Computer-aided quality assurance: A critical appraisal. *Archives of Internal Medicine, 147*, 1297–1301.

Jones, T.V., Lindsey, B.A., Yount, P., Soltys, R., & Farani–Enayat, B. (1993). Alcoholism screening questionnaires: Are they valid in elderly medical outpatiens? *Journal of General Internal Medical, 8*, 674–678.

Lohr, K.N. (1994). Guidelines for clinical practice: Applications for primary care. *Internal Journal of Quality Health Care, 6*(1), 17–25.

Meltzer, H.Y., Cola, P., Way, L., Thompson, Bastani, B., Davies, M.A., & Snitz, B. (1993). Cost effectiveness of clozapine in neuroleptic-resistant schizophrenia. *American Journal of Psychiatry, 150*, 1630–1638.

Overall, J.E., & Gorham, D.R. (1962). The brief psychiatric rating scale. *Psychological Reports, 10*, 799–812.

Reid, W.H., Mason, M., & Toprac, M. (1994). Savings in hospital bed-days related to treatment with clozapine. *Hospital and Community Psychiatry, 45*, 261–264.

Stewart, A.L., Hays, R.D., & Ware, J.E. (1988). The MOS short-form general health survey. Reliability and validity in a patient population. *Medical Care*, *26*, 724–735.

Taube, C., Lee, E.S., & Forthofer, R.N. (1984). DRGs in psychiatry. An empirical evaluation. *Medical Care*, *22*, 597–610.

Wilson, G.A., McDonald, C.J., & McCabe, G.P. (1982). The effect of immediate access to computerized medical records on physician test ordering: A controlled trial in the emergency room. *American Journal of Public Health*, *72*, 698–702.

13
Treatment Planner: A VA Blueprint for Managed Mental Health Care
Kenric W. Hammond

The ubiquitous Mental Health Treatment Plan originated in the *Wyatt v. Stickney* decision (1971) that established that involuntarily hospitalized patients in the state of Alabama had a "right" to treatment (*Wyatt v. Stickney*, 1971). Among the judicial prescriptions to protect this right was a general format for treatment plans (*Wyatt v. Stickney*, 1972). The decision applied only to Alabama, but it set national standards for treatment of involuntary patients, and by extension, psychiatric patients in general. The Wyatt treatment planning standards are essentially those enforced by accrediting bodies today. A *written* plan must document the condition treated, communicate the method, frequency, intensity, duration, and expected outcome of treatment, and do so within a specified time frame. Enforcement varies somewhat with the treatment setting. Free-standing and state psychiatric hospitals apply most of the Wyatt criteria under the Joint Commission on Accreditation of Health Care Organization's Mental Health Manual standards (JCAHO, 1992); psychiatric units within general medical hospitals follow somewhat more flexible hospital accreditation guidelines. The Health Care Financing Agency applies similar standards for Medicare certification.

Currently, written treatment plans function mainly to *certify* treatment, documenting and communicating a promise about the treatment to non-clinical entities outside the treatment setting. Treatment plans in charts are vital for accreditation, and most insurance carriers request copies of treatment plans before they pay for care. Accreditation and payment are essential, of course, but there is little sense that written treatment plans (in contrast to *planning* treatment) have major clinical impact. Treatment plan writing tends to receive low priority except in the weeks and months before inspections. The clinical utility of written plans is inconsistent and usually less than satisfactory. Intended or not, strict plan-writing requirements imply that those who care for patients cannot be trusted. This negative element may reinforce a perception that treatment plan writing is peripheral busywork that is counterproductive when it interferes with seeing patients.

This unpopular reputation warrants a cautious approach to the subject of automating treatment plans. Promising too much risks disappointing an audience seeking relief, but promising too little begs a question of "Why trouble at all?" if the result is mere chartsmanship. Sobered by these risks, a team of Department of Veterans Affairs (VA) mental health clinicians recently completed specifications for a computer-based treatment planning system. The decision to proceed ultimately rested on the fact that treatment planning was required, and would remain so. The chief design task was to determine how best to reduce the labor of plan creation, while optimizing the clinical utility and relevance. The group began with five goals:

1. Improved compliance with treatment planning requirements,
2. A more uniform treatment planning process,
3. Reduced effort to create acceptable plans,
4. Using computer communications to make plans accessible, and
5. Integrating the treatment plan with existing information resources.

State of Mental Health Care in VA

VA is the largest "single payer" health care system in the United States, and possesses exceptional depth and breadth in its mental health services. VA provides general psychiatry services at 171 medical centers and has many special programs for posttraumatic stress, alcohol and drug dependence, geriatric psychiatry, clozapine treatment, intensive community care and an array of vocational rehabilitation services. In addition, it supports community-based Veterans Outreach Centers and administers an extensive system of contracts with private providers in outlying geographic areas. Although it is a single organization, VA's mental health programs are not highly coordinated. Improved continuity of care may be one of the more tangible benefits of information technology. Even *within* many VA medical centers erratic coordination of clinical programs results in duplication or omission of services. Similar fragmentation plagues the patchwork of private, community, and governmental providers that constitutes the United States' mental health services delivery system.

VA Market for Treatment Planning

A 1991 survey of VA Psychiatry and Psychology services identified treatment planning as a top priority for development of new mental health computing capability, and created an opportunity to plan a long-desired addition to existing mental health applications. It also posed a significant challenge, given the diversity of VA clinical programs. Since then, health care reform initiatives, continued pressure to shrink government agencies, and research demonstrating the value of continuity of care for the chronically mentally ill have further defined the challenge. The VA market is demanding tools for quality management, cost-effective treatment, and restructured service delivery emphasizing primary care, case management, and community-based care. At the same time there is a need to reduce fragmentation of services both within the VA and at the VA/community interface. This increases the importance of patient care information exchange among and between caregivers and resource managers. Still, ability to meet specific needs of local programs remains the prerequisite for acceptance by potential clinical users. Because treatment plans are required, and in theory summarize patient assessments, interventions, and outcomes, considerable interest has developed in devising a system that will also produce aggregate cost and effectiveness data.

Duplicating the current paper-based system was not believed to be enough of an improvement to successfully entice or warrant mandating adoption of a new system. However, forces of change in the VA system have combined with increasingly capable computerized patient record (CPR) technology to recast the treatment plan as a tool to manage individual patients as well as institutions by linking clinical outcomes to utilization while promoting uniform standards of care. Shifts in VA's management strategy spurred by health care reform initiatives include:

1. Rewarding capitated enrollment, not unit workloads,
2. Encouraging links to, rather than duplication of community resources,
3. Applying quality standards to populations as well as to individuals, and
4. Greater accountability to deliver satisfactory outcomes, not just revenue.

Our explicit goal was to finesse busywork by easing the development of treatment plans, and at the same time create data bases useful for tracking the clinical and institutional aspects of continuing care in a distributed service network. The direction taken was based on an assessment that VA's Decentralized Hospital Computing Program (DHCP) possessed the capabilities needed to make these goals attainable.

VA Information Systems

The VA's commitment more than a decade ago to adopt homogeneous programming, language, and hardware standards has yielded a steady flow of clinical and administrative applications supporting all phases of patient care and agency management (Andrews & Beauchamp, 1989). Communications utilities have evolved for central reporting of inpatient and outpatient workloads and electronic transmission of patient data between medical centers. Today's DHCP consists of central micro-computer clusters at each medical center that serve up to several thousand text-based video terminals. The configuration permitted rapid deployment of significant computing power at low unit cost, but in recent years has dulled in user appeal because it does not fully take advantage of the visual programming environments, wide-area communications, and data capture technologies of the 1990s. Despite royalty-free availability, DHCP software, except for a few notable installations in government health facilities here and abroad, has mainly existed to serve the VA. It is now accepted the VA's "proprietary" system must evolve toward an open architecture enabling connectivity with external health care information systems and commercial microcomputer software products. A new direction in information technology complements greater emphasis on community-based care of defined populations.

The DHCP Mental Health System was the first VA clinical application to support patient records with a history, physical examination, Diagnostic and Statistical Manual (DSM) diagnosis, problem lists, progress notes, and patient-interactive tests and interviews; but it did not include a treatment planner (Hammond & Gottfredson, 1984). Present interest is strengthened by new technical capabilities that permit planning systems to integrate with the broader information environment by exchanging information between remote data bases. Belief that treatment planning should evolve from being a fetish for passing inspections to true usefulness in supporting continuous, accountable care informed every step of the design process.

Current Treatment Planning Practice

Treatment plans are required in the mental health wards and clinics of accredited hospitals, including VA medical centers. Community providers may not routinely produce outpatient treatment plans if they do not need JCAHO accreditation. When plans are required, paper forms are almost always used. Paper-based plans take time and energy to produce. To the extent that they duplicate previously captured information or fail to add value to care, paper-based treatment plans waste resources. They are produced because they are required.

A good written plan concisely justifies treatment by stating the patient's problems, and for each one, describes planned goals, interventions, and outcome measurements. It makes clear who is responsible for specific elements by listing staff and professional titles, and notes the physician with overall responsibility. When the JCAHO mental health standards are operative, patient strengths are also noted. Often programs use the plan to communicate compliance with administratively required treatments, such as the educational, vocational, recreational, nutritional, and spiratal components of the Joint Commission's "biopsychosocial" standard. In inpatient settings an initial plan is required within a few days of admission to care and in outpatient clinics within several visits or weeks of the initial contact. Inpatient plans must be updated every few weeks, but no precise schedule is spelled out for outpatient services.

The forms most often used for writing plans are fill-in-the-blank documents or checklists. They produce a formally complete plan that is rarely succinct, carrying less information per page than a hospital summary, and are not very portable. Checklists do compensate for inconsistent staff writing skills. When sufficient numbers of timely, individualized plans meeting guidelines are found in surveyed charts, the treatment program passes review. The written plan is a "ticket" to reimbursement and accreditation, but its ability to support ongoing clinical decision making is limited.

The chief flaw of a paper-based plan is not the information it contains, but its unavailability once it is filed in a chart. Its summary of problems, interventions, and responsibilities is exactly the information needed when a psychiatric patient, at a time when the treatment alliance is often weakest, presents in an emergency. Unfortunately, even when records can be located, relevant information from the most recent "master" treatment plan risks being outdated or is buried in bulky checklists and "boilerplate." Paper forms do not facilitate updating plans when transfers of care occur, either. Because the "master" plan must remain with the inpatient record, a new plan in a separate chart location must be written, if required, when a patient transfers to out-patient care. These shortcomings reinforce the opinion that written treatment plans are administrative ballast. This is a legacy of a judicial remedy intended to protect patients' civil rights in an archaic custodial system, not to support continuity of care in integrated service networks.

The best work on the actual process of writing treatment plans is *Fundamentals of Psychiatric Treatment Planning* by James Kennedy (1992). It acknowledges the administrative significance of treatment planning, and insists that treatment plans should be relevant to patient care. Kennedy urges use of simple language and routine outcome rating scales to track treatment results. The manual provides sample forms to create plans, pays attention to the need to leave room for updates on master plans, and describes how to set up the forms with commercial word processors. These are excellent guidelines for computerized treatment planning projects, especially on inpatient units.

Using computers to fill out electronic forms should become a popular alternative to the multipage checklist. Computer output is legible and compact and allows remote retrieval and recycling of the plan for updates. Numerous electronic systems are marketed. Most are designed for stand-alone computers, but inexpensive local area network technology can extend single user applications to multiple users. Psychiatric hospital chains and some managed care concerns use computer-assisted treatment plans to reduce the labor of plan production, mainly in-house. These systems have the potential to use the planning system to disseminate treatment guidelines across a large organization.

Word processors supporting "mail merge" fields and "macro" programming are suited to developing electronic-form-based treatment planning systems. The advantage is local control of form and content, but lack of standardized content and portability is a drawback. Better for standardization are systems that build plans using hierarchical menus or pick lists linked to data bases of diagnoses and clinical terminology. These may have restricted vocabularies and difficult user interfaces that make them less expressive and individualized than free-text systems. Taintor's foreword to Kennedy's book notes that menu-based systems can be more time consuming and complex than the paper forms they replace. Promoters of such systems cite rapid retrieval of stored plans, but this is mainly possible when the plan resides on the computer system that created and stored the plan. The chief disadvantage of all commercial and developmental treatment planners reported to date is the inability to transmit updatable plans *between* computer systems.

VA Treatment Planning Project

The VA group* established to meet the broad need for computer-based treatment planning immediately faced the challenge of providing utility to a geographically and philosophically diverse clinical community. It was concluded that a free-form word-processing approach would produce too small an improvement over the current system of paper forms to warrant a major effort. Left open was the question of how to improve compliance with mandatory aspects while increasing the value of treatment planning to clinicians and managers.

Several pilot efforts provided instructive experience. At the Tampa VA Medical Center, Girgenti and others adapted VA's Nursing Care Plan package to write treatment plans on a psychiatry unit using a hierarchical narrative-builder known as Text Generator to create plans from menus (Girgenti & Mathis, 1994). At the Salt Lake City VA Medical Center, Weaver, Christensen, and Sells developed a microcomputer-based system for a local area network using a terminology system based

---

* The task group consisted of: Kenric Hammond, M.D. (Tacoma), chairman; Dale Cannon, Ph.D. (VA Central Office); Allan Finkelstein, Ph.D. (Albany); Kathleen Kusel, RN (North Chicago); Joyce Girgenti, RN and Dennis Brightwell, M.D. (Tampa); Martha Banks, Ph.D. (Cleveland); D. Robert Fowler, M.D. and Timothy Shea, MSW (Dallas); Frank Backus, M.D. (Seattle); Jeffery Sells, Ph.D. (Salt Lake); Lawrence Andreassen and Mark Devlin (Dallas VA Information Systems Center).

on DSM-III-R (Weaver et al., 1994). This system also produced patient activity schedules and teaching handouts. Hammond et al.'s experience with menu-driven record systems for geriatric outpatient records and mental health treatment plans provided other views of what might be effective in the VA's clinical information environment (Hammond, Prather, Date, & King, 1990).

It was evident that a single system could not satisfy everyone. Those accustomed to a graphical interface would be reluctant to return to text-based systems, but others might not be able to afford the computers needed for networked graphical workstations. Concern arose over un-coordinated development of systems incapable of communicating with each other and with the standard VA system, sacrificing not only rapid access to treatment plans over DHCP's 80,000 data terminals, but also integration with an information environment containing pharmacy, laboratory, order entry, and problem data bases.

Summary of Requirements

Below is a broad summary of requirements generated by the group, with details of each following. Attention was paid to structuring the system to support anticipated VA agendas for service delivery reorganization, quality and resource management, and information technology. The system has not yet been implemented, but encouraging pilot efforts and experience with the current distributed and integrated elements of VA's DHCP portend success.

1. To satisfy clinicians, treatment plans must be:
   a. easy to produce,
   b. supportive of multidisciplinary inputs,
   c. clinically relevant, and
   d. readily available at any DHCP terminal.
2. To satisfy program managers Treatment Planner data bases must:
   a. support standards of care,
   b. support quality management and continuity of care, and
   c. meet accreditor and third party payer standards.
3. To satisfy strategic managers the system should
   a. support networked care delivery.
4. To satisfy Information Systems Managers Treatment Planner software must:
   a. operate on multiple platforms,
   b. permit exchange of information between platforms, and
   c. integrate with other data in the institutional information system.

Clinician Requirements

For clinicians, the fundamental requirements are ease of use and availability, assuring that treatment plans can be readily produced and retrieved whenever and wherever they are required. Key factors include:

1. Content appropriate to the treatment setting,
2. Ability to consolidate contributions of multiple team members,
3. Support for authentication of the plan by a psychiatrist, and
4. Ability to conveniently update prior plans.

Computer data entry is slower than hand entry, but updating an existing plan stored on a computer is faster than rewriting a plan. Taking full advantage of this requires that significant numbers of prior plans be available to update. This requires moving computer plans from one location to another, and in a compatible format. Provision must be made for multidisciplinary staff to draft separate contributions, using the team meeting to assemble the overall document.

Central to these capabilities is a standard skeleton capable of organizing and importing basic treatment plan elements, including document and patient identifiers, treatment locale, treatment team and team membership, multiple problems, goals and interventions, problem-specific and global outcome measures, and authentication.

Development and system-wide distribution of VA's Problem List data base has assisted greatly. This CPR component supports a *single* patient problem list expressed in a *controlled vocabulary*. Creators of a plan will be able to view and edit the current patient problem list. Problem orientation allows linking treatment plan information to other CPR components referencing problems, including progress notes, visits, orders, results, and billings. Problem List employs the VA Clinical Lexicon, a terminology standardized to support passing problem data between sites as well as between software applications (Lincoln, Weir, Moreshead, Kolodner, & Williamson, 1994). Clinical Lexicon is based on the National Library of Medicine's Unified Medical Language System (Lindberg, Humphreys, & McCray, 1993) and encompasses a number of widely used controlled terminologies, including the International Classification of Diseases, ninth edition, clinical modification (ICD-9-CM), the Systematized Nomenclature of Medicine (SNOMED), DSM III-R, and DSM-IV (World Health Organization, 1995; College of American Pathologists, 1993; American Psychiatric Association, 1987, 1994).

The clinical content of the treatment planner is being refined by the development group, drawing on several older sources, including systems developed at the Salt Lake, Loma Linda, and Tampa VA medical centers. The content distributed with the package will be modifiable at local sites. Altering Problem List nomenclature will be discouraged to avoid degrading the patient data base with multiple synonymous terms and to preserve consistency when patient records migrate from one setting to another.

Identification of treatment teams and individuals is supported by existing data structures in the DHCP. Through these, team information can be linked to a physical location, as well as individual staff information derived from personnel, clinical privileging, and payroll data bases. Also, Treatment Planner will have the capability to define a "super" team, consisting of a combination of two or more defined teams, to coordinate jointly shared care. The treatment plan data base will reference the patient's primary caregiver and case manager when either is defined.

Program Management Features

Many of the data elements that support treatment team function will be useful for those who manage clinical resources and track staff and program performance. Examples include analysis of problems treated in a population, caseload analyses, and tracking of primary care assignments. Data elements to support quality management are also specified. The most important of these are:

1. Ability to embed standards of care and "clinical pathways" in the plan,
2. Problem-specific and global patient outcome measurements, and
3. Tracking timely treatment plan completion.

Reduction of variation in patterns of care is a rewarding quality and cost-containment strategy. When an objectively validated treatment standard exists, it is easier for clinicians and managers to work in partnership toward a common goal of providing effective, consistent care. Dissemination of standards for the treatment of mental disorders remains an infant science, but rapid progress is being made, as exemplified by the publication of the Agency for Health Care Policy Research's Guidelines for Treatment of Depression, and similar American Psychiatric Association guidelines for treatment of depressive disorder (Depression Guideline Panel, 1993; American Psychiatric Association, 1993). VA has recently instituted an External Peer Review Program to assess compliance with a number of treatment standards. The program is still formative, but it is a significant first attempt to measure clinical performance uniformly at all VA medical centers. The content of the treatment planner interventions and goals segments will be adapted to address critical elements of emerging standards.

Reproducible and valid measurements of clinical status have suported mental health research for many years, and are increasingly applied to patient populations enrolled in managed care. Clinical support data bases (e.g., pharmacy, laboratory, and medical record systems) are valuable, but are not specifically designed to systematically track outcomes. Outcome measuring instruments permit assessment of program effectiveness and identification of opportunities to improve systems of care in ways that retrospective case reviews do not. Joint Commission standards for treatment planning do encourage expressing treatment goals in "objective language," but paper-based systems permit neither aggregation nor systematic follow-up of outcome attainment. Computer-based systems storing outcome and cost data can furnish a continuous view of a delivery system's cost effectiveness to strategic planners. To support this, the proposed system allows specification of problem-specific and global outcome measures. Organizations requiring and regularly practicing computer treatment planning will be able to systematically gather problem-oriented outcome measurements at little additional effort.

The planning group has not specified which outcome instruments will be used with the treatment plan, but there is a strong possibility that VA's central management will endorse specific assessment tools. Currently, the Brief Psychiatric Rating and Abnormal Involuntary Movement Scales are used to track patients treated with clozapine. Other possibilities include the Short Form (SF)-36 medical outcome scale, the Beck Depression Inventory, and DSM-IV's Axis V (Guy, 1976; Stewart, Hays, & Ware, 1988; Beck, Ward, Mendelson, Mock, & Erbaugh, 1961). Kennedy's treatment planning manual presents an *anchored* adaptation of Axis V that is suitable for routine clinical use.

Strategic Management Support

Under almost any imaginable scenario, the VA health care system will drastically change in the next two decades. Reduction of federally funded health services and a dwindling and aging veteran population may force VA to compete with alternatives such as Medicare and the private sector. To survive, the agency will need to be responsive to its patients, and convince taxpayers that it offers high quality care at the right price. VA will likely increasingly resemble other large managed care organizations. More care will be delivered in outpatient settings, contracts with community providers will increase, and centralized management will wane. In some areas, such as Washington State, consortia of VA medical centers will propose to qualify as a state-certified health plan for veterans and their families, delivering services at their traditional campuses, in satellite clinics, and through contract providers. The architects of change will require population-based data to guide strategic planning, distributed patient information systems that support a variety of service delivery packages, and population-based quality management tools.

Psychiatric services in the VA compare favorably with those available in most communities, and represent a potential source of competitive advantage for the agency in the forthcoming health care shakeout. To preserve this capacity, and to better project it upon community-based networks, the new treatment planning system must facilitate coordination, preserve continuity, and assure consistent quality of care at all levels. This implies the ability to support production of treatment plans in multiple settings, to easily move them about, and to aggregate data. Software capable of running on small and large systems, with communications support and a common data base architecture will be required.

Information Systems Management Considerations

Those who plan and support clinical information systems are key stake-holders in any CPR project. Their endorsement will hinge on technical feasibility that is a product of simplicity, modularity, and economy. Fifteen years of clinical computing in VA have taught that the most durable component of an information system is the data organization and that decisions affecting data architecture have a far-reaching impact. To maximize options the specifications requires:

1. Data elements common to all platforms,
2. Production of treatment plans on stand-alone as well as networked systems, and
3. Transmission of treatment plans to Medical Center data bases.

These will be accomplished stepwise. The first phase will concurrently involve installing a treatment plan storage data base on DHCP hospital systems and building a plan-writing system to be implemented on clinical workstations running Microsoft Windows, along with a specification for bidirectional data exchange. The common data set to be used is described below. Theoretically, the data interchange gateway between DHCP and microcomputers will permit *any* software developer to write a program to the specification, and to modify functionality and clinical content without sacrificing interchange capacity. Data packaging standards, exemplified by the Health Level 7 (HL7) specification for laboratory data transmittal, and work of other standards groups, has rapidly progressed, necessitated by the proliferation of software products and platforms (Cahill, Holmen, & Bartleson, 1991). The first version of the treatment planner will support transmitting data, along with standard patient and document identifiers, as an ASCII text stream, via the Telecommunications Protocol/Interconnect Protocol (TCP/IP). Succeeding iterations will tag treatment plan components with problem identifiers from the VA Clinical Lexicon, and eventually an HL 7-style packaging format will be applied.

Specifications Summary

Structure

Below are the essential data elements of the VA Treatment Plan. Those present in the current DHCP data structure are indicated with an asterisk.

Table 1. Formal Structure of VA Treatment plan Data Base

Treatment Plan	Problem	Expected Outcome	Interventions	Manifestation	Outcome Measurement
Creation date/time	Creation date/time	Creation date/time	Creation date/time	Creation date/time	Creation date/time
Creator	Creator	Creator	Creator	Creator	Creator
Patient	Patient	Patient	Patient	Patient	Patient
Current (y/n)	Current (y/n)	Current (y/n)	Current (y/n)	Current (y/n)	
Status	Status	Status	Status	Status	
	Treatment plan	Intervention	Manifestation	Intervention	Intervention
	Expected outcome	Manifestation	Outcome measure	Outcome measure	Manifestation
	Intervention	Outcome measure	Start date		Outcome measure
	Manifestation	Expected achievement date			
	Outcome measure				
	Expected resolution date				

	Resolution date	Achievement date	Stop date	Rating (numeric)
Authentication date/time				
Responsible team			Responsible person	Hospital location
Case manager			Hospital location	
Primary therapist				
Authenticated by				
Last editor				
Last edit time				
Edit history	Edit history	Edit history	Edit history	Edit history

1. Identity of patient * and document:
   a. patient name* and Social Security Number*;
   b. document type as treatment plan;
   c. the status of the treatment plan (e.g., active, inactive, past due);
   d. an (optional) global outcome measurement, such as Axis V;
   e. patient's case manager;
   f. patient's primary therapist;
      identification of the physician* approving the treatment;
   h. status of document as *draft* or *authenticated*;
   i. dates of creation and authentication; and
   j. review date.
2. Identity of treatment team:
   a. team name* and location*; and
   b. team members* and professional titles*.
3. Problem list:
   a. restricted to a workable set of major syndromes*;
   b. expressed in Clinical Lexicon controlled vocabulary*; and
   c. problem status as active or inactive*.
4. Manifestations of each problem:
   a. brief summary statements of component symptoms.
5. Expected outcomes (goals) for each problem:
   a. time frame expected for accomplishment of outcome; and
   b. an (optional) measurement standard for the outcome.
6. Interventions planned for each problem:
   a. joint and specific responsibilities for implementing interventions; and
   b. indication of the frequency and intensity of the intervention.
7. An audit trail of edits.

A listing of patient strengths as specified in the Consolidated Standards is not included in this specification. While not irrelevant, the concept of "strength", unlike "problem," does not translate well to other elements of the CPR and most VA settings do not address strengths in their treatment plans. Table 1 summarizes the data elements in a normalized matrix of formal components. Figure 1 diagrams the organization of the information structure.

Figure 2 illustrates the central position of a treatment plan to other data flows in health care. Computer-based treatment planning has only recently become feasible thanks to evolution of patient record and organizational data bases supported in VA's DHCP, in particular the Problem List. Development of modular plans has been possible for a number of years, but the technical barriers to transporting updatable plans between programs and sites have hindered integrated implementation. Partial implementations of planning systems are problematic because computer-stored plans generated at a site rapidly lose synchrony

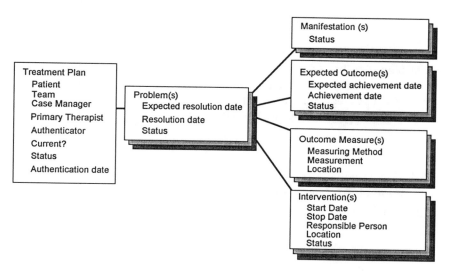

Figure 1. Block diagram of treatment plan data elements and relationships. The figure shows the relationships of data elements presented in Table 1. A treatment plan is associated with a specific patient and treatment team. Each problem it addresses contains one or more manifestations, expected outcomes, interventions, and outcome measurements. Elements are date stamped with an audit trail. Problems, etc. may reference a future date for status review (e.g., problem resolution). Data transport tools will permit moving plans that follow this data structure between sites.

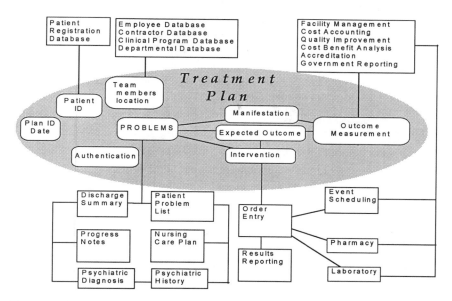

Figure 2. Central position of the treatment plan in organizational data flow.

with subsequent program plans stored on paper or inaccessible computer media.

Figure 3 illustrates linkages allowed by a networked, distributed treatment plan data base. The key capability for supporting continuity of care in a heterogeneous mental health care delivery system is the ability to exchange updatable treatment plan information between data bases, permitting the plan to migrate from one care setting to another along with the patient.

Content

In a pilot effort begun in 1980, Hammond and Munnecke chose to organize problem-oriented treatment around syndromes, because symptom clusters, goals, and interventions appeared to naturally organize together

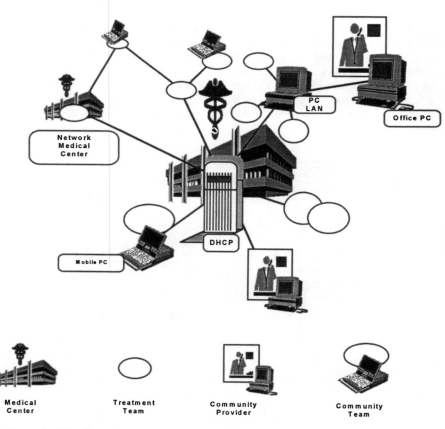

Figure 3. Distributed treatment planning for networked care delivery.

(Hammond & Munnecke, 1984). Examples included depressive and psychotic syndromes, and so on. The finer grained categories of the DSM system were not especially useful for laying out a treatment plan. Kennedy also endorsed this approach in his manual, noting that extensive nomenclature risked fragmenting treatment themes, and suggested limiting topics covered in any one plan to no more than a half-dozen. The VA system will offer about 30 general syndromes for working up specific patient needs, and allow users to relabel the general syndrome name with a more specific problem name from the Clinical Lexicon, if desired.

Planning will proceed by choosing a syndrome, relabeling it if necessary, and then selecting manifestations, expected outcomes (goals), and interventions from lists built for the syndrome. The development group's current approach to writing content is to strive for brevity, clarity, and consistency, not exhaustive detail. From a user perspective, it is annoying to scan more than about seven choices on a pick list. It is also confusing, when choices branch to subchoices, to exceed three levels of branching. The development group continues to refine the content. Domain experts tend to be more generous with complexity than caregivers want, and it will be paramount to avoid excessive data entry time and wordy documents. The current intention is to furnish a sparse set of basic content, and allow users to add terms for manifestations as they wish, and allow free text entry. It will also be possible to develop a plan without menus at all, yet the plan will remain storable in the defined data structure as long as it is referenced by a problem identifier. To promote consistency across the data bases of separate systems, the VA plan will enforce the standard problem nomenclature maintained in its Clinical Lexicon.

The favored prototype for a system to write treatment plans is the microcomputer system developed by Weaver, Sells, and Christensen at the Salt Lake City VA Medical Center (Weaver et al., 1994). This runs under Microsoft Windows. A character-based entry system using existing DHCP "mainframe" software is feasible, and if developed will adhere to the common data dictionary. Treatment Plans will be displayable on both workstations and DHCP text terminals, and be editable, at minimum, with a text editor.

Despite menus, writing treatment plans on a computer will be slower than on paper. Experience with stand-alone systems has demonstrated that advantages of updating machine-stored plans and other documents are rapidly dissipated if the computer system is not consistently used. Most pilot treatment planning systems described in the literature have been restricted to single sites. This limits plan creation, retrieval, and updating to one place, and poses a barrier to wider usage. It is our hope that a computerized treatment plan available in all venues over a course of care will yield the "critical mass" of usage that encourages wide adoption.

Summary

We have outlined an approach designed to overcome the most important barriers to installing computerized treatment plans in complex mental health care delivery environments. The aim is to maximize flexibility for users, yet assure the consistent content and rapid access to a current plan that supports continuity of patient care. The essential features are:

1. a standard data dictionary supporting diverse planning systems on many platforms;
2. modular content, allowing physically separate members to contribute to a single plan;
3. authentication procedures for review, approval, and locking of drafted plans;
4. transportable plans, freed from the chart, available at any workstation;
5. use of a Lexicon to name problems and link to order entry and CPR components;
6. a uniform content core consistent with established standards of care; and
7. support for specification, storage, and tracking of clinical outcome measurements.

While VA challenges and priorities may not be identical to those of the wider mental health care community, we doubt that the problems of fragmentation and nonportability of the treatment plan are unique to the VA. It is our hope that the solutions proposed for VA's vision of distributed care will apply generally to the ongoing task of providing high quality, well-managed, and integrated mental health care.

References

American Psychiatric Association. (1987). Diagnostic and statistical manual of mental disorders (3rd ed., rev.). Washington, DC: American Psychiatric Association.

American Psychiatric Association. (1993). Practice guideline for major depressive disorder in adults. *American Journal of Psychiatry, 150*(Suppl.), 29.

American Psychiatric Association. (1994). *Diagnostic and statistical manual of mental disorders: DSM-IV.* Washington, DC: American Psychiatric Press.

Andrews, R.D., & Beauchamp, C. (1989). A clinical database management system for improved integration of the Veterans Affairs hospital information system. *Journal of Medical Systems, 13*, 309–320.

Beck, A.T., Ward, C.H., Mendelson, M., Mock, J., & Erbaugh, J. (1961). An inventory for measuring depression. *Archives of General Psychiatry, 4,* 561–571.

Cahill, B.P., Holmen, J.R., & Bartleson, P.L. (1991). Mayo Foundation Electronic Results Inquiry, the HL 7 connection. *Proceedings of the Fifteenth Annual Symposium on Computer Applications in Medical Care* (pp. 516–520). New York: McGraw-Hill.

College of American Pathologists. (1993). In R.A. Cote, D.J. Rothwell,J.L. Palotay, R.S. Beckett, L. Brochu (Eds.), *SNOMED international: The systematized nomenclature of human and veterinary medicine* (3rd ed.). Northfield, IL: American College of Pathologists.

Depression Guideline Panel. (1993). *Depression in primary care: Detection, diagnosis, and treatment* (AHCPR Publication No. 93-0552, Quick Reference Guide for Clinicians, Number 5). Rockville, MD: U.S. Department of Health and Human Services, Public Health Service, Agency for Health Care Policy and Research.

Girgenti, J.R., & Mathis, A.C. (1994). Putting psychiatric nursing standards into clinical practice. *Journal of Psychosocial Nursing and Mental Health Services, 32*, 39–42.

Guy, W. (Ed.). (1976). *ECDEU assessment manual for psychopharmacology: Publication ADM 76-338* (pp. 534–537). Washington, DC: U.S. Department of Health Education and Welfare.

Hammond, K.W., & Gottfredson, D.K. (1984). The VA mental health information system package: Version 1. *Computer Use in Social Services, 4*, 6–7.

Hammond, K.W., & Munnecke, T. (1984). A computer-assisted psychiatric treatment plan. *Hospital and Community Psychiatry, 35* 160–163.

Hammond, K.W., Prather, R.J., Date, V.V., & King, C.A. (1990). A provider-interactive medical record system can favorably influence costs and quality of medical care. *Computers in Biology and Medicine, 20*, 267–279.

Joint Commission on Accreditation of Healthcare Organizations. (1992). *MHM, 1993 accreditation manual for mental health, chemical dependency, and mental retardation/developmental disabilities services.* Oakbrook Terrace, IL: Joint Commission on Accreditation of Healthcare Organizations.

Kennedy, J.A. (1992). *Fundamentals of psychiatric treatment planning.* Washington, DC: American Psychiatric Press.

Lincoln, M.J., Weir, C., Moreshead, G., Kolodner, R., & Williamson, J. (1994). Creating and evaluating the Department of Veterans Affairs electronic medical record and national clinical lexicon. *Proceedings of the Eighteenth Symposium on Computer Applications in Medical Care* (p. 1047). American Medical Informatics Association.

Lindberg, D.A.B., Humphreys, B.L., & McCray, A.T. (1993). The unified medical language system. *Methods of Information in Medicine, 32*, 281–291.

Stewart, A.L., Hays, R.D., & Ware, J.E. (1988). The MOS short-form general health survey. Reliability and validity in a patient population. *Medical Care, 26*, 724–735.

Weaver, R.A., Christensen, P.W., Sells, J., Gottfredson, D.K., Noorda, J., Schenkenberg, T., & Wennhold, A. (1994). Computerized treatment planning. *Hospital and Community Psychiatry, 4*, 825–827.

World Health Organization. (1995). *ICD-9-CM: International classification of diseases* (9th rev.), *Clinical modification* (4th ed.). Los Angeles, CA: Practice Management Information Corp.

Wyatt v. Stickney, 325 F. Supp. 781, 785 (1971).

Wyatt v. Stickney, Appendix A, 1972, F. Supp. 373, 379 (1972).

14
Automated Methods of Clinical Quality Management
Chris E. Stout

You don't have to do this.
Survival is not compulsory.

W.E. Deming

The concept of quality management methods has existed for at least the last 40 years. The late W. Edwards Deming is considered to have been the originating and driving force behind what many call Total Quality Management (TQM) or Continuous Quality Improvement (CQI). (In this chapter TQM will generally refer to both concepts.) The TQM concepts have caught fire and are currently quite in vogue with most companies, management seminars, books, and business schools. Yet, even with such exposure and concomitant enthusiasm, TQM principles have not yet been embraced by most mental health professionals. TQM concepts are on their way, however. The Joint Commission on Accreditation of Healthcare Organizations (JCAHO) endorses numerous TQM ideals and thus, many approved psychiatric facilities are working to better understand and utilize them. This chapter broadly covers the key aspects of TQM philosophy and specifically provides two detailed actual examples of procedures using such principles, demonstrating how automated methods expedite the system.

Paradigm Shift/Culture Shock

Perhaps one of the primary difficulties that TQM has had in making the translation from manufacturing management globally to health service management in general, and behavioral healthcare management in particular, is its lexicon. Many clinicians are not used to, or may initially consider it inappropriate, to refer to patients as customers or care as a product. Many consider this as "commoditizing" the all important doctor–patient relationship. With the exception of pro bono or volunteered help, professionals receive a fee for such services or products. Thus, even though most professionals are not drawn to psychiatric care by profits but instead with the goal to help others, there is, nevertheless, the reality of having to be paid in order to be able to actually do so. Psychiatric practice is a business—be it a facility, group, or even a solo practice. As such, it is incumbent upon leaders, owners, or whomever serve as decision makers, to know as much about spreadsheets as they do bedsheets. That is, the business/fiscal/personnel management issues weigh equally with the clinical aspects of patient care. If one cannot stay in business, one cannot provide *any* service or care. And, if a practice or facility support or clinical staff are inappropriate or inefficient, it becomes impossible to provide good or high quality care.

This aspect provides a good transition to the basic TQM tenet of improving quality with a focus on outcome (also known as product). TQM terms such as empowerment, nonblaming perspectives, solution-focused goals, data-based (less biased) decision making, working with teams, soliciting others' input, and so forth, should ring positively in clinicians' as well as administrators' ears.

Managed Care's Impact and Impetus

Any practitioner and administrator in practice or operation today has likely been impacted by managed care. In health care, managed care's initial goal was to help reduce the costs associated in care provision. The presumption was that there were costs from unnecessary types, venues, or durations of behavioral healthcare. Therefore, within this hypothesis, managed care organizations spawned the growth of utilization management services.

Recently, these groups have begun to examine patient outcomes. Automated, integrated TQM systems allow practitioners and facilities to conduct their own studies providing internal methods to improve themselves. Improving clinical outcomes within a cost-effective system is a noble (and attainable) ideal. Initiating such should not be cause for systemic-chaos or operations upheaval. There is a learning curve, but it is typically a short one. As the old cliché goes, "If you don't have the time to do it right the first time, how can you have time to do it over?" This is especially true for patient care. If you were a manufacturer and you had a flaw in your widget, you could scrap the run, suffer the loss, and retool to correct the defect. In healthcare, no one can have an error tolerance that is acceptable below 100%. The goal then becomes consistent high quality that providers, patients, and payors can all afford. TQM procedures, especially those enhanced via automation, will be key.

A Closer Look at TQM

There are volumes of books, articles, tapes, and seminars on TQM principles. (Many top selections appear in this chapter's concluding bibliography.) So, any brief overview of TQM in this format is bound not to do it justice. Nevertheless, a little coaching and exposure may be useful.

The Chicago Community Trusts' Government Assistance Project has delineated nine Quality Principles and Processes that succinctly capture the essence of TQM (Howick & Gray, 1992). First of all, *Focus on Internal and External Customer Expectations*. What do your customers want beyond quality, affordable care? Perhaps convenient hours, baby sitting, close locations, well-lit parking, nonfrustrating voice mail? What do your staff/clinicians want? Up-to-date equipment, less paperwork, job security, stimulation, and challenge at manageable levels? *Solve Problems Through Teams*. No one likes a dictator or autocrat. Team members bring in slightly different perspectives as to what the problem is, its causes, and thus, its possible solutions. Remember, we are all smarter together than anyone of us alone. Third, *Analyze Problems Comprehensively*. Impulsive solutions often beget a new additional set of problems. Iatrogenic solutions are oxymorons. Teams need to use time appropriately, not taking too long, but also not creating solutions that only deal with the superficial aspects of the problem.

Next is *Improve Work Systems That Effect the Delivery of Services*. A blood test is only useful if it is timely. The same is true for a psychological battery. Managed care has taught us to be prompt in the provision of services. *Make Data-Based Decisions*. Clinical psychologists trained within the scientist–practitioner model will readily understand and assimilate this deceptively simple point. Too often decision makers fool themselves into thinking that their views are unbiased or that somehow *they* have the rare ability to see their own blind spots. (This goes in tandem with working with a team to mitigate individual biases.)

Innovators *Develop Action Plans With Responsibilities and Performance Measures*. Teams need to be wary of the phenomenon of "diffusion of responsibility." That is, specific members need to volunteer or be appointed to do specific tasks, and these specific tasks need to be measurable and measured. This also provides for data-based decision making, not presumption, not bias. *Work on Continuous Improvements*, not end goals, per se. The idea is not to miss reaching a target, to avoid becoming jaded, or be tempted to rest upon laurels. Advancement, betterment, and growth are believed to result from ongoing modifications and refinements.

It is recommended that we should *Measure Progress Against an Established Baseline*. We can establish our own "internal" baselines; most of us already have by default. For example, what is the average length of stay in an inpatient facility, or average number of out patient sessions for a certain diagnosis, or how many days does it take to turn around a psychological test battery? These can serve as internal pre-TQM baselines. We can also seek out noncompetitors with whom we share similarities and make mutual, collegial arrangements to share data on certain specific measures of quality performance. And finally, a *Focus on Quality Saves Money*. And saving money is a good thing. It does not matter if your facility is for profit or not for profit. Not exploiting an opportunity for a savings is tantamount to waste, pure and simple. All administrators have an ethical mandate to exercise fiscal responsibility. It makes little difference how the resultant savings is then managed, be it to plow directly back into the practice or facility to expand services, reduce rates, make capital expenditures, or simply make shareholders happy. Greed is indeed bad and different from savings; however, within most all mores, saving money is a virtue.

Clinicians will hold an affinity to the scientific approach (Howick & Gray, 1992) that TQM methods champion. These include making decisions based on data, not hunches; an investigation of root causes of problems; a drive to seek permanent solutions in lieu of traditional quick fixes (that are often more problem causing than problem solving). Also, many behavioral health care clinicians can apply TQM's systemic perspective to their organizations, regardless of type. Focusing on functions, departments, or units as discrete, distinct, or noninterdependent can create micromanagement problems. Visionary leadership rarely springs forth from this perspective. Similarly, it is quite helpful to conceptualize all work duties as a series of interrelated processes that should be studied and improved. Complexity usually yields inefficiency; therefore, simplicity should improve efficiency. Of additional appeal to clinicians are the concepts noted by Howick and Gray (1992) in the 85/15 Rule and 95/5 Rule of "systemic" management. By definition, within the 85/15 Rule, 85% of a facility's or practice's problems can be solved by improving the *system*, whereas only 15% of a facility's/practice's problems are within control of *individuals* within the system. Thus, if you tinker and improve the functioning of the system instead of blaming the staff, then the majority of your problems will be taken care of.

The 95/5 Rule posits the position that organizational success will result if you deal directly, honestly, and fair handedly with 5% of your staff and modify existing policies and procedures to communicate such trust for the 95% of remaining employees. The point is similar to that of the 85/15 Rule in that staff function at their optimum when trusted, and that the majority of staff come to work (be it a clinic, facility, agency, practice, or any type of setting) wanting to do a good job (regardless of their duty).

Methodologically, the concepts of "Plan-Do-Act-Check" aid to operationalize what has been discussed herein. For example, *Planning* would involve the determination of goals and targets for the current project/task at hand. Additionally, developing methods with which to reach these goals would also occur. *Doing* would incorporate engagement in any needed educational or specialized training necessary and then initiating and conducting the work. *Checking* would simply involve evaluating the effects of implementation and lead to *Acting*, or taking whatever type of appropriate action is necessary.

Another fundamental aspect of TQM processes is the mission statement. Although this may seem unnecessary or superfluous to some, it can actually serve as an excellent guide to decision making, especially the difficult decisions, and serve as a public statement as to what a facility or practice stands for. Ideally, it should be developed by all members of the group; but if this is not practical or possible, it should then be composed by a group representative of a diverse, heterogeneous cross section of the organization or practice. It is very important that the mission statement be understood and supported by the staff (Howick & Gray, 1992). It should have meaning to both those inside and outside of the system or facility. An example of a mission statement developed by a privately owned behavioral health care system is as follows:

> It is the mission of "ABC" Health Systems to provide an innovative, high-quality, comprehensive continuum of mental health services to our customers and the community.

As alluded to early in this chapter, there are no current nationally recognized models of excellence in behavioral health care's use of TQM principles. This does not mean, however, that there are not any such components in operation. For example, Choice Health in Colorado has been instrumental in designing TQM methods and ideals into their procedures. Their model represents one of the more forward-thinking models in the country. Their system is fully automated and dependent on computerized data scoring and management. Additionally, Forest Health Systems in Illinois has also developed procedures based on TQM principles. These case examples shall be examined in detail, two of which are predicated on the utilization of various automated systems.

Case Example I: Decreasing Psychological Report Turnaround Time

In a moderately sized psychiatric inpatient hospital a TQM team was developed to decrease the time it took to have a full psychological testing battery be placed in the patient's chart. First of all, the Director of Quality Management solicited a team of volunteers who were representative of all the "stakeholders" (i.e., someone involved in the process). The team included: the Director of Quality Management (as coach and mentor); a representative unit secretary (person who routes psychological testing orders); the Director of Staff Development (to better orient staff); a representative of the Medical Records Department (they process psychological reports when complete, log them in, and route them to the patients' charts); a representative testing psychologist (to note his needs and presumably other psychologists' as well); and the Chief of Psychology (whose responsibility it would be to monitor and evaluate the new mechanism when developed). Ideally, a patient's input would have been used too, but it was impractical for this task.

The initial meeting included a discussion on the TQM procedure to be utilized, an exploration and common articulation of the problem, and an explanation of how each member normally carried out their role or function. The program and staff roles were graphically drawn using a fishbone diagram. Brainstorming was used to develop potential ideas and procedures. A prototype procedure was derived with group consensus. It was explicitly written and met with the group's approval who then agreed on a 6 week pilot test. A meeting was set at the end of the 6 week trial with the option for the team to meet earlier if necessary. That meeting could be called by *any* team member.

At the 6 week trial's end the team reconvened. A few problems were noted and methods to deal with them were developed by the team. The revised procedure then was tried for another month. At the conclusion of that trial, the team met again. They were unanimously satisfied, the new procedure was formally adopted into the Hospital's Quality Management Plan and Policy and Procedure Manual, and the team was dissolved. However, periodic "fine-tunings" occur as needed and anyone can identify such a need to the Chief of Psychology and/or Director of Quality Management.

Case Example II: Quality Improvement Methods

As TQM principles dictate data-based decision making, an inpatient facility wished to link quality management concerns to patients' opinions (Stout, 1993a). As a result, a patient satisfaction survey was modified from a previous patient report card on the hospital. Data are collected just prior to discharge that yields 70% to 95% of the monthly report rates. (This procedure compares quite favorably to that of mailed surveys that yield only 2% return rates, thus providing *no* generalizability.)

The survey data are manually entered into *FoxPro*™ (a Microsoft, Inc. data base program for Windows and DOS operating environments). The results are then tabulated and monthly reports of "comment data" (i.e., verbatim patient responses to survey items) are compiled and routed to appropriate administrators, directors, and department heads. Numeric data are generated from Likert scale items. On an annual basis from a prior year's aggregate findings, a mean monthly average ($\bar{x}$) and standard deviation (SD) can be calculated. These averages are used to create an expected range one standard deviation ($\bar{x} \pm 1\,\mathrm{SD}$) above and below the mean. Each quarter's current or real time data is compared with last year's benchmark. If a quarter's data falls within the range, the expectation is met. If it drops below the lower range limit of the standard deviation (an indication of patient satisfaction), then it is cause for celebration and an exploration of what is being done to account for this improvement. If it exceeds the upper range (i.e., higher patient dissatisfaction), then it is recommended that a helpful, nonblaming, solution-focused team be formed to help determine the problems and experiment with solutions. The required statistical procedures are carried out by exporting the data base to a statistical package such as SPSS/PC$^+$ or MINITAB.

This data-based procedure guards against the not uncommon circumstance of "Oh, our department is always in trouble because so-and-so doesn't like us" or the corollary of "That department always gets what they want because they're favored, not because of their performance." For department heads, such systems seem to mitigate anxieties around favoritism, antagonism, turf, or politics, because it is the departments' *own* data, from the patient's perspectives, concerning what is important. And usually it is each department that is in the best position to improve their performance (Hinton & Stout, 1992). A sample patient satisfaction survey appears in Figure 1.

Current refinements of this system are to use optical scanning and "bubble" sheets for rapid data entry. Future possibilities include direct on-line entry of patient opinion via notebook computers or hand-held pen-based systems with character recognition capabilities and direct downloading to the data base.

Case Example III: Automated Outcomes Management Model

The key to the model's success is its manifold utility. It offers improved quality of care, improved methods to market; and competitively (and more safely) bid for capitated contracts, and improved practice management in terms of business and clinical supervision. All methods described are managed with relatively easy to use computerized data bases (or spreadsheets) and statistical packages.

Three components to fully integrated outcome management systems are included in this model: patient satisfaction; patient outcome (i.e., symptomatic resolution pre- versus posttreatment); and patient follow-up (i.e., treatment functioning, usually for 6–12 months after treatment's end).

All types of patient study, even an opinion survey, are best preceded by the patient's informed consent. From this point, a basic TQM patient satisfaction survey is the first component in this model. It may be administered at the end of any treatment episode, in any setting. One example of this was detailed in Case Example II.

Patient outcomes are measured using pre-and posttreatment brief, self-administered symptom rati-g forms. The Symptom Checklist-90-Revised (SCL-90-R) and Brief Symptom Inventory (BSI) are both popular in the behavioral health field (Derogatis, 1977, 1994). Both are available in computer-scorable forms from NCS Assessments. Such data, when used

PATIENT SATISFACTION SURVEY IV

The quality of care provided by ABC Hospital is evaluated on an ongoing basis. We therefore ask that you take a few moments to tell us how we can improve. Your opinion will help us know how we may best serve our patients and community. Thank you for your time and consideration.

Completed by: Patient _____ Parent _____ Guardian _____

Date Completed: _____ / _____ / _____ Unit Name: _____ House Case - YES
                                                                                 - NO
Staff responsible for completion _____

....

How did you hear about our facility?

_____ 1.	present psychiatrist		_____ 8.	school personnel
_____ 2.	family physician		_____ 9.	courts / probation officer / police
_____ 3.	family		_____ 10.	TV ad
_____ 4.	friend		_____ 11.	radio ad
_____ 5.	psychologist		_____ 12.	paper / magazine ad
_____ 6.	social worker		_____ 13.	insurance company
_____ 7.	addictions counselor		_____ 14.	crisis line
			_____ 15.	other _____

How would you rate the following:
(Please circle your answer and comment specifically on items rated (3) or (4). Comments on items rated (1) or (2) would be appreciated).

	strongly agree	mildly agree	mildy disagree	strongly disagree	not applicable
1. ADMISSION OFFICE: (Admission to the hospital)					
a. The Admission staff member was pleasant and courteous.	1	2	3	4	5
b. The Admissions Officer was helpful in explaining the papers I signed.	1	2	3	4	5
Comments: _____					
2. ADMISSION BY UNIT STAFF: (Admission to the unit)					
a. During my Admission onto the unit, unit staff treated me with consideration and respect.	1	2	3	4	5
Comments: _____					

MISCO12   1/93   REV.: 12/93
Z212

Figure 1. Patient satisfaction survey IV.

	strongly agree	mildly agree	mildly disagree	strongly disagree	not applicable
3. QUALITY OF CARE:					
a. The care provided by my psychiatrist was beneficial.	1	2	3	4	5
Comments: _____					
b. The care provided by my psychologist was beneficial.	1	2	3	4	5
Comments: _____					
c. The care provided by my certified alcohol counselor was beneficial.	1	2	3	4	5
Comments: _____					
d. The care provided by my social worker was beneficial.	1	2	3	4	5
Comments: _____					
4. UNIT STAFF (Nurses and Techs):					
a. The staff was courteous and helpful.	1	2	3	4	5
b. The care was beneficial.	1	2	3	4	5
Comments: _____					
5. ACTIVITY THERAPY DEPARTMENT (e.g., Leisure Education, Workshop, Teams Challenge Course):					
a. The staff was courteous and helpful.	1	2	3	4	5
b. The care was beneficial.	1	2	3	4	5
Comments: _____					
6. TUTORING SERVICES (school; adolescents and children only):					
a. The care was courteous and helpful.	1	2	3	4	5
b. The care was beneficial.	1	2	3	4	5
Comments: _____					
7. LAB / X-RAY / EEG / STAFF					
a. The staff was courteous and helpful.	1	2	3	4	5
b. The staff treated me in a professional manner	1	2	3	4	5
Comments: _____					
8. FINANCIAL SERVICES:					
a. The Business Office staff was helpful and efficient in providing assistance in financial matters.	1	2	3	4	5
Comments: _____					
9. ACCOMMODATIONS:					
a. The community areas (i.e.; dayroom, TV room) were attractive, clean and comfortable.	1	2	3	4	5
b. My individual room was attractive, clean and comfortable.	1	2	3	4	5
Comments: _____					

Figure 1. *Continued*

with an appropriately worded consent, also may be very helpful in treatment planning.

Patient follow-up studies may be best executed with data collection via the telephone, as opposed to mailed, self-addressed stamped envelopes

	strongly agree	mildly agree	mildly disagree	strongly disagree	not applicable
10. FOOD SERVICE:					
a. The food service was of high quality.	1	2	3	4	5
b. The food was served in sufficient quantity.	1	2	3	4	5
c. Dietary staff were courteous.	1	2	3	4	5
Comments: _____					
11. DISPOSITIONAL / DISCHARGE PLANNING:					
a. If needed, Vocational Counseling was provided and beneficial.	1	2	3	4	5
b. If needed, I was assisted in planning for living arrangements after discharge.	1	2	3	4	5
c. Arrangements were made for follow-up counseling after discharge.	1	2	3	4	5
12. Overall, my stay was beneficial.	1	2	3	4	5
Comments: _____					
13. Friends and relatives were treated in a courteous and professional manner when they visited or phoned.	1	2	3	4	5
Comments: _____					

14. If a friend needed this facility, I would recommend it. _____

15. What were the most helpful experiences, activities, or therapies during your hospital stay? _____

16. What did you dislike about your hospitalization? _____

17. What would you recommend to improve our facility and services? _____

18. Is there any Doctor/Therapist you feel deserves special recognition? _____

19. Is there any employee you feel deserves special recognition? _____

20. General Comments? _____

Thank you for your input.

Please return this survey to staff.
(Staff: Return to Research Mailbox.)

Figure 1. _Continued_

and survey forms. Mailings, although a boon to maintaining the confidentiality of respondents, have typically poor response rates, and may waste time and materials. Telephone calls improve response rates at the possible cost of subject frankness in reporting. Such procedures should be conducted with confidentiality in mind. Instruments for telephone data collection should be tailored for a practice's needs rather than being purchased from a vendor. Of course, adding symptomology measures provides rich data, but doing so may decrease subject compliance.

These data may easily and efficiently be maintained in such data base programs as Borland's dBase or Microsoft's FoxPro, or spreadsheets such as Lotus 1-2-3 or WordPerfect's Quattro Pro. These are available, as are comparable others, in most computer software stores and catalogues. Some of these also may adequately address reporting needs. If not, Stat Pack, SPSS/PC$^+$, or MINITAB may do the statistical trick.

There are also consultants and service bureaus that can aid in establishing a system to actually running it via a turnkey product. Costs vary according to need. Depending on volume, complexity, and the number of reporting periods, costs can range from $7 to $35 per patient per complete episode of care.

In behavioral health care, the future is now. Electronic billing for Medicare is already in place, and there soon will be financial disincentives if a practice uses the old-fashioned paper methods. For example, electronic billings can now be paid in as few as 15 days as compared to 30 or more days for paper-based filing, which provides a drastic improvement in practice cash flow. Three major managed care organizations are planning similarly automated systems, and it is expected that many more will follow suit.

Future advances in this area will be made in the form of expedited data entry, using touch-tone phones and other in-home interactive technologies (Stout, 1993b). Expansion of other psychometric tools to assess broader levels of functioning (e.g., Health Status Questionnaire 2) and severity of symptoms will improve diagnostic accuracy. Computer-aided testing (CAT) will also help improve psychometric refinement.

Conclusions

It is this author's thesis that TQM has much to offer in improving behavioral health care and its various delivery systems. To summarize, the merits include: empowerment and involvement of staffs within a team/system focus; blame free problem resolutions; more impartial/less biased data-based decisions; administrative efficiency; improved clinical and administrative supervision; and the most important bottom line— improved patient care. Of course, there are costs, too. For example, data are demanded and many will need systems to collect and use this information; integrating departments and personnel in TQM teams may rock some corporate cultures; there can be an associated stigma with being "evaluated"; there are initial costs associated with training and concomitant time; and, as noted earlier, we still do not set have any great models of excellence to emulate in behavioral health care (Stout, 1994).

TQM is something that an entire system must use. TQM pockets or islands simply cannot work.

The long-term benefits of TQM outcome management systems are that you can develop improved referral and triage based on an intervention of various patient factors (e.g., diagnosis, culture, demographics, etc.) in tandem with clinician factors (e.g., experience, specialty, culture, demographics, clinical performance data, etc.) combined within an empirical model (*not* just checklists or at random). It also provides for systems that prioritize patient needs/care, aids in management via clear quantifiable indications, and yields control of care with fiscal responsibility.

For those practices that stay current, the future need not be dim. The keys are an integration of TQM principles (however basic) along with automation, good data collection methodologies, a knowledge of market trends, and a spirit of quality patient care within a vision of cost-effective clinical performance.

References

Derogatis, L.R. (1977). Symptom-Checklist-90: Administration, scoring, and procedure manual. Towson, MD: Clinical Psychometric Research Press.

Derogatis, L.R. (1994). Case story: Use of the SCL-90-R within a hospital TQM program. Minnetonka, MN: National Computer Systems, Inc.

Stout, C.E. (1993a). Is TQM right for you? *Chicago Medicine, 97*, 25–26.

Stout, C.E. (1993b). Empirically based decision-making for managed care transitions. In D.H. Ruben & C.E. Stout (Eds.), *Transitions: Handbook of managed care for inpatient to outpatient treatment.* Westport, CT: Praeger Publishers.

Stout, C.E. (1994). *Managing capitation and outcomes in mental health.* Nashville, TN: Business Network, Inc.

Hinton, J., & Stout, C.E. (1992). Patient satisfaction. In M.B. Squire, C.E. Stout, & D.H. Ruben (Eds.), *Current advances in inpatient care.* Westport, CT: Greenwood Press.

Howick & Gray, Inc. (1992). *Team member training for continuous improvement* (Manual) (pp. 10, 20). Madison, WI: The author.

Bibliography

Special Publications

Carnevale, A.P. (1991). *America and the new economy.* Baltimore, MD: The American Society for Training and Development and the U.S. Department of Labor Employment and Training Administration. To order, call 410/516-6949.

Magaziner, I.C. (Chair). (1991). *America's choice: High skills or low wages.* Washington, DC. National Center on Education and the Economy. To order, call 716/546-7620.

Parisi, A.J. (1991). The quality imperative. *Business Week, October 25* (Special ed.). To order, call 800/635-1200.

General Books

Crosby, P. (1979). *Quality free: The art of making quality certain*. ASQC Quality Press.

Crosby, P. (1984). *Quality without tears*. Miluaukee, WI: ASQC Quality Press.

Deming, W.E. (1982). *Out of the crisis*. Cambridge, MA: Massachusetts Institute of Technology, Center for Advanced Engineering Study.

Glasser, W. (1990). *The quality school: Managing students without coercion*. New York: Harper & Row.

Imai, M. (1986). *Kaizen: The key to Japan's competitive success*. New York: Random House.

Juran, J.M. (1988). *Juran on planning for quality*. New York: Free Press.

Juran, J.M. (1989). *Juran on leadership for quality: An executive handbook*. New York: Free Press.

Kanter, R.M. (1983). *The change masters: Innovation for productivity in the American corporation*. New York: Simon & Schuster.

Levine, D.U., & Leqotte, L. (1990). *Unusually effective schools*. Madison, WI: The National Center for Effective School Research and Development.

Peters, T. (1987). *Thriving on chaos*. New York: Harper & Row.

Scherkenbach, W.W. (1988). *The Deming route to quality and productivity— Road maps and roadblocks*. Washington, DC: Mercury Press.

Senge, P.M. (1990). *The fifth discipline: The art and practice of the learning organization*. New York: Doubleday Currency.

Townsend, P.W., & Gebhardt, J.E. (1986). *Commit to quality*. New York: Wiley.

Walton, M. (1986). *The Deming management method*. New York: Perigee Books.

Whiteley, R.C. (1991). *The Customer Driven Company*. Reading, MA: Addison Wesley.

Leadership

Bennis, W.G. (1989). *Why leaders can't lead—The unconscious conspiracy continues*. San Francisco, CA: Jossey–Bass.

Berry, T.H. (1991). *Managing the total quality transformation*. New York: McGraw–Hill.

Byham, W.C. (1988). *Zapp!* New York: Harmony Books.

Cheany, L., & Cotter, M. (1990). *Real people real work: Parables on leadership in the 90's*. Knoxville, TN: SPC Press Publications. To order, call 615/584-5005.

Gordon, T. (1977). *Leader Effectiveness Training*. New York: Bantam Books.

Harvey, J.B. (1988). *The Abilene paradox, and other meditations on management*. Lexington, MA: Lexington Books.

Miller, L.M. (1989). *Barbarians to bureaucrats*. New York: Ballantine Books.

Schlechty, P.C. (1990). *Schools for the 21st century: Leadership imperatives for educational reform*. San Francisco, CA: Jossey–Bass.

15
Monitoring Certification of Independent Providers of Alcohol and Drug Abuse Services

Bruce W. Vieweg, Robert McClain, and Doris Pickerill

This chapter describes a computer program application that has assisted the Missouri Division of Alcohol and Drug Abuse to fulfill its statutory responsibilities in certifying DUI (driving under the influence) intervention programs.

In 1983 Missouri statute established DUI intervention programs and designated the Division of Alcohol and Drug Abuse as the state agency responsible for developing standards and certifying that each DUI intervention program met such standards. In brief, the standards require that each DUI offender receive a screening assessment and participate in a 10 hour education program as a condition of driver's license reinstatement or as may be ordered by the court. It is also possible for the offender to meet requirements by completing a more extensive treatment and rehabilitation program for substance abuse. The DUI intervention program is named ARTOP, short for Alcohol or Drug Related Traffic Offenders Program.

In 1988 a further state statute created a distinct intervention program for minors. The statute known as Abuse and Lose, established sanctions (including loss of driver's license) and an intervention program for any minor found in possession of alcohol or drugs or for any minor found driving with any blood alcohol level whatsoever. The intervention program

AAIMS development was supported in part under a contract with the Missouri Department of Mental Health, Division of Alcohol and Drug Abuse, the Missouri Department of Highway Safety, and by the Missouri Institute of Mental Health. Copies of the software may be requested from the senior author. Much of this work was done when the senior author was on the faculty at the Missouri Institute of Mental Health in St. Louis. Mr. Vieweg and Mr. McClain are now with the Missouri Department of Mental Health, Mr. Vieweg with the Office of Information Systems and Mr. McClain with the Division of Alcohol and Drug Abuse. Ms. Pickerill is with the Missouri Institute of Mental Health in St. Louis.

established under this statute was nicknamed ADEP, short for Alcohol and Drug Education Program.

Each agency and individual requesting certification to be a provider of ARTOP or ADEP services must follow these certification processes:

1. *Agencies*: An application must be submitted by the agency that descibes its organization, staff, assessment methods, and program schedule. A site survey is conducted and includes interviews with both adminstrators and clinicians, a tour of the facility, a review of student satisfaction and feedback questionnaires, and a review of student records. A report of the findings is submitted to the Division of Alcohol and Drug Abuse (ADA) that includes certification status (full, probationary, or denial). Full certification is for 2 years.
2. *Individuals*: An application must be submitted that documents the education, experience in the ADA field, and completion of the ARTOP and/or ADEP training program. Full certification is for 5 years.

By 1990 more than 25,000 offenders were entering this intervention system each year. The intervention system created under these two statutes had grown to 55 agencies operating 90 ARTOPs and ADEPs at more than 125 program sites. The agencies also had approximately 400 staff (most of whom worked on a part-time basis) conducting screening assessments and providing educational classes. ADA was responsible for certifying each of the programs every 2 years and for certifying that each of the assessors and instructors met certain qualifications.

The state statutes authorized only one staff position to monitor these programs. In addition, the Division reassigned the equivalent of a second staff member to other duties. The responsibility for certifying programs and coordinating the intervention system became difficult and demanding with a total of only two staff. One of the strategies for meeting these administrative responsibilities was to increase efficiency through a computer program application that came to be known as AAIMS (ARTOP and ADEP Information Management System).

Prior to the development of AAIMS, data were maintained in many paper files and in multiple word processing documents. Each time a change occurred with a single agency or individual assessor/instructor, multiple word processing documents had to be changed and updated. Clearly there was a need for a system where each change was made only one time.

Staff had difficulty keeping track of where each agency stood in the certification process, for example, which agency needed to be sent a renewal application this week, which surveys needed to be scheduled for next month, which assessor applications were pending, etc. All management reports had to be compiled from scratch. An annual report summarizing certification activity and also the number and characteristics of DUI offenders had proven particularly time consuming for staff to compile.

Any questions about a particular intervention program required searching through paper files or else relied heavily on the knowledge and experience of individual staff members. However, if an individual left, all of the personal experience and knowledge of that individual was lost.

Given these circumstances, the design and development of AAIMS was directed toward the following goals:

develop a tracking and reminder system regarding all certification activities and steps;
automatically generate routine directories and listings that are provided to interested individuals across the state;
improve access to basic data about each program and each assessor/ instructor; and
an ability to compile special management reports through a query module.

AAIMS includes information about the number and characteristics of offenders that entered each intervention program, but it was not designed as a client-based information system. Composite data could be generated such as, how many offenders are referred by municipal courts or how many offenders report a prior DUI offense in the last 5 years.

At the heart of AAIMS is a tickler or reminder mechanism that throughout the production of a task report, notifies certification staff when recertifications, and the tasks associated with recertifications, are coming due. Additional monitoring is provided for new agencies and new individual clinician applications as well as for agencies that have provisional or probationary status. A special monitoring routine, with other deadline dates and tasks, is provided for those agencies that have been denied certification. The rules that drive the reminders consist of carefully delineated time tables for tasks that are related to the specific certification status being monitored. For example, Table 1 presents the due date rules associated with the six specific tasks that are monitored for each agency undergoing routine recertification. Similar tables of rules, together with specific tasks, have been explicitly defined for each condition requiring monitoring.

Table 1. Tickler Rules

Action	Due Date Rule
Application sent	120 days before certification expires
Application returned to ADA office (date)	30 days after application sent
Site survey (date)	60 days after application sent
Surveyor(s) assigned	60 days after application sent
Report issued	120 days after application sent
Rating form sent	150 days after application sent

AAIMS requires that the entry and updating of the specific monitoring informaiton be completed in a timely fashion or the tickler report mechanisms will not present accurate information and the weekly task report will quickly lose its utility. A single task will appear on the task report continuously until the system is informed of its completion. In implementing AAIMS, division staff have had to remember to briefly log the completion of each activity. The actual data entry has taken 1 to 2 hours per week.

System Requirements

AAIMS will operate on any IBM-PC or compatible microcomputer, with one floppy and one fixed disk drive, running MS or PC DOS, version 5.0 or greater, and Microsoft Windows version 3.1. The application requires, at minimum, an 80386 based microcomputer. Because of its sophisticated Graphic User Interface (GUI), a color monitor and/or high resolution monitor is recommended. For full functionality a Microsoft compatible pointing device, mouse, or trackball is required. A minimum of 2 MB of working memory is recommended.

AAIMS is programmed in Borland C++ Version 3.1, with the added support of several commercially available tool boxes including CodeBase Version 4.5 that provides access to the dBASE IV data bases. All data are stored in dBASE IV version 1.5 data base files.

Enter/Edit Module

Separate entry/edit routines are provided for agency and individual staff information. All data entry in AAIMS utilizes a forms approach. The following figures show typical data entry screens for agency data in Figure 1, and for individual data in Figure 2.

Additional entry/edit forms to enter certification information, to link individual certified staff members with the agencies, to track or monitor the agency status, to enter agency complaints, to enter specific organization information, to enter information about the specific program sites that offer the programs, and to enter any free text agency notes or comments are accessed by pressing one of the buttons located along the top of this main data entry screen for agencies. Additional entry/edit forms for individual clinician information is also available behind each button located along the top of the main data entry screen. Help is available from each screen by pressing ⌐F1⌐ or by pressing the special Help button.

Report Module

Many preprogrammed reports are available as a selection from a menu of available reports. All reports were developed using R&R Report Writer

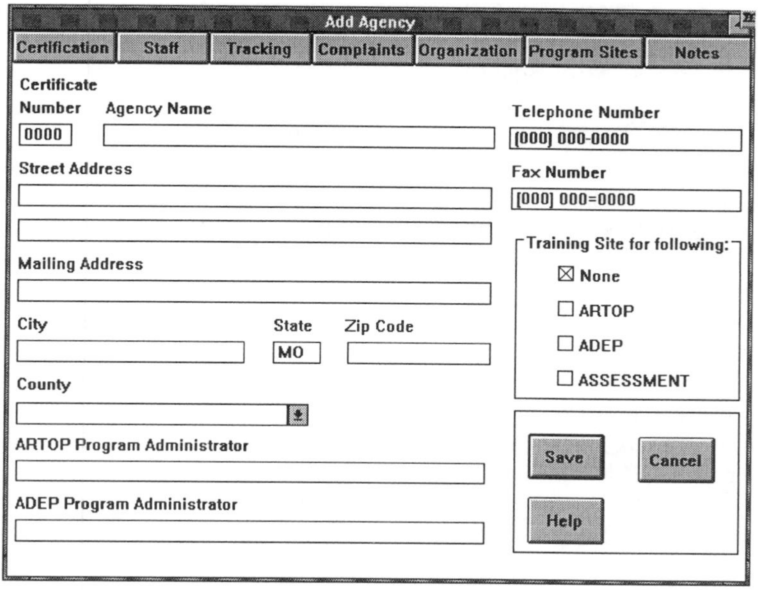

Figure 1. Main data entry screen for agency information.

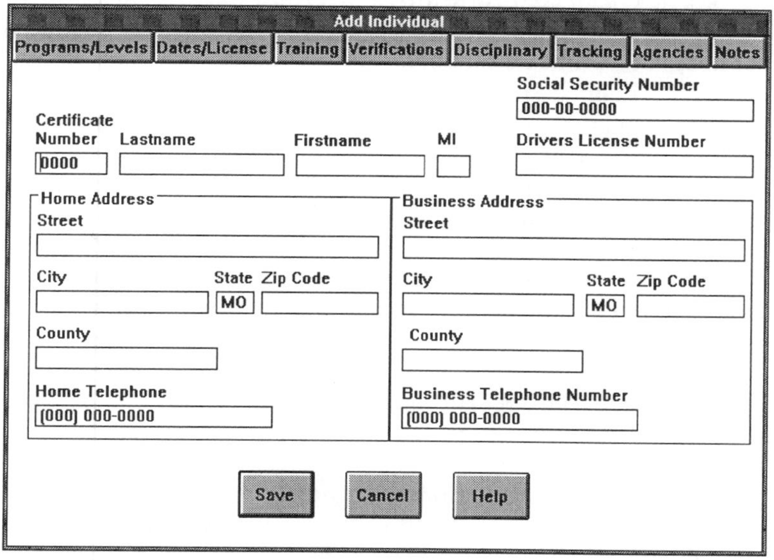

Figure 2. Data entry screen for individual clinician information.

for Windows and linked to the application within the AAIMS executable file. Each of these reports can be directed to the printer, to the computer screen, or to an electronic file.

Agency or Individual Tasks: Provides detailed tickler reminders of all tasks that are due for a single individual or agency and the current status of the tasks.

Agency or Individual Tracking Summary: A summary report of all tracking that is currently active for either agencies or individuals.

Agency Program Administrators: This is a simple listing of all program administrators, together with their agency name, ordered alphabetically by administrator last name.

Agency Profiles: This report presents all information about an agency in a structured report.

Listing of all Agencies: This is a simple listing of all agencies that were ever certified by the Division.

Directory of All Agencies: This is listing of all relevant information about certified agencies, including information about each of the related program sites. Also included is the county location, the date that the certification will expire, and the current certification type if different from full 2 year certification.

Agency Mailing Labels: Mailing labels may be printed by program type or for all programs.

Individual Clinician Profiles: All information about certified individuals listed on a single page formatted report.

Listing of All Qualified Instructors and Professionals: This is a simple listing of all individual clinicians that includes name, qualification, programs, and certificate numbers.

Listing of All Trained Individuals: This is a simple listing report of all individuals who received training in ADEP or ARTOP but who have not applied for certification.

Special Letters Notifying Agencies/Individuals of Their Recertification: These letters use a standardized text with unique agency or individual information added. They can be printed for all agencies or individuals whose certification expiration data is within a selected month.

Certificates of Certification: This option will print all certificates of agencies or individuals whose certification expiration date fall within a selected month.

Frequency Counts: This report summarizes information about agencies or individuals. Summary aggregate information for agencies is provided for number of agencies by certification status, number of programs by program type; or number of program sites by program type. Summary aggregate information about individuals includes current certification status, number of qualified instructors; number of qualified professional and number of qualified trainers by program type.

Figure 3 shows the first screen of the AAIMS Task Report. Each report that is printed to the screen presents the same tool bar at the top.

Annual Statistics Module

Each agency that is certified by the ADA must submit aggregate utilization information about their program sites and clients at the end of each fiscal year, usually in June or July. Data are entered separately by program type (ADEP or ARTOP). Figure 4 represents the first data entry screen for the ARTOP program.

Aggregate data collected form each site include client/student demographic information (sex, race, age, marital status, income, employment status, living arrangements); total number of students; number of students by referral type; total number of courses given; and prior DUI/DWI (driving while intoxicated) offenses.

Associated with these aggregate statistics are a series of preprogrammed reports that summarize the individual agency aggregate information. An additional report lists all those agencies for which no, or incomplete information has been provided.

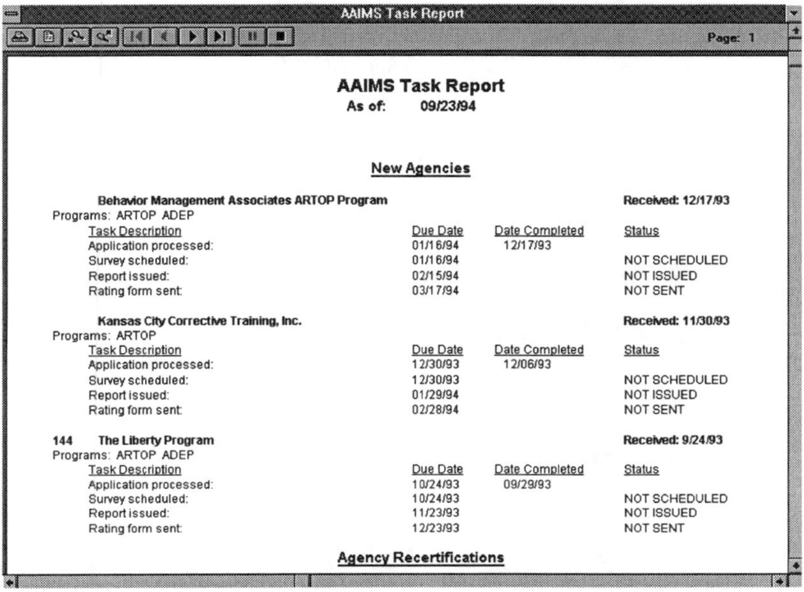
AAIMS Task Report

Page: 1

AAIMS Task Report
As of: 09/23/94

New Agencies

Behavior Management Associates ARTOP Program — **Received: 12/17/93**
Programs: ARTOP ADEP

Task Description	Due Date	Date Completed	Status
Application processed:	01/16/94	12/17/93	
Survey scheduled:	01/16/94		NOT SCHEDULED
Report issued:	02/15/94		NOT ISSUED
Rating form sent:	03/17/94		NOT SENT

Kansas City Corrective Training, Inc. — **Received: 11/30/93**
Programs: ARTOP

Task Description	Due Date	Date Completed	Status
Application processed:	12/30/93	12/06/93	
Survey scheduled:	12/30/93		NOT SCHEDULED
Report issued:	01/29/94		NOT ISSUED
Rating form sent:	02/28/94		NOT SENT

144 The Liberty Program — **Received: 9/24/93**
Programs: ARTOP ADEP

Task Description	Due Date	Date Completed	Status
Application processed:	10/24/93	09/29/93	
Survey scheduled:	10/24/93		NOT SCHEDULED
Report issued:	11/23/93		NOT ISSUED
Rating form sent:	12/23/93		NOT SENT

Agency Recertifications

Figure 3. AAIMS Task Report.

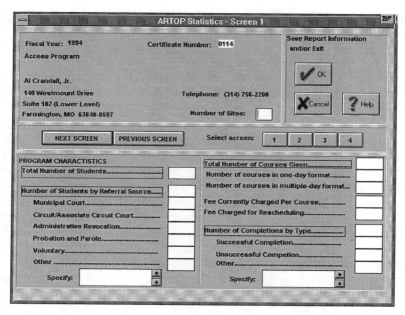

Figure 4. Data entry screen for annual statistics data, ARTOP program.

Query Module

The Query Module supports the development of user-defined search strategies and the generation of reports of selected data items from the results of those searches. Query can search both agency or individual clinician information. Figure 5 provides an example of a query. A query is built one statement at a time. In this example, we are looking for all

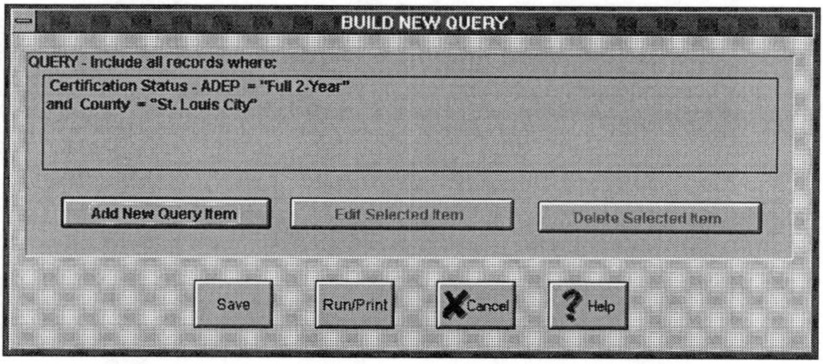

Figure 5. Sample query statement.

agencies that provide ADEP services that have a full 2 year certification and are located within St. Louis City. When the Run/Print button is pressed on the above screen, the user is prompted to select the items to print from the results of the query. This is done by checking off the desired fields from the list of available print fields as shown in Figure 6. An identical process is followed when querying the individual clinician information. Each query can be saved with a unique name for later retrieval and use.

Final Comments and Observations

This application is used extensively by certification staff within the ADA. This windows-based application has proven to be user friendly, attractive, and a sophisticated approach to microcomputer-based applications. The most significant limitation is that it does not support multiple users. To accommodate more than one user, it is necessary to copy the program and its data bases to a shared drive and have each staff member copy the program and data bases to their own microcomputer. A multiuser network version of the software would be an excellent modification. Experience has also shown that a small, ongoing budget item for additional computer programming time is important. The DUI intervention system is not static and new goals and legislative mandates wait just beyond the immediate horizon. The computer applications must also be able to evolve.

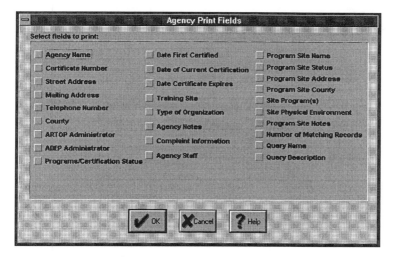

Figure 6. Print field selection screen.

Reference

Vieweg, B.W. (1993). *ADEP and ARTOP reference manual and users' guide.* Unpublished technical manual. St. Louis, MO: Mental Health Systems Research Unit, Missouri Institute of Mental Health.

16
Impact of Managed Care on Automation
Bruce W. Johnson

During the past few years managed care and health care reform have had a significant impact on management information systems (MISs) and will continue to do so over the balance of the decade. The initial impetus for health care reform and the rapid expansion of managed care in the behavioral health care market has been the spiraling cost of health care.

Although the American Health Securities Act was never passed, employers and various state and local agencies are implementing their own health care reform plans by designing cost containment strategies that employ some form of managed care. Concurrently, and partially in response to managed care, other accreditation bodies and regulatory authorities have been developing new guidelines for managing utilization and monitoring quality. Further, structural and functional changes in service delivery mechanisms are changing how providers work with one another and create new requirements for sharing information. All of these forces in the market place tremendous demands on the behavioral health care provider for detailed and timely information.

Managed care techniques may have been designed to reduce costs to payers, sponsors, and enrollees, but in the process they have dramatically increased administrative costs for providers. Thus, many behavioral health care organizations are faced with the prospect of adapting to increased administrative and clinical costs with reduced reimbursements. The only effective way to combat these escalating information management requirements and the resultant administrative costs is through the implementation of an integrated MIS.

In today's fast paced rapidly changing business environment, older proprietary batch-oriented data processing systems that simply report historical information for a specific accounting period are no longer adequate. The CEO and departmental managers of the 1990s require contemporaneous information that can only be provided by an on-line, real time, MIS. During the late 1970s and 1980s many providers were satisfied to track patient services and produce first and third party billings. Today, the behavioral health care provider needs a sophisticated set of software that fully integrates the patient accounting, financial accounting, and clinical records applications. This chapter will address the various aspects of managed care from the perspective of the provider and the corresponding information required to prosper during the next decade.

Health Care Costs

During the end of the 1980s health care spending accounted for almost 12% of our gross national product. At that time the Department of Commerce projected that this percentage would continue to grow at a rate of 10 to 14% annually (U.S. Dept. of Commerce, 1989). Over 10% of these health care dollars were being spent on mental health and substance abuse services (Goran, 1992). With the cost of health care in general and mental health in particular growing at an alarming rate, it is no wonder that health care reform became an important topic for debate in state and federal legislatures.

Health Care Reform

In 1993 the Clinton Administration proposed its Health Care Reform Plan that was followed by the American Health Security Act released on October 27, 1993. The Plan was not only designed to guarantee comprehensive health coverage for all Americans, but also made very specific recommendations on reimbursement mechanisms and requirements for automation. An important component of the plan was to implement a managed care model for reimbursing health care providers. After a year of vigorous debate and unprecedented lobbying by affected industries, the 103rd Congress announced that there was no hope of passing health care reform legislation in 1994.

Although Health Care Reform has stalled at the Federal level, both the states and private sector are rapidly moving toward managed care. In the public sector health care reform is being led by the restructuring of state Medicaid programs including funding for mental health and substance abuse services. In fact, most states are either planning or implementing managed care models for reimbursements. Managed care mechanisms of funding are also being employed by the county community mental health boards. In the private sector managed care organizations (MCOs) are being formed by insurance companies, providers, and employers to maintain a competitive edge in the market place. A study by the Health Insurance Association of America (Gabel, Di Carlo, Fink, &

de Lissovoy, 1989) estimated that more than 70% of Americans with employer-sponsored insurance are enrolled in managed care plans.

Managed Care

Unfortunately, managed care is not a well-defined single entity. There is no universal set of standards by which it is defined. However, the organizations and reimbursement models that comprise managed care systems share the objective of reducing cost through the reduction of reimbursements and by controlling utilization and referrals. In general managed care can be defined as a diverse, constantly changing set of interrelated policies and procedures designed to manage the accessibility, quality, utilization, and cost of health care services. Each of these areas will be explored and its implications for automation discussed.

Managed Care Reimbursement Models

Reimbursement models refers to the methods by which a provider is compensated for the services delivered under a managed care contract. These arrangements provide a combination of financial incentives and disincentives to modify the cost and utilization of services. The reimbursement methodology has a major impact on the type, volume, and quality of services delivered by the provider. Models that are commonly employed in managed mental health services include fee for service, discounted fee for service, capped fee schedule, capped fee schedule with withhold, primary care capitation and full capitation, per diem charge, and per case payments. The two primary reimbursement mechanisms used by managed care organizations are fee for service and capitation. Each method has special requirements for automation.

The fee for service reimbursement method refers to the use of a predetermined fee or discounted fee for a specific service or procedure. In a capitated arrangement a payment is made to the provider as a fixed monthly amount per member or per capita. Payment is made to the provider whether or not services are delivered. With full capitation, the provider is 100% liable for all services. In other capitation arrangements the managed care organization shares the risk with the provider.

Each reimbursement mechanism carries its own special set of requirements for information. In the fee for service model, it is important for the organization to have a good grasp of what it costs to provide specific services before contracting for set fees. A system for implementing and monitoring cost controls should also be in place. Applications that are helpful with these processes are an integrated set of financials (purchasing, accounts payable, general ledger, budgeting, payroll, and cost accounting). Because fee for service arrangements also typically have benefit limits and conditions built into the contract, it is important that the billing and accounts receivable have a contract management function.

In the capitated model, providers must control their own utilization and costs. This is done through various utilization management functions, contract management software, and cost accounting. All of these will be discussed in greater detail.

Management Information Systems

Virtually all areas of mental health software have been influenced by managed care. In accounting applications the three programs that are the most useful for managed care contracts are general ledger with budgeting, cost accounting, and billing/accounts receivable. If the organization is a publicly funded mental health board or community based nonprofit agency, a fund accounting general ledger is also useful. Of the three, the billing and accounts receivable programs have received the most attention.

In the clinical applications, there are two general areas of interest: basic charting functions and clinical management functions. The charting functions include client registration, assessments, treatment plans, progress notes, and medical information. The clinical management functions include quality assurance, utilization review, and clinical staff administration. Automation of these applications furnishes the behavioral health care provider with the information necessary to evaluate and control accessibility, quality, utilization, and cost.

Accessibility/Availability

Accessibility and availability refer to the ease with which patients can avail themselves of programs and services at a specific facility or offered by an individual provider. They include the ability of a patient to contact the provider, schedule an appointment, arrange for transportation, obtain assistance with finding financial aid, as well as the availability of appropriate personnel and services. Some of the measures that provide an index of accessibility include:

1. Number of phone calls required to make contact with intake personnel;
2. Length of time between initial contact and intake interview;
3. Length of time on waiting list for outpatient services;
4. Length of time between appointments;
5. Zip code analysis comparing residence of patient with location of facility;
6. Percent of patients seen by a temporary therapist;
7. Number of referrals to outside organizations;
8. Discharged inpatients failing to receive service within a specified period of time;

9. Number of persons on waiting lists for residential facilities; and
10. Number of persons on waiting lists for specialized services, for sample substance abuse.

To answer these questions it may be necessary to expand the patient data base and develop custom reports to track the appropriate information. These measures can also be developed into quality improvement indicators as described below. Examples of reports that are useful in evaluating accessibility/availability criteria include:

1. *Applicant Latency Report*: A cross-tabulation report (2-dimensional table) used to evaluate the latency between the patient's initial contract and the first appointment. The time frame required for the first appointment is displayed along the x axis and risk level along the y axis, with the number and percentage of clients for each cell.
2. *Contact Frequency Report*: A cross-tabulation report to monitor frequency of contacts by level of risk. It lists the contact frequency along the x axis and risk level along the y axis, with the number and percentage of occurrences for each cell.

Provider Networks

Frequently, managed care companies seek to contract with a vertically integrated provider network that can provide its enrollees with continuity of care. They prefer to contract with a single provider or network that can provide a full spectrum of services from inpatient to outpatient programs, in a variety of settings with varying levels of intensity. Few organizations can provide all of these programs and services equally well, so many organizations have begun to form strategic alliances with other providers, creating functional service networks. When multiple organizations are integrated in a single network, there are additional data processing requirements. Because patients may be referred to a therapist in any of the participating organizations, it is advantageous to have a communications link connecting all of the entities. Communication and coordination are facilitated when a central access point coordinates the referral process and begins the intake with a telephone interview. Ideally, the data collected should be entered directly into a computer, while the caller is on the phone. In the not too distant future, the telephone and computer industries will integrate their products and merge the telephone and computer terminal. Another function that needs to be shared among all practices is the checking and scheduling of appointments. When a central access point is used to coordinate intakes, the staff member needs access to a centralized scheduling system so that the schedules can be checked and appointments made for all therapists in the network. A centralized system requires a common data base and a single master patient index. A unique case number should be assigned and used by all providers. With a common data base that can be accessed from all locations, the intake worker or case manager can begin the patient registration process during the initial telephone interview. This information should be immediately available at any location. A centralized access point and a coordinated staff and patient data base can simplify registration and improve patient access to the provider network.

A case manager at the central access point who also authorizes services will need on-line access to utilization criteria, carrier contract information, benefits, prior treatment, and at least some limited clinical information. He or she will also need to check on present authorizations as well as annual or lifetime limits. Access to a central data base of providers and staff credentials is also useful for case assignments.

Quality Assurance (QA)

Quality Assurance refers to activities designed to prevent and/or correct problems with quality. This implies altering the behavior of providers and practitioners. It may include screening for poor quality care, e.g. peer reviews, attempting to modify aberrant practice patterns, retrospective reviews of individual cases, chart audits of clinical performance, and various systematic monitoring and evaluation of specific treatment and charting practices (Berlant, 1992).

Many fear that the advent of managed mental health care and its attendant administrative oversight and financial controls will compromise the quality of patient care. One role of providers and various regulatory authorities and accreditation bodies is to assure that cost controls and constraints on access and utilization do not adversely impact the quality of patient care. MCOs are also continually monitoring accessibility, utilization practices, and client information against standards to determine the appropriateness, quality, timeliness, and efficacy of care. Some of the areas that are evaluated as part of the QA process include:

1. Organizational needs assessment to determine service requirements;
2. Patterns of use to analyze utilization;
3. Client satisfaction;
4. Client outcome, reviewing individual and aggregated records when the desired outcome is not achieved;
5. Demographic analysis to project need; and
6. Level of need in market area.

QA systems can help improve an organization's operations both retrospectively and proactively. The best way to correct a deficiency is to prevent it. A good QA system will produce tickler reports as reminders of specific clinical and documentation activities including dates for completion, follow-up review dates, and case review schedules. QA linked to a patient record system can help with retrospectively checking patient records. Completeness of records can be tested to assure that required elements pertinent to a problem or diagnosis are present. Further, the system can determine if the documentation was entered in a timely manner. High risk or difficult cases can be selected by the computer. Alert flags and various clinical criteria can be tested, and records selected for review. Indicators of critical events or conditions can be surveyed when threshold values are exceeded and the system can flag a record for more detailed review.

If a system does not have a dedicated utilization review (UR)/QA module it is still possible to set up a simple documentation checklist for UR/QA staff. When clinical documentation is not on-line, some general purpose programs will allow the user to create simple checklists for recording the results of documentation reviews. Figure 1 shows a sample checklist for evaluating patient care documents.

When the results of the review recorded with a checklist are not derived automatically by the system, the user has several options. The survey can be kept in the central MIS or PC data base, spreadsheet, or statistical package. This is not the ideal method of automating the QA/UR process, but it does provide the department with an on-line record of the review. These data can then be correlated with other program, staff, and client related variables.

Other types of QA reports that are useful include the following:

1. *Complaint by Type Report*: Used to evaluate the frequency of different types of patient complaints. It is a cross-tabulation report (2-dimensional matrix) with the type of complaint along the y axis and the various locations and/or programs along the x axis.
2. *Incident by Program Report*: Used to evaluate major incidents by program. It is a cross-tabulation report with the type of incident along the y axis and the various locations and/or programs along the x axis.

Outcome Measurements

In today's managed care environment sponsors and payers are demanding that providers demonstrate the efficacy of their treatment protocols. They are asking for demonstrable proof that the patients' level of functioning and quality of life are improving. This may be measured by the staff, the patient, and significant others, including employers. Outcome studies are used by the payers and plan sponsors to identify efficacious practice patterns as well as cost-effectiveness of providers and clinicians.

Payers are interested in measures of cost, length of stay, and recidivism, while sponsors (employers) are interested in client satisfaction and level of functioning, particularly with respect to on-the-job performance.

Unfortunately in mental health and substance abuse treatment areas there are no clearly defined *standards* for quality based on outcome

Assessments:	Y/N	**Progress Notes:**	Y/N
Please indicate the information documented in the intake assessment:		Please indicate the information documented in the progress notes:	
Presenting problem:	____	Progress notes documented for each service :	____
Rule out diagnosis :	____		
Previous mental illness :	____	Notes relate to treatment goals :	____
Substance abuse :	____	Notes document the response to treatment :	____
Total deficiencies:	____	Total deficiencies:	____

Psychosocial history:

Please indicate which information was documented in the psychosocial history:

Interpersonal relationships :	____
Education :	____
Family history of mental illness :	____
Complete within X days of admission:	____
Total deficiencies:	____

Individual Plan of Service:

Please indicate which of the information was documented in the IPOS:

IPOS indicated a problem, with related goals and objectives :	____
IPOS was reviewed every X months :	____
Total deficiencies:	____

Discharge Summary:

Please indicate which of the information was documented in the discharge summary:

Summary prepared within X days of termination :	____
Summary included the level of functioning:	____
Summary included diagnosis :	____
Summary included the reason for discharge :	____
Summary included the service summary :	____
Summary included any referrals :	____
Total deficiencies:	____
Grand total of all deficiencies:	____

Figure 1. Clinical record review checklist.

measures. Accreditation bodies such as the Joint Commission on Accreditation of Health Care Organizations (JCAHO, 1990–1992) and Commission on Accreditation of Rehabilitation Facilities (CARF) publish guidelines on how to internally develop indicators of quality, but do not make specific recommendations as to what these indicators should be, nor do they recommend or require any specific outcome measures. Absent any formal standards, a myriad of different systems for monitoring and analyzing quality data has evolved over the years.

The dearth of universal standards provides the therapist with several options. One alternative is to internally develop an outcome measurement instrument. The advantage to this approach is that it can be custom tailored to meet specifications. The disadvantage is that it takes considerable effort to develop a set of reliable outcome factors that are orthogonal with respect to one another. It may also take several years to build a large enough data base to conduct meaningful research.

Another option is to purchase a third party commercial product. Benefits of this approach include the fact that the design and testing of the instrument has been completed. Typically a large pool of data has been collected using the survey as a reference point. With some of the more sophisticated psychometric tests, the vendor will provide scoring, analysis, and interpretation services. The disadvantage to this method is the cost. If the researcher is lucky, a well-documented and researched instrument may be found in the public domain, which eliminates royalty fees.

Finally, there are outcome evaluation consulting firms that will conduct research. They will do a professional, independent, and objective job and most have their own data base for comparisons. Regardless of the method employed for monitoring, measuring, and analyzing outcome, the measures should be standardized among all staff members and providers participating in the project.

Outcome indices must be consistently applied by all staff. A management information system can assist by providing the therapist with standardized assessment tools regarding the patient's history, presenting problems, behavior, mentation, emotions, etc.

Quantitative Analyses

The evaluation of clinical data at most facilities is complicated because treatment in a real life setting involves no experimental controls. Confounding variables not under the control of the therapist or even the treatment milieu may skew results and limit conclusions made from statistical analysis. This disadvantage can be partially overcome by developing a large historical data base of treatment and outcome data. The larger the sample size and the better its consistency, the stronger the case that can be made for a casual relationship between treatment and effect. One way to increase sample size is to pool data with other providers. This may be done by developing a common data base with other providers in a network, among providers that receive significant revenue from the same funding source, or through a commercial utilization review and outcome monitoring consulting firm. The assessments can be conducted verbally or using a written instrument, or entered directly into the program. The entire assessment instrument can be kept on-line or summary indices can be entered.

The various outcome measures can then be correlated with interventions, clinicians, programs, and provider organizations to determine clinical effectiveness. Predictability can be improved through increasing sample size and by controlling for variables that influence the dependent measures. By comparing treatment parameters with outcome measures a dose–response relationship may be established. Dose–response relationships of treatment intensity and length of stay with outcome for a specific diagnostic category can be identified.

The system can be used to help determine which treatment protocols are most beneficial and determine the optimal treatment time for specific presenting problems and diagnostic categories. With a fully integrated system, treatment cost can be determined and cost benefit analyses conducted.

If multiple providers are going to use a central data base it is important to apply standardized terminology and methods. The same instruments should be administered in the same way, at the same time, etc. Definitions of treatment, diagnostic, and outcome categories and codes should be standardized across all participants. Feedback mechanisms to adjust assumptions and treatment models must be in place. Some of the basic clinical parameters that are typically collected include:

1. Diagnostic and Statistical Manual of Mental Disorders (DSM-IV) diagnosis, all axes;
2. Presenting problem;
3. Level of functioning;
4. Status of goal attainment;
5. Miscellaneous outcome measures; and
6. Client satisfaction measures.

The treatment parameters that should be monitored include:

1. Program,
2. Service,
3. Clinician,
4. Level of intensity of service,
5. Length of stay/treatment,
6. Number of services,
7. Treatment goals, and
8. Treatment objectives.

Some of the demographic variables that are typically collected include:

1. Age,
2. Gender
3. Ethnicity, and
4. Education.

Quality Improvement

Over the past few years there has been an expansion of the areas of quality assessment and QA into one of Quality Improvement (QI), also known as Continuous Quality Improvement (CQI) or Total Quality Management (TQM). CQI as described by JCAHO (JCAHO, 1992) "is a process which [is] used to monitor, assess and improve service. High priority aspects of care and service are selected, and a methodology is developed to monitor these aspects of care and service . . . Standards are developed for the indicators so that they can be evaluated based on programmatic and outcome goals." The JCAHO manual states that the usefulness of these data will depend on the use of "valid performance measures and the application of reliable data collection techniques and statistical methods." (JCAHO, 1992). The indicators can be outcome, process, rate-based, or sentinel events. These can be used to evaluate domains of care such as accessibility, appropriateness, continuity of care, effectiveness of care, efficacy of care, efficiency of care, customer satisfaction, safety, and timeliness.

Ideally the QI system should work with clinical, demographic, service, and accounting data. The clinical indicators should be developed by clinical staff for each program and service. The accounting and organizational indicators can be designed by the management team.

Policies and procedures should be developed for the data collection and reporting process. Standardized reports should be prepared at predetermined intervals and reviewed by the QI Team. Software should provide an easy method of running and displaying the reports including a link to a graphics program. It is also an advantage to be able to report changes in indicators over time. If a dedicated QI system is not available in an organization's software, some of these functions can be performed by a sophisticated report writer, even without a QI program. However, this method of developing a QI system is significantly more challenging.

UR

The current UR of mental health providers by MCOs is typically based on a "med/surge" model in which claims are reviewed against criteria established by the payer. Specific protocols and criteria are used to compare various demographic, clinical, and benefit data to determine the medical necessity of an admission, discharge, termination, continued stay, etc. According to Berlant (1992), "Utilization Review focuses on third party determination of the medical necessity for treatment at a particular level of care or for a particular procedural intervention . . ." Medical necessity is defined differently from payer to payer. It varies by program and diagnosis and the criteria may even be applied inconsistently within the same organization.

UR is conducted by payers, third party administrators (TPAs), and UR companies as a mechanism for reducing inappropriate claims and thereby helping to control costs. Because the payers are using these systems it would make sense that all providers would develop parallel systems of their own to help reduce the number of claims rejected. Mistakes and incomplete records can be caught before they are submitted to the payer. Ideally, a system should also be in place to manage utilization before services are delivered, a process referred to as Utilization Management, which will be discussed in greater detail in the next section. It is our recommendation that a provider have a system in place that supports both concurrent and retrospective review of utilization.

MCOs are not only verifying enrollee claims to check them for accuracy and completeness, but many are also reviewing the client clinical profile and service history before authorizing services. To facilitate this process many MCO case managers are requesting more client clinical information to evaluate the need for services. This will necessarily increase the administrative costs of the contract. If the MCO can accommodate it, the data can be transferred electronically via magnetic media or modem.

Retrospective utilization review at the provider level uses the computer to identify records that fail to meet specific criteria for the above processes. Deficiency reports should be prepared that identify activities that are already overdue or areas of the record that are incomplete or inappropriate. In addition to retrospective utilization review practices, a good MIS will provide the behavioral health care provider with tools to help avoid charting deficiencies before they occur. One mechanism for accomplishing this goal is to prepare tickler reports and schedules for various clinical and documentation activities.

UR systems should have the capacity to develop statistical norms, length of stay for example, based on historical data. The data from individuals' cases can then be compared to the range, median, mean, and standard deviations of the defined treatment population. When combined with payer and organizational protocols, these data can help case managers and reviewers recommend the appropriate providers, practitioners, and treatments. The managed care contract manager can use these data when requesting approvals or extending authorizations. Records sampled for each program and service provided may be reviewed applying utilization criteria, and those exceeding norms for admission, continued stay, frequency of service, or discharge criteria can be reviewed in greater detail to explain variances and identify opportunities to improve efficiency.

Ideally providers should have access to the same claims editing software that is used by the MCOs they contract with. Frequently, a billing department is not aware of problems with a claim until it is rejected and a denial is received. By the time the rejected claim is received, corrected, and reprocessed, several months may have passed. Payers, when setting up a UR system, should be able to furnish providers with UR criteria for mental health and substance abuse programs and services.

These criteria can be translated into specific edits and reports to be run against the active patient file. If designed correctly, these parameters will help the billing department identify and correct coding errors, clinical errors, utilization parameter violations, incorrect relationships between procedures and diagnoses, violations of key payer regulations, etc. An effective UR system, because it must apply criteria to data that come from both billing/accounts receivable and clinical modules, requires a closely integrated information system.

Utilization Management. Utilization management (UM), a prospective approach to controlling utilization and costs before they occur, is rapidly replacing retrospective UR of services that have already been delivered. UM is defined by the Institute of Medicine as a set of techniques to manage health care cost by influencing patient care decisions on a case-by-case assessment of the appropriateness of care prior to its provision. Such techniques as readmission screening, preauthorization of services, review of continued stay, and recertification are employed (Gray & Field, 1989).

UM is particularly important to MCOs with fee-for-service contracts and to providers assuming risk under capitated contracts. Automation is the most cost-effective way to implement utilization management.

Currently there is disagreement as to whether a payer's criteria for medical necessity should be made available to providers. Some MCOs publish protocols specifically for their provider network, while others keep them a guarded secret. When no clear set of standards for defining what services are appropriate for a particular diagnosis is available, it is difficult to develop a UR system. Under this scenario, a *denial* management system can be of benefit to the provider. When utilization criteria are closely held, actual claims and denials can be analyzed by payer and service to determine the utilization criteria employed.

Some characteristics of a good UM system include the ability to build utilization criteria for specific payers and plans, and to cross-reference claims data with payer files. The system should also be able to generate reports with dates for UM procedures. In more sophisticated systems UM decision trees are incorporated into software that assists professionals in placing the patient or in reviewing services delivered. An automated UM system can improve the speed, accuracy, and consistency of claims. Among the different analyses of interest in a managed care contract are:

1. Length of stay/treatment by diagnosis,
2. Length of stay/treatment by severity of illness,
3. Length of stay/treatment by clinician,
4. Number of admissions by therapist, and
5. Number of referrals by therapist.

Referral Management. Another important component of a UM system is a referral management function. When a provider's captitated risk includes costs of services delivered by outsiders, it is essential to track these costs. A referring organization should be able to project its costs based on diagnosis, level of functioning, and services recommended. These data will affect the capitation budget.

An organization that subcontracts with many providers will benefit from a data base of cost and outcome data for each contractor. Summaries of outcome measurements by diagnosis can be tracked. On-line access to practitioner-specific information relating to expertise, credentials, training, and education is helpful when one interfaces with networks of providers and practitioners.

Basic Charting Functions

A fully automated QA and UR system requires on-line clinical functions as well. In addition to the basic patient registration functions that support them, traditional clinical applications that will provide the QA and UR programs with data for reviews include:

1. Treatment/service planning;
2. Progress notes;
3. Assessments; and
4. Client abstracts.

Depending on the desired level of automation, a system may actually prepare this documentation on-line or simply provide a format for noting the presence or absence of the activity or documentation. Fully automated patient information systems greatly simplify running UR and QA reports because on-line patient records can be checked by a computer program.

Treatment Planning. Most mental health software developers have integrated treatment plan modules into their client information management systems. These are often generic so they can be adapted to prepare a variety of treatment, education, rehabilitation, and other types of individualized service or care plans. Typically, this software establishes a hierarchy of problems, goals, and objectives for a client and monitors progress toward achieving them. The system selected should be adaptable to the terminology used by the organization and its programs. Users should have the capability to change the output names of the plan, problem, goal, and objective fields to accommodate various requirements. For example, a treatment plan may be referred to as a individualized client plan, or individualized service plan, individualized habilitation plan, or individualized education plan.

The systems typically have the capability of creating as many plans as required for an individual client. Many planners are hierarchical and relational by design. For example, the highest level of the hierarchy could be the problem or skill area(s) to receive attention during treatment. The next level of the hierarchy related to the problem would be the long-term treatment goals. There may be one or more goals related to the problem. The third level of the treatment plan is the objective. The short-term objectives may be specific steps, processes, issues, or actions that need to be taken.

Typically, there are multiple objectives associated with each long-term treatment goal. It is also helpful to have a status code associated with the objective. This can be used to track how close a client is to achieving his objectives and goals. Some systems also allow therapists to record barriers to completing goals and objectives. Ideally, a treatment planning function should be integrated with service notes, client registration, abstracts, QA, UR, scheduling, and accounts receivable modules.

Assessments. It is recommended that the central MIS be used for simple, limited assessments and that third party products be purchased for more sophisticated applications. Numerous commercial automated tests and questionnaires are available to supplement an automated client record. These programs may be integrated with the basic record or used as stand-alone packages running on a microcomputer. When these data are standardized and coded, they can be used to build a data base of clinical information for clinical studies and statistical reports. A large number of interviews and instruments are available for assessing social, psychological, psychoneurological, and medical conditions. Potential problem areas evaluated include religion, family, education, marriage, personality traits, sex, military experiences, employment, crime history, alcohol and drug abuse, and medical illnesses. Some systems produce an index of the type and severity of the problem and others produce narrative reports that supplement observations of clinical staff.

Systems can be set up for direct client administration on the computer, while others use a hard copy questionnaire that is then transcribed by support staff. For self-report interviews, ability for therapists to annotate patient responses is desirable. Some programs are designed to automate specific psychological tests, and others permit users to define their own question items.

The ability to support user-added questions and new questionnaires is very valuable, especially when combined with the customized reports. When statistical analysis is required and content analysis is not available, there are a number of excellent survery programs developed for marketing that can be applied to mental health.

Service Notes. Several mental health information management systems include word processing systems with clinical modules. These systems allow users to transcribe progress or service notes associated with treatment interventions. When the text processor is integrated with the clinical software, clinical notes are accessible to other analyses.

One should beware of word-processing-based systems that simply jump back and forth between the clinical information system and a word processing document. If this approach fails to establish links to events recorded in the information system, the ability to integrate the progress record with other aspects of the information system is lost. Linking allows associating notes with specific areas of treatment plans and assessments. Progress notes should be able to link notes to specific services and be secured from modification when closed. Other features that are attractive in a progress notation system include electronic signatures, code table lookups, glossaries, merge features to insert text from other areas of the client's record, and macro programming. All notes should be date and time stamped and linked to other variables that can be searched for easy retrieval.

Client Abstract. Regardless of clinical functions that are performed on-line, a patient abstract system should be set up in the clinical MIS. This will summarize the various demographic and clinical information recorded. It should support a variety of on-screen and printed reports that summarize salient clinical and treatment history. In addition to the basic summary, additional detailed information as required should be available as well.

Financial and Accounting Functions

Managed care has also had a significant impact on accounting. In the past it has been adequate to report a financial position for a previous accounting period. Many public entities operated on a cash-based receipts and disbursements system. Cost accounting, if done at all, was calculated on a program basis, or services were costed out at the end of the year by dividing the number of services delivered into the program cost. In today's "real time environment" such retrospective historical analysis is not always adequate. Organizations require current cash flow projections, that is, program cost calculations from the previous month based on *actual* staff time worked in a program. Cost calculations down to the individual service level are essential for internal cost management. These requirements are driven by the absolute necessity of having accurate and current cost information with which to negotiate fee-for-service and capitated contracts. Computer programs for scheduling, billing and accounts receivable, contract management, budgetary accounting, cost accounting, and quality improvement are essential to a provider's ability to monitor and control financial performance.

Design Considerations

When implementing a system it is critical that the information systems department work with the clinical staff to design the clinical and demographic measures to apply to UR and QM. All of the staff who will be using the system should participate to some degree in its design. Without their input, it is doubtful that practitioners will buy into the new technology. It is also vitally important to the success of a project to provide continuous, useful clinical feedback to staff for their practice. Of particular value are useful on-line displays and printed reports available at any time.

A mental health MIS must strive to minimize the data collection and processing burden of employees. Data for reporting and analysis should be a by-product of normal business and clinical operations. This has been done for many years in business areas with integrated accounting systems. Information entered into the purchasing system, for example, updates the accounts payable module, which in turn posts to the general ledger making it available for budgeting and cost accounting. In clinical areas this integration has been lacking. It is difficult to find fully functional clinical software where all clinical applications are integrated. There are even fewer programs available that fully integrate clinical and accounting applications.

Summary and Conclusions

In the past few years managed care has had a significant impact on the design and implementation of mental health MISs. These changes include expansion and modification of existing programs and the development of new applications. This has also led to the integration of applications software developed for other markets with current mental health programs.

Despite an increase in administrative expense, adaptation to managed care is having some positive effects on provider organizations and their MISs. First, it forces business operations to run more efficiently through strategic application of technology. Second, it entices vendors to expand their present software and to develop new applications, particularly for clinical records. Many providers may not survive the transition to managed care. Those that do will depend more than ever on automation. In the opinion of the author, automation is no longer a luxury for mental health providers. It is a necessity for survival in the 1990s.

References

Berlant, J.L. (1992). Quality assurance in managed mental health. In S. Feldman (Ed.), *Managed mental health services*. Springfield, IL: Charles C. Thomas.

Gabel, J., Di Carlo, S., Fink, S., & de Lissovoy, G. (1989). Data watch: Employer-sponsored health insurance in American health affairs.

Goran, M.J. (1992). Managed mental health and group health insurance. In S. Feldman (Ed.), *Managed mental helath services*. Springfield, IL: Charles C. Thomas.

Gray, B.H., & Field, M.F. (Eds.). (1989). Controlling costs and changing patient care? The role of utilization management. Washington, DC: National Academy Press.

JCAHO (Joint Commission on Accreditation of Health Care Organizations). (1990). *Primer on Indicator Development and Application: Measuring Quality in Health Care.*, Oakbrook Terrace, IL: JCAHO.

JCAHO (Joint Commission on Accreditation of Health Care Organization). (1992). *The transition from QA to QI: Performance based evaluation of mental health organization*, Oakbrook Terrace, IL: JCAHO.

U.S. Department of Commerce. (1989): *U.S. Industry Outlook.* (30th ed.) (51-1–51-6). Washington, DC: GPO.

17
VA National Mental Health Microcomputer Data Base System
Allan S. Finkelstein

In the late 1980s the U.S. Congress and the Department of Veterans Affairs (VA) Central Office developed several projects including the Enhanced Substance Abuse Project and PostTraumatic Stress Disorders Clinical Teams (PCT) to expand mental health care in the VA. Moneys were specifically earmarked for these programs as part of the nation's "war on drugs" and a continuing focus on the special problems of combat veterans. Along with these funds was a mandate to track how the dollars were spent, and on whom. It is extremely important to know both the clinical and administrative features of treating these patients because controversy abounds both in the clinical and political arenas about just who the patients are, how they are treated, their prevalence in the general population, and rates of recidivism.

The National Mental Health microcomputer Data Base System (NMHDS) is a comprehensive program for providing computer support in Mental Health throughout the VA. Several nationwide ADP systems exist to support clinical and administrative functions. The NMHDS was developed to enhance data collection and analysis from a clinical perspective in mental health. The need for a microcomputer system to fill holes left by the other systems is the focus of this chapter. It both describes the NMHDS system and its features and provides a case study in designing and implementing such a project.

"Customers" for this project were diverse and therefore the scope of the design was multifaceted. There was a great need at the hospital program level for general computer support. Word processing, spreadsheets, and other basic computing needs were lacking and unavailable for local purchase. Other needs were for support of administrative reporting. For many years the VA Central Office has expected numerous labor intensive quarterly reports that give relatively little feedback or useful information to the programs that produce them. Despite the number, none of the reports could tell the Central Office whether the additional moneys for clinical enhancement were leading to increased services for veterans. Typical of bureaucracy, the push for increased funding and staffing was budget based rather than results oriented. The value of outcome measurement was agreed upon by all, but lack of a precise and standardized methodology for measuring outcome stalled the impetus to conduct adequate evaluations.

The NMHDS project was expected to provide some solutions to these problems, primarily to give control of their data to program managers and clinicians. VA hospitals' core systems have been downsized from minicomputers to clustered microcomputers over 15 years, and control of core computing resources has consistently remained (as it should) with the information resource management service (IRM). IRM has responsibility for the hospital information system and data integrity. Ad hoc reports, data "fishing," and the clinical perspective have taken a back seat to the daily demands of automating support services like laboratory, pharmacy, and purchasing departments. The desktop perspective of NMHDS was intended to give data access and control back to clinical program managers. Centralized reporting continues, but NMHDS supports this from a perspective that allows administrative reports to flow directly from patient encounters.

Goals for Automation

Reduction in Resource Use

Computer usage necessitates new skills in clerks, managers, and other staff. Added reporting requirements also place burden on the clinical staff. Because of this, a reduction in overall resource use was a primary design concern. A careful study of the minimal data set required was made along with measurements of the time necessary for data input by a trained clerk. These findings were carefully fed back into the design phase.

Attempts to lessen the time required for data input were successful to a degree, but it became clear that paper-and-pencil forms would always be quicker than logging on a microcomputer, entering the demographic information, and then entering the individual data points. The difference between paper-and-pencil times and computer entry times were minimized but remained significant. Overall time per patient was on the order of 10 to 15 minutes but this was time needed to *transcribe* data into the computer from forms distributed with the NMHDS documentation. The forms were designed to closely follow the computer screens with an eye to easing transcription. While automation could not outperform simply placing completed forms into medical records, other benefits achieved, including reduction in reporting burden due to careful design of data sets, would need to be figured in the overall costs and benefits equation.

Comparability Across Sites

A wise saying goes, "Once you've seen one VA hospital, you've seen one VA hospital." There are large differences in hospital size, patient populations, staffing, and even philosophy. At the program level these differences are magnified geometrically. To gather comparable data across these differing sites, a high degree of standardization is required. Computerization assured that all sites were collecting the same information. Standardization in this project came from a single program manual, the definition and style features of which fostered a high degree of consistency. The computer maintained a totally consistent environment over time and site. This permeated down to the level of question wording, question order, and the look and feel of the forms and screens. Without standardization, divergence would have been nonrandom across differing sites, making it more difficult to draw valid conclusions.

Consistency of Data Collected

Beyond the comparability across sites, the data must be internally consistent. If the data do not meet internal validity standards, errors abound. For example, no World War II veteran could have been born after 1930, but errors of this kind are often seen in the transcription process between form and computer. Nontypographical errors also occur. Patients may give contradictory answers that are not challenged, referential consistency rules may be broken and simple clerical mistakes can occur when recording information in patient charts. With a computer program it is possible to build in error checks and validity rules like the one listed above. Other techniques involve restricting allowed answers to discrete sets and preventing clerks from skipping vital information segments (i.e., no null responses to exam dates). Illegibility, a major problem in medical records, produces errors as well, and moving away from handwritten records to minimize this was a major step in and of itself. NMHDS applies internal consistency checks immediately, permitting the clerk to correct a problem in real time. This has led to a degree of data integrity not otherwise available. Error trapping improves the quality of the outcome data gathered, with fewer rejected incomplete records.

Ease of Access and Analysis

Arguably, the purpose of the medical record is to provide a historical basis for continuity of patient care, but easy access to these records is paramount. Low cost fast retrieval is what a computer data base is all about. Records can easily be retrieved by date, program, staff, patient, or other attributes. Reports for individual patients across all data points are easily generated, and reports based on individual attributes, such as program discharge date, are also available through simple menu selection. Security features are built into both the local and national data bases and include timing out with inactivity, multiple level passwords, and data audit trails that comply with VA-wide security policy.

Data analytic capabilities go well beyond canned reporting. Reporting implies predetermined output with predetermined templates and formats, and the consistent look and feel of NMHDS reporting capabilities are formidable and comprehensive. For ad hoc analyses, statistical manipulation, and hypothesis testing, more sophisticated data management methods are also required. NMHDS exposes data to analysis in many ways. By supporting traditional Standard Query Language (SQL) queries and exporting data to Microsoft Excel spreadsheets based on user-selected sorts and searches, data are available to most of today's analytical tools. This makes powerful data analysis possible at the local level.

Multiple Data Views

The project required both a desktop and a national perspective. NMHDS local sites regularly upload their data to the national data base. This mandated a national data base to mirror the local sites as well as to allow a global view comparing programs around the country. The national data base serves as a "backup of last resort" as well, allowing a local data base to be reconstructed as of the last national data upload. A multiple data view design allows the use of ad hoc SQL data base querying and construction of an executive decision support system. This decision support tool is based upon customer-defined cross tabulations and totalizations. The dual view of the data supporting local desktop systems and a unified national repository was central to the design and key to the ability to meet both local program management and Central Office information needs.

Information Gathered

The information gathered by NMHDS is intended to reflect both the status of the clinical program and to describe the patients served. A summary of the NMHDS data points gives a clear indication of the areas surveyed and the intent of the project. NMHDS collects a minimal data set and is in no way intended to be an exhaustive review of patient characteristics or VA care. The structure of the national network is one of relational tables in an SQL structure. The local data structure is pictured in flow chart form in Figure 1.

Treatment Program Information

A description of each clinical program surveyed is required before the first data transmission can occur. The hospital with which each program is

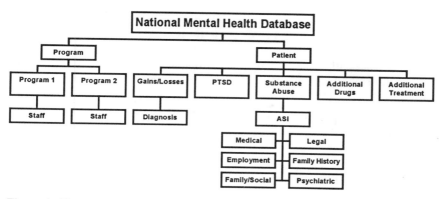

Figure 1. Data map.

affiliated is specified and information such as program type and batch reporting requirements is entered. A description of the program in free text format is also requested. Each program is named and its inpatient or outpatient status is specified. Program director and contact information is collected. This contact information includes computer modem lines, voice phone numbers, and "snail" mail addresses.

Program Staffing

The pivotal resource in any mental health program is staffing. The number of admissions, patient demographics, substance abuse types treated, and most other data are meaningful only in relation to resources expended, most particularly staffing. NMHDS asks that each staff member of a surveyed program be named and described by degree and job title. Full-time employment equivalents (FTEE) and used to indicate how much time each staff member spends in each program. Many staff are part-time or are split over multiple programs. This FTEE specification corrects patients to staff ratios to reflect this fact.

Patient Demographics

To clearly identify individual patients, complete demographic information is necessary. Full name, social security number, date of birth, and gender are the primary identifiers. Other information such as address, race, and religion are added. Veteran-specific data such as period of service and eligibility status are also collected.

Psychiatric Diagnosis

Many of our patients have substance abuse and another psychiatric disorder concurrently. These dual diagnosis patients traditionally present the most difficult treatment problems. NMHDS asks for full Diagnostic and Statistical Manual of Mental Disorders-III-Revised (DSM-III-R) diagnosis. Selections are made either by DSM-III-R code or through a pick list of categories and titles. This ensures recording of a full and specific diagnosis that conforms directly with DSM and International Classification of Diseases-9th ed. (ICD-9). Junk diagnoses such as "rule out depression" are therefore precluded. A primary diagnosis is also specified and only a single primary diagnosis is allowed. Data validation is immediate and precise.

Addiction Severity Index (ASI)

The ASI was chosen as the major instrument to measure types and levels of substance abuse. ASI is a standard in the field and has been normed in many varied settings (Stoffelmayr, Mavis, & Kasim, 1994). It was originally developed in a VA medical center and VA population norms for the last 15 years are available. ASI was first used to measure treatment outcomes over a wide variety of settings. Its questions survey a broad range of areas that affect outcome. NMHDS uses the ASI substance abuse section as the primary determinant of the severity of substance abuse and to survey the range of abuse. The other six areas assessed by ASI are medical, legal, employment, family history, family/social, and psychiatric. Levels of severity are found for each and composite scores may be computed. The ASI was constructed both to touch on all major areas that affect treatment outcome and to serve as a minimal data set that can be generated at low cost by trained technicians. The ASI's publication record attests to the acceptance of its validity, ability to measure need for treatment, and ability to aid matching patients with treatment settings.

Post Traumatic Stress Disorder (DTSD) Treatment Screening Form

Dr. Robert Rosenheck of the VA Northeast Program Evaluation Center and the National Center for PTSD has responsibility for evaluating and monitoring the PCT programs. One of the measures created by this center was the PTSD Screening Form. This data collection tool enjoys wide usage throughout the VA and predates our project. NMHDS uses it to collect information on military history, psychiatric/substance abuse history, and problem areas needing treatment. Items focus on combat experience and war related stress. Previous treatment, legal background, and employment status are also surveyed. NMHDS faithfully reproduced this form, down to its batch coding marks and internal codes. The use of the well-established form, while not optimized for computer presentation, improves comparisons with data collected from other programs using the PTSD Screening Form.

Hardware and Software Platform

Over 250 programs were either created or expanded and received computer hardware. Each program was sent two microcomputers, an Intel based MS-DOS PC and an Apple Macintosh. This mixed computer environment was selected for nontechnical reasons and created software design considerations that we were only partially successful in addressing. The data base system was developed using the data management package, Omnis 7, from Blythe Software Inc. Omnis 7 was selected to allow joint development on both the PC and Macintosh because the resulting code is compatible at the binary level. Its support of SQL queries underlies the local data/wide area network configuration. Omnis 7 has a completely visual interface and is event driven at its core. This allows full integration with the Windows and Macintosh graphical user interfaces. Furthermore, the good security features and strong programming tools that it offers are built in and not just added on.

Attempts were made to have the data base run on both machines simultaneously. Unfortunately, the major company supplying peer-to-peer Apple-PC networking left the field just as we were implementing this system. A decision was made to focus the data base on the PC Windows platform and to continue supporting the office automation functions of both platforms. Each system was shipped with Microsoft Office (containing MS Word, the Excel spreadsheet, and the Powerpoint presentation package). These packages were then used as containers for NMHDS data.

NMHDS is coordinated by Dr. Dale Cannon for the VA Central Office Mental Health and Behavioral Sciences Service and the author is responsible for software development. Mr. Keith Cosgrove manages the Remote Systems Support Center in Pittsburgh, PA. This center houses the Help Desk, the national server, and provides hardware repair and maintenance. The National Server consists of an Oracle data base running on a UNIX system. Sixteen telephone lines are available for data transmission. User questions and problems are handled by Help Desk staff who are in close contact with the clinical program managers and the software development team.

User Interface

The local data base runs under Windows 3.× and is graphical by its very nature. To enter data, navigate through the application, or enter and leave the program, the user uses the mouse to select menus and "push buttons." The user moves back and forth between the mouse and keyboard entry. To facilitate training and speed data entry, a consistent interface and screen makeup is presented across the application. A tour of a representative screen follows. Understanding this screen generalizes across the entire package.

Figure 2 shows a Windows 3.× screen that will serve as our example. At the very top of the screen are the standard Windows control buttons, along with the title and a pull-down menu bar. The Applications and Patient menus are used to navigate through the data base. Menus remain constant across the screens.

From the Applications menu, the user may select either a Patient or a Program area (Fig. 2). Under the menu bar are one or more windows for data entry and display. Figure 2 has two of these windows, each with its own title: Patient and Gains/Losses.

The lower third of each screen contains buttons for NMHDS retrieval and editing commands. Find selects and displays a desired record. The Insert, Edit, and Delete buttons actually change the data. Insert is used to enter new records. Edit is used to change existing records. Delete is used to remove data. When it is not permitted to delete data this button does not function. In edit mode, the button area is used to OK or cancel a data base command. A user must confirm data, editing, or deleting data.

When a selection is to be made from a predefined list, a picklist or scrolling window that displays the list of choices will appear. Items are selectable by button click or keyboard.

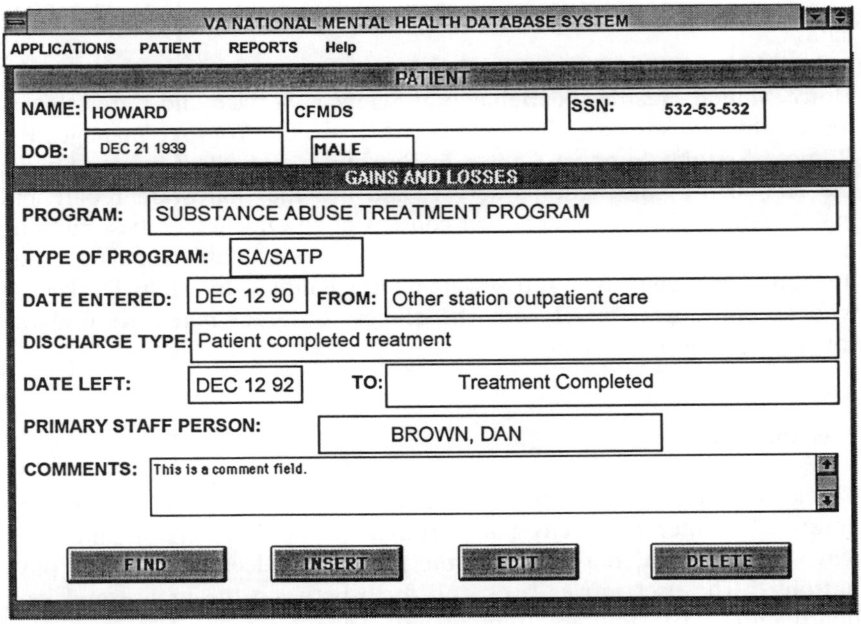

Figure 2. Gains/Losses screen.

When the Program Screens Assessment, Gains/Losses, Diagnosis, Substance, or PTSD screens are displayed, the top window indicates the current patient. Depending on the context, the program shows and removes or "grays out" unavailable button and menu choices. The graphical Windows interface makes each screen rich with information and possible user actions, but despite the complexity improves user efficiency.

Standard Windows Help is available at all times via the Help menu option. An overview of the system, Help Desk information, and sample screens are fully documented for on-line referral and assistance. Additionally, each screen provides a brief description of each entry field.

NMHDS Reports

NMHDS offers many report options. Some are administrative in nature, showing how many total records are in a data base or presenting a clinician by clinician list of current patients. Direct patient reporting suitable for charting is a simple menu choice as are the abilities to list data by data or patient, or to list all data for a specific patient.

Some of the more complex reporting options in NMHDS are reported below. For example, the Automated Management Information System section of the Extended Reports application provides a useful tool for compiling the substance abuse data reported monthly to the VA's Austin, Texas Data Processing Center. It should be made clear that actual key-punch type reports are not produced here on the system. But ability to easily extract the data from the NMHDS greatly simplifies reporting and saves a great deal of time and effort over previous manual tallying methods. This is an example of a reporting option developed to mirror an older reporting requirement.

Cross Tab

The Extended Reports application provides the capability for cross-tab reports up to 15 columns wide by any number of rows. When the selected data exceed 15 columns, a simple summary report with subtotals is produced instead. Output can be a printed report, a graph, or an Excel file. The Cross Tabs screen is shown in Figure 3.

Cross-tab fields can be selected from any of the available NMHDS files by clicking the appropriate "radio" button at the bottom left of the screen. After selecting a primary file, a field is selected from a simple picklist. Once a primary field has been chosen, a Primary/Secondary push button appears, allowing selection of a secondary file and field in the same manner. When it is necessary to select a subset of the data, a Search Condition push button allows choosing a single-field search condition. Any field can be selected for this search, but only from the primary file.

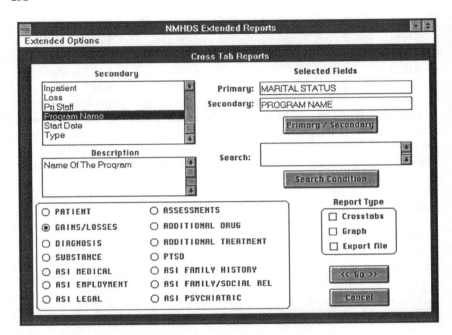

Figure 3. Cross Tab Report.

More involved searches are conducted using the Multiple Search reporting option. After selecting a report type, pressing Go begins the report generation process.

The first type of report, a standard cross tabulation, is normally printed to the screen. Aso available are Graph, and an Export option that produces a comma-delimited file, GENERIC.CSV, containing the key field, the selected field from the Primary file, and the selected field from the Secondary file. This file can then be imported into Microsoft Excel or any other application supporting the file format.

Ad Hoc Reports

This option allows users to design their own custom reports or to run reports distributed separately by the Software Development Center in Albany, NY. Nine sample reports are distributed with the application, and can be modified or used as a basis for developing custom reports at each site. Omnis 7 provides extensive on-line help for use with the ad hoc report generator.

Multiple Search

This is the most general-purpose and flexible reporting option in the Extended Reports application. Fields can be selected from any single

NMHDS file, combined with those from the main patient file, and searches can be constructed using multiple fields, ANDs, and ORs to narrow down the data to exactly that needed. Output can be directed to a scrollable browse window, a printer, an export file, a graph, or to a mail merge document in Microsoft Word.

The opening screen for the Multiple Search option (Fig. 4) contains a group of radio buttons identical to those on the Cross Tabs screen, one for each file in the NMHDS data base. Selection of a file makes available all fields in that file, plus all fields in the Patient file, for searching and reporting. The window at the bottom of the screen shows the search conditions currently in effect, and initially displays All Records. To the right of this window are the search push buttons: AND, OR, Undo Last, and Reset. Only buttons that apply at any given time are displayed for use. Initially, only the AND button is shown, and is used to enter the first search condition as outlined below. At the top right of the screen, the number of records meeting the current search conditions is displayed and updated as the search conditions are changed. The initial value represents the total number of records in the selected file. Below this number are the View and Cancel push buttons. Cancel returns to the main Extended Reports menu screen, while View is unavailable until a file is selected and the number of records passing the search conditions is nonzero. Selecting View opens another window allowing selection of fields to be displayed and selection of the report mode as described above.

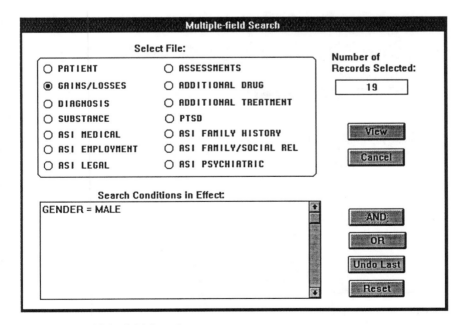

Figure 4. Multiple-field Search.

Entering Search Conditions

When an NMHDS file is initially selected, the search window displays All Records, and the record count represents the entire file. At this point, only the AND button is available to initiate a search. Selecting AND opens the window shown in Figure 5. The picklist at the upper left of the screen is shows all fields in both the selected file and the Patient file, all of which are available to construct a search condition. A brief description of each field is also provided. Radio buttons allows the selection a search comparison operator. Values to be compared are entered in the Comparison Value box. When this box is left empty, a field content of NULL is assumed. Pressing the OK button returns the main Multiple Search screen where the current search condition and record count are displayed. AND and OR can continue to be used to build a more elaborate search. To undo the last search condition entered, a user presses the Undo Last button. The Reset button removes all search conditions.

Viewing Query Results

At any time during the construction of the search, the currently selected records can be browsed or directed to any of the other available output formats by selecting the View push button (Fig. 6). The title at the top of the screen shows the files currently selected, and the field picklist allows selecting multiple fields from these files for display or other output. Double clicking on a field in the picklist places an asterisk next to it

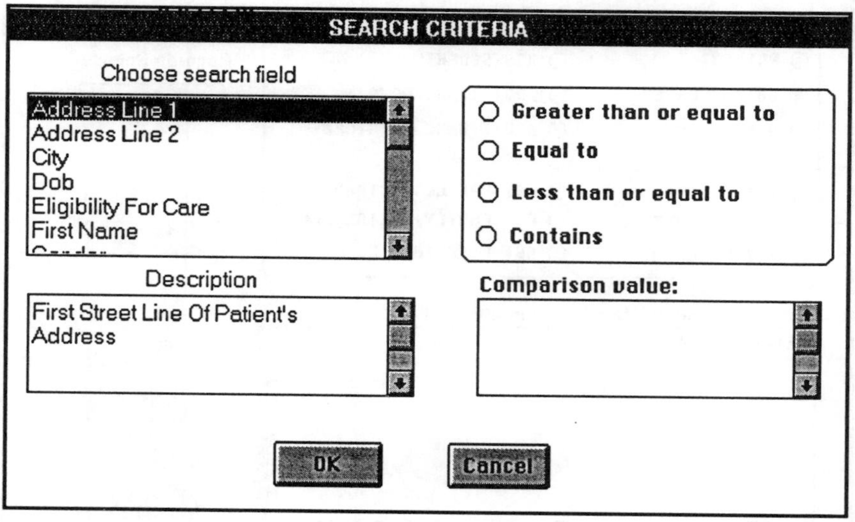

Figure 5. Search Criteria.

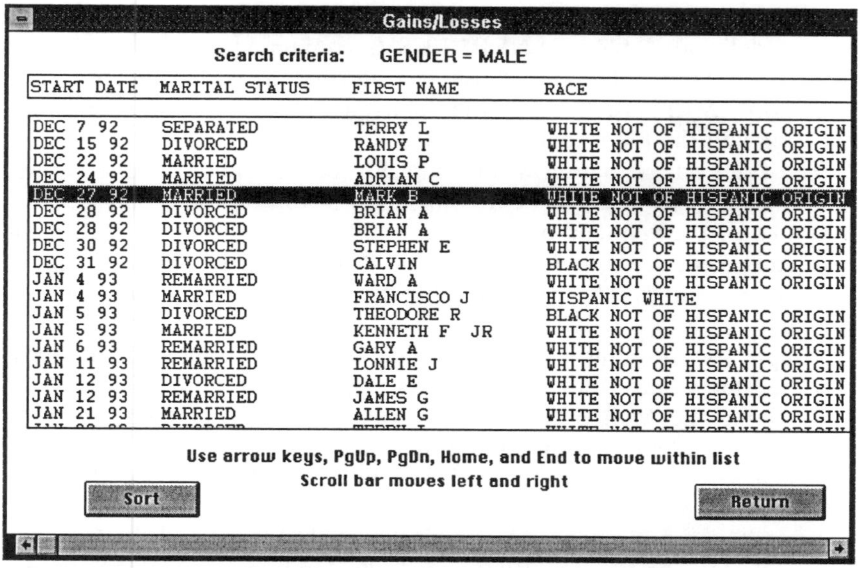

Figure 6. Sample output screen.

indicating it has been selected, and the current field count is updated at the bottom of the screen. Clear selected deselects all fields and resets the field count to zero. Go processes the currently selected records and fields and produces an output type selected using the radio buttons at the lower left. Cancel returns to the main Multiple Search screen, and leaves search conditions and field selections intact for further manipulation.

Five different output options are available for the records and fields selected in the Multiple Search section of the Extended Reports application. If the Browse output option is selected, a window opens for display of the selected data, similar to the one shown below. The window title shows the file selected. Directly beneath it the search criteria in use are displayed. Field titles are shown along the top of a scrollable browse window, allowing viewing of all the data selected. There is a practical limit to the number of fields that can be displayed in this window, depending on the widths of the fields selected. A vertical scrollbar is available at the extreme right of the data displayed, but keyboard scrolling is probably preferable in most cases. The horizontal scrollbar at the bottom of the screen is used for movement to the left or right.

The Sort push button displays a picklist of all fields selected, and allows sorting of the displayed data on one of the selected fields. This local sort option does not affect the order of the records in other output options selected subsequently. Return simply returns to the field and output selection screen.

Selecting Excel as the output option will result in the generation of a comma-delineated file, GENERIC.CSV, containing the selected fields from the NMHDS files for those records that met the current search conditions. Microsoft Excel is then started from within the current application and the file is loaded for use.

The Print output option will prompt for a sort field as did the Browse option. Only this selected field is included in the report produced, with subtotals of the number of occurrences of each value contained in the field (divorced, separated, married, etc.). The report is initially sent to the screen, but can be printed using the P at the top of the vertical scrollbar.

Graph also prompts for a sort field, and then produces a pie chart based on the values contained in the selected field.

Selecting the Mail option automatically selects eight fields from the Patient file related to addressing a mail merge letter in Microsoft Word. Other fields can be selected individually as well. A Word data file, GENERIC.TXT, is created for use with a standard Word mail merge document, a sample of which is included as MAILMRGE.DOC. Other fields selected can be similarly inserted into the body of the letter to give it a customized personal appearance. Microsoft Word is automatically opened with MAILMRGE.DOC as the current document, so a user-created document that is used often can be renamed to MAILMRGE.DOC for automatic access from within the current application. Similarly, once created, GENERIC.TXT can be renamed and reused as a Word data file.

Current Status. NMHDS is currently in production in over 120 different programs. Over 40,000 different patients are represented in the data base. Extensive upgrades to the software allowing more efficient reporting and entry have just been shipped. Staff training at the local level is now the most pressing problem. The graphical nature of the data base and Windows system makes training more manageable. Also helpful is the ever expanding number of clinicians who use computers in their daily work. However, significant staff turnover, particularly at the data entry level, makes training an ongoing concern. Attempts to increase informal communication channels with the field through the fax and modem capabilities of the computers are becoming central for the software development team.

The newest feature is an Executive Decision Support package that is clearly client–server in nature. National decision makers have real time access to the national data base, but all interface and query building activity is performed on the desktop. The server acts on the query and sends back only the results. Output formatting and charting can be conducted locally. This setup maximizes the strength of the national SQL data base yet minimizes transmission time. The Decision Support package focuses on cross tabs, and date-related totals are designed "on the fly" by the user.

NMHDS places computer power in the hands of local programs while leveraging a national effort. The national roll-up furnishes current data and ad hoc querying support to national program managers while production data useful to local management remains local where it is also useful. Software development, Help Desk functions, and equipment maintenance are nationally supported. The distributed architecture of this versatile and flexible program data management system overcomes the disadvantages of one-way reporting and simultaneously encourages local maintenance of clean data that brings benefit both locally and nationally.

Reference

Stoffelmayr, B.E., Mavis, B.E., & Kasim, R.M. (1994). The longitudinal stability of the Addiction Severity Index. *Journal of Substance Abuse Treatment, 11*, 373–378.

Part III
Knowledge Management

18
Computer-Based Education for Patients and Professionals
Steven Locke and Marcia E.H. Rezza

An important frontier for computer applications in mental health is the use of computers for the education of patients and professionals. Although computer-based training has been used extensively in industry, the introduction of computer-based technology to the field of mental health has been slow. Efforts to protect the core of humanistic values essential to mental health practice, coupled with technophobic avoidance, have delayed the acceptance of computers by mental health professionals as an important educational adjunct. The remarkable ability of the computer to manipulate information in novel ways can lead to increased understanding and new learning for both patients and caregivers. We are on the threshold of an explosion of creative applications of educational technologies. These advances will revolutionize how we learn and lead to greater patient empowerment and demystification of the process of treatment. In this chapter we will review the state of computer-based applications in mental health education and provide readers with an extensive list of electronic resources for professional and patient education.

History

The use of computers in psychiatric education dates from the early 1960s. Slack and his colleagues demonstrated the effective use of computers for medical interviewing (Slack, Hicks, Reed, & Van Cura, 1966; Slack & Slack, 1972). They further demonstrated that under some conditions computers were superior to clinicians or written instructions when used for interactive patient education (Fisher, Johnson, Porter, Bleich, & Slack, 1977). Others followed with special mental health applications in the areas of automated psychological testing, computer-based psychiatric interviews, computer-assisted diagnosis, decision support software, computer-aided instruction, and even computerized treatment interventions. Elwork and Gutkin, writing in 1985, predicted that computers were likely to have a major impact on society in general and on psychology, psychiatry, sociology, and related behavioral sciences in particular (Elwork & Gutkin, 1985). In the same year, Hedlund et al. reported that while automation had been most successful with self-report measures, there was limited success with the automation of free-form projective assessment tools. Progress in the computerization of clinical tests of cognitive function fell somewhere in between. Agreement between clinical and computer-derived psychiatric diagnoses was reported to be good (Hedlund, Vieweg, & Cho, 1985).

The 1980s saw a surge of projects that used the computer to teach special subjects, including statistical design, cognition, and perception, Schwartz (1988) reviewed this literature and concluded:

1. an enormous amount of work was needed before computers could simulate human intelligence;
2. text-based systems would not achieve student acceptance, do not lend themselves to the teaching of nonverbal behavior or emotion, and are too different from the live clinical encounter to permit adequate transfer of skills;
3. computer simulations of psychopathology require consensus among experts about the basic phenomenology being simulated; and
4. computer-based educational projects must have the potential for widespread distribution to justify the time, effort, and expense needed for development.

Schwartz maintained that the phenomenological orientation of the Diagnostic and Statistical Manual of Mental Disorders-III-Revised (DSM-III-R) and the development of systems that permit the display of human behavior, interspersed with computer-aided instruction, created new opportunities for mental health education. He also predicted that acceptance of computers in psychiatric education would occur more easily in the field of behavioral medicine because of its emphasis on measurable behavior and its close ties to other medical specialties where computers have earned greater acceptance (Schwartz, 1988).

In considering the future impact of computer-based education, Schwartz (1988) predicted:

1. that students would learn better and faster and would achieve greater uniformity of knowledge and skills;
2. that faculty would find it easier to evaluate and grade students, using more objective performance criteria;
3. wider use of computer data bases;
4. wider availability of computer-based consultation and decision support;
5. clarification of the educational niches in which computer-based training would be superior to traditional methods;

6. expanded use of interactive video in psychiatric education;
7. greater use of computer-based resources by mental health professionals who used computers during their training.

Barriers to Utilization

In 1986, the leading annual index of medical software, The Burgess Directory, listed only 14 psychiatry applications out of a total of over 1,000 commercial medical software products. this dearth of applications documented the delay in introducing computer applications into psychiatry and mental health. One explanation for the delay was the concern that patients would find computers threatening or difficult to use. Research indicated, however, that patients enjoyed using computers both as data gatherers and as teaching devices (French & Beaumont, 1987; Hedlund et al., 1985; Mathisen, Evans, & Meyers, 1987; Slack, 1984). Thus, there is no support for the idea that the delay in introducing the use of computers in mental health practice is due to patient resistance. Rather, it has been the resistance of clinicians and institutions to the use of computers for collecting and providing mental health information that has slowed the introduction of information technologies into the field.

Resistance to the expansion of the role of computer-based education is due to issues related to cost and distribution; resistance is strengthened by the requirement for special skills in the courseware developer. Authoring courseware requires both pedagogic and artistic skills, and is more like producing a feature film than authoring a textbook. While many faculty can serve in the role of content experts, far fewer have the talent or ability to produce well-crafted computer-based instructional materials. As Schwartz (1988) put it, "Traditional teachers will not, in general, welcome the computer revolution. The use of computers requires skills they often do not have and do not choose or have the time to develop. Computer usage generally moves upward through the faculty ranks and its full acceptance does not come until a new generation of faculty, comfortable with computers, reaches senior positions."

During the past decade, sophisticated software applications that permit educators to author "courseware" have become widely available (Petty, Lynch, & Rosen, 1993; Politser, Gastfriend, Bakin, & Nguyen, 1987). In addition, new "expert" systems for displaying knowledge may enhance decision making and improve diagnosis. These educational and decision support software tools can help clinicians to cope with the exponential increases in information that tax their ability to keep current with new scientific knowledge.

One unexplored area that has emerged is the use of computer-based tools in mental health nursing care. It is evident that the increased use of computer technology in health care settings is having an impact on the

nursing profession (Lacey, 1993). Although computers are being increasingly incorporated into the psychiatric nurse's working environment,
there is little research about their attitudes toward computerization.
Understanding nurses' attitudes toward and experience with computerization is essential to the successful expansion of the use of clinical computing in
mental health settings.

Therapists' resistance to the greater use of microcomputer technology
in their practices has been studied by Levitan and Willis (1985). They
found that among psychologists and psychiatrists surveyed, the barriers to
greater use were lack of knowledge, cost, time, and the subjects' belief
that their practices were too small to justify computer use. They also
reported that practitioners generally did not recognize the degree to
which they rely on information as a resource for conducting their clinical
and administrative tasks (Levitan, Willis, & Vogelgesang, 1985).

Patient Education

Several trends are converging to create the growing need for patient
education materials in both primary care and specialized mental health
settings. These trends include the movement toward patient-centered
care, the growing demands of health care consumers to participate in
their own care, a need to increase the quality of informed medical decision
making, the emphasis on quality improvement and reduction in health
care utilization, and cost-containment strategies in the managed care
environment. These trends have created an opportunity to expand the
role of informtion technology in mental health. Examples of these opportunities include:

1. home health references;
2. office or institution-based health references;
3. interactive risk assessment tools (e.g., HIV risk: Locke et al., 1992;
   Be Well™ health risk appraisal: Slack, Safran, Kowaloff, Pearce, &
   Delbanco, 1995);
4. interactive screening tools (e.g., the AUDIT or the Michigan Alcohol
   Screening Test);
5. interactive informed consent;
6. psycho-education resources:
   a. tailored messages, either disease-specific or treatment-specific, for
      example, drug side effects (Morss, Lenert, & Faustman, 1993);
   b. electronic information resources, for example, the Lithium Infor-
      mation Center (Carroll et al., 1986).
7. behavioral medicine applications:
   a. preparation for surgery;
   b. health promotion and disease prevention;

c. risk assessment (Locke et al., 1992; Paperny, Aono, Lehman, Hammar, & Risser, 1990; Schneider, Taylor, Prater, & Wright, 1991);
8. rehabilitation applications;
9. genetic counseling.

Professional Education

Applications for professional education, both graduate and postgraduate, include the classifications in the following sections.

Administrative Applications

Software systems have been developed to assist in class scheduling and to track trainee performance and grading. Examples: EM-PSYCH, a training program scheduling data base (Inderbitzin, Tadros, & Swofford, 1993); and The Electric Resident, a computer system for training psychiatry residents (Powsner & Byck, 1989).

Quality Improvement Education

Computer programs have been developed to monitor exceptions to standards of care and to flag cases for clinical review (Molnar & Feeney, 1985). As managed care organizations and other health care provider systems move toward an electronic record, it will become easier to develop methods for monitoring quality of care and adherence to clinical guidelines. Such systems may then be used to identify providers whose patterns of care may suggest the need for continuing education. Automating quality improvement procedures can lead to improved care while reducing costs. Such monitoring, if combined with individually tailored continuing education programs, should eventually lead to system-wide reductions in malpractice premiums.

Teaching Clinical Problem Solving (Simulations)

Interactive computing permits modeling clinical decision making through the use of patient simulations, for example, CAMPS (Computer-Assisted Medical Problem Solving) (Diserens, Schwartz, Guenin, & Taylor, 1986; Mackenzie, Popkin, & Callies, 1985). In one study a computerized, simulated encounter with an alcoholic patient was used to assess the performance of a randomly selected sample of primary care physicians in diagnosing alcoholism. Only 32% of the physicians diagnosed alcoholism with high certainty. One third of the doctors misinterpreted symptoms of alcoholism and erroneously made other psychiatric diagnoses, chiefly anxiety or depression (Brown, Carter, & Gordon, 1987). Use of simulations offers an opportunity to provide clinicians with ongoing education and self-assessment of their clinical skills.

Searching Clinical Data Bases for Medical Education

Searching tools have been developed to permit exploration of patient clinical data bases for research and pedagogic purposes. These utilities permit testing clinical hypotheses on large patient populations. Examples: ClinQuery (Safran et al., 1990) and CLINFO (Strain, Norvell, Strain, Mueenuddin, & Strain, 1985).

Delivery Systems

There are many electronic offerings commercially available or distributed for free on the Internet. Educational software can also be downloaded from computer bulletin board systems (Miller, 1994). The Internet also serves as a community of experts who exchange information via electronic mail distributions, news groups, and online forums. In addition to resources for professionals, there are numerous specific support groups for individuals in need. The Appendix describes access methods and lists some of the more important resources. For nonnetworked applications, CD-ROM and laser disk are popular distribution media for reference tools and course ware. Selected resources are listed and described in the Appendix.

Academic Course Ware

Since Schwartz's review in 1988 (Schwartz, 1988) authoring systems and microcomputers have become more powerful and accessible. Growing numbers of faculty with computer experience are developing academic course ware that use computers to teach educational topics formerly taught only in the traditional classroom format. Crosbie and Kelly (1993) reported their use of a microcomputer-based "personalized system of instruction" to teach applied behavioral analysis in a psychology department in Australia. Although the study was uncontrolled, all but 4% of the students acquired proficiency in the material and the vast majority reported enjoying the experience (Crosbie & Kelly, 1993).

Self-Assessment and Examinations. It is expected that self-assessment tools for practitioners like the PRITE (an examination published by the American College of Psychiatrists) will become available in electronic form. Already publishers in the mental health field have begun to expand the development of electronic teaching tools for the mental health field. One example is a psychopharmacology education software package developed using Multiple Choice, a HyperCard-based software application that facilitates the simple preparation of stand-alone computerized testing (Gitlow & Tanner, 1991). In addition, such authoring systems can be used to create examinations for performance evaluation. Eventually, examinations may be administered interactively over computer networks, including the use of digitized full-motion vignettes of patient interviews.

Psychopathology. Computer-based methods for teaching psychopathology and diagnosis have been described (Stout, 1988). In the near future, interactive multimedia will be an important method for supplementing the classroom or bedside teaching of psychopathology. An important advantage of interactive multimedia is the ability to illustrate several examples of the pathology being highlighted. Students in mental health specialties could use an interactive "electronic textbook of psychopathology" as a laboratory for the refinement of diagnostic skills. In addition, vignettes from feature films may be used to illustrate psychopathology, as well as to teach the mental status examination (Hyler & Bujold, 1994).

Decision Support

Systems developed for decision support can assist the psychiatric clinician or student in diagnosis and treatment decisions. Such software applications address both clinical and educational issues. There are numerous such expert systems described in the literature (JAMA, 1987; Biczyk do Amaral, Satomura, Honda, & Sato, 1993; Bronzino, Morelli, & Goethe, 1989; Coler & Vincent, 1987; Copeland, Dewey, & Griffiths–Jones, 1986; Erdman, 1985, 1987a, 1987b, 1988; Erdman et al., 1987; Erdman, Greist, Klein, & Jefferson, 1987; Erdman, Klein, & Greist, 1985; Feinberg & Lindsay, 1986; First, 1994; First et al., 1993; Gelernter & Gelernter, 1986; Greist, 1987; Hardt & MacFadden, 1987; Hedlund & Vieweg, 1987; Hedlund, Vieweg, & Cho, 1987; Hrabal & Ticha, 1991; Johri & Guha, 1991; Kohri, 1993; Lewis, 1992; Lewis et al., 1988; Lundsgaarde, 1987; Maurer, Biehl, Kuhner, & Loffler, 1989; Miller, M. 1987; Miller, R. 1987; Morelli, Bronzino, & Goethe, 1987; Moreno & Plant, 1993; Murphy & Pardeck, 1988; Overby, 1987; Plugge, Verhey, & Jolles, 1990; Servan–Schreiber, 1986; Sherman, 1989; Stein, 1994; Werner, 1987; Wilkinson & Markus, 1989a, 1989b).

Reference Applications

Bibliographic Searching. Although exhaustive manual searching has higher specificity and sensitivity than computer-based bibliographic searching (Bareta, Larson, Lyons, & Zorc, 1990), computerized searches are fast and relatively inexpensive (Horowitz, Jackson, & Bleich, 1983). Furthermore, as the electronic medical record becomes the standard, the ability to integrate electronic bibliographic searching into clinical information systems will become more widespread (Powsner & Miller, 1992; Safran, Slack, & Bleich, 1989; Strain et al., 1990) Bibliographic searching can be performed using commercial on-line networks (e.g., PaperChase on CompuServe) or CD-ROM (e.g., Aries Systems' Knowledge Finder, or Silver Platter).

Other Reference Applications. Other electronic reference applications include electronic data bases available on-line or on CD-ROM and include such examples as the Physicians Desk Reference and the DSM-IV. These are listed and described in the Appendix.

Summary and Conclusion

Psychiatric informatics is an expanding frontier. The informational needs of patients and clinicians in mental health settings will stimulate the creative development of many new applications for patient and professional education. Interactive multimedia is an educational medium especially well suited to addressing these educational needs. As the bandwidth of networked information sources to the clinic and the home expands, the opportunities for improved educational resources will increase geometrically. These technologic advances, which have developed more slowly in psychiatry than in other areas of medicine, will revolutionize the delivery of mental health services. There is a pressing need to electronically link managed care organizations, hospitals, insurance companies, and providers. Economic and administrative pressures on clinicians are creating networks of mental health information upon which most clinicians will depend. These networks will offer interactive credentialing, case management, utilization review, psychological testing, consultation, and on-line continuing education. Even technophobic clinicians will find the advantages of being connected to these emerging information resources compelling. The resulting enhancement of educational resources will lead to improved clinical care at lower cost and help patients become better informed.

References

Bareta, J., Larson, D., Lyons, J., & Zorc, J. (1990). A comparison of manual and MEDLARS reviews of the literature on consultation-liaison psychiatry. *American Journal of Psychiatry*, *147*, 1040–1042.

Biczyk do Amaral, M., Satomura, Y., Honda, M., & Sato, T. (1993). A design for decision making: Construction and connection of knowledge bases for a diagnostic system in medicine. *Medical Informatics (London)*, *18*, 307–320.

Bronzino, J., Morelli, R., & Goethe, J. (1989). OVERSEER: A prototype expert system for monitoring drug treatment in the psychiatric clinic. *IEEE Transactions in Biomedical England*, *36*, 533–540.

Brown, R., Carter, W., & Gordon, M. (1987). Diagnosis of alcoholism in a simulated patient encounter by primary care physicians. *Journal of Family Practice*, *25*, 259–264.

Carroll, J., Greist, J., Jefferson, J., Baudhuin, M., Hartley, B., Erdman, H., & Ackerman, D. (1986). Lithium Information Center: One model of a computer-based psychiatric information service. *Archives of General Psychiatry*, *43*, 483–485.

Coler, M., & Vincent, K. (1987). Coded nursing diagnoses on Axes: A prioritized, computer-ready diagnostic system for psychiatric/mental health nurses. *Archives of Psychiatric Nursing*, *1*, 125–131.

Computer programs to support clinical decision making. (1987). *Journal of the American Medical Association*, *258*, 2374–2376.

Copeland, J., Dewey, M., & Griffiths–Jones, H. (1986). A computerized psychiatric diagnostic system and case nomenclature for elderly subjects: GMS and AGECAT. *Psychological Medicine*, *16*, 89–99.

Crosbie, J., & Kelly, G. (1993). A computer-based personalized system of instruction course in applied behavior analysis. *Behavior Research Methods, Instruments & Computers*, *25*, 366–370.

Diserens, D., Schwartz, M.W., Guenin, M., & Taylor, L.A. (1986). Measuring the problem-solving ability of students and residents by microcomputer. *Journal of Medical Education*, *61*, 461–466.

Elwork, A., & Gutkin, T.B. (1985). The behavioral sciences in the computer age. *Computers in Human Behavior*, *1*, 3–18.

Erdman, H. (1985). The impact of an explanation capability for a computer consultation system. *Methods of Informatics in Medicine*, *24*, 181–191.

Erdman, H. (1987a). A computer consultation program for primary care physicians. Impact of decisionmaking model and explanation capability. *Medical Care*, *25*, S138–S147.

Erdman, H.P. (1987b). A computer consultation program for primary care physicians: Impact of decisionmaking model and explanation capability. *Medical Care*, *25*, 138–147.

Erdman, H.P. (1988). Computer consultation in psychiatry. *Psychiatric Annals*, *18*, 209–216.

Erdman, H.P., Greist, J.H., Gustafson, D.H., Taves, J.E., et al. (1987). Suicide risk prediction by computer interview: A prospective study. *Journal of Clinical Psychiatry*, *48*, 464–467.

Erdman, H.P., Greist, J.H., Klein, M.H., & Jefferson, J.W. (1987). A review of computer diagnosis in psychiatry with special emphasis on DSM-III. *Computers in Human Services*, *2*, 1–11.

Erdman, H.P., Klein, M.H., & Greist, J.H. (1985). Direct patient computer interviewing. *Journal of Consulting & Clinical Psychology*, *53*, 760–773.

Feinberg, M., & Lindsay, R. (1986). Expert systems in psychiatry. *Psychopharmacology Bulletin*, *22*, 311–316.

First, M. (1994). Computer-assisted assessment of DSM-III-R diagnoses. *Psychiatric Annals*, *24*, 25–29.

First, M., Opler, L., Hamilton, R., Linder, J., Linfield, L., Silver, J., Toshav, N., Kahn, D., williams, J., & Spitzer, R. (1993). Evaluation in an inpatient setting of DTREE, a computer-assisted diagnostic assessment procedure. *Comprehensive Psychiatry*, *34*, 171–175.

Fisher, L., Johnson, T., Porter, D., Bleich, H., & Slack, W. (1977). Collection of a clean voided urine speciment: A comparison among spoken, written, and computer-based instructions. *American Journal of Public Health*, *67*, 640–644.

French, C., & Beaumont, J. (1987). The reaction of psychiatric patients to computerized assessment. *British Journal of Clinical Psychology*, *26*(Pt. 4), 267–278.

Gelernter, D., & Gelernter, J. (1986). Expert systems and diagnostic monitors in psychiatry. *Medical Informatics*, *11*, 23–28.

Gitlow, S., & Tanner, T. (1991). Psychopharmacology education software. The first of a series. *Proceedings of the Annual Symposium on Computer Applications in Medical Care* (pp. 945–946).

Greist, J.H. (1987). Aids to diagnostic decisionmaking. *Medical Care*, *25*, 153–156.

Hardt, S., & MacFadden, D. (1987). Computer assisted psychiatric diagnosis: Experiments in software design. *Computers in Biology and Medicine*, *17*, 229–237.

Hedlund, J.L., & Vieweg, B.W. (1987). Computer generated diagnosis. In *Issues in Diagnostic Research* (pp. x, 349). New York: Pergamon Press.

Hedlund, J.L., Vieweg, B.W., & Cho, D.W. (1985). Mental health computing in the 1980s: II. Clinical applications. *Computers in Human Services*, *1*, 1–31.

Hedlund, J.L., Vieweg, B.W., & Cho, D.W. (1987). Computer consultation for emotional crises: An expert system for "non-experts." *Computers in Human Behavior*, *3*, 109–127.

Horowitz, G., Jackson, J., & Bleich, H. (1983). PaperChase. Self-service bibliographic retrieval. *Journal of the American Medical Association*, *250*, 2494–2499.

Hrabal, A., & Ticha, M. (1991). Prospects of expert systems in psychiatrus diagnostics. *Acta Universitatis Palackianae Olomucensis Facultatis Medicus*, *129*, 229–233.

Hyler, S.E., & Bujold, A.E. (1994). Computers and psychiatric education: The "Taxi Driver" mental status examination. *Psychiatric Annals*, *24*, 13–19.

Inderbitzin, L., Tadros, A., & Swofford, C. (1993). EM-PSYCH: A training program scheduling database. *Journal of Medical Systems*, *17*, 97–102.

Johri, S., & Guha, S. (1991) Set-covering diagnostic expert system for psychiatric disorders: The third world context. *Computer Methods and Programs in Biomedicine*, *34*, 1–7.

Kohri, S. (1993). On a probabilistic set covering model for diagnosing psychiatric disorders. *Journal of the Academy of Hospital Administration*, *5*, 13–17.

Lacey, D. (1993). Nurses' attitudes towards computerization: A review of the literature. *Journal of Nursing Management*, *1*, 239–243.

Levitan, K.B., & Willis, E.A. (1985). Barriers to practitioners' use of information technology utilization: A discussion and results of a study. *Journal of Psychotherapy & the Family*, *1*, 21–35.

Levitan, K.B., Willis, E.A., & Vogelgesang, J. (1985). Microcomputers and the individual practitioner: A review of the literature in psychology and psychiatry. *Computers in Human Services*, *1*, 65–84.

Lewis, G. (1992). Computerized assessments of psychiatric disorder using PROQSY: Discussion paper. *Journal of the Royal Society of Medicine*, *85*, 403–406.

Lewis, G., Pelosi, A., Glover, E., Wilkinson, G., Stansfeld, S., Williams, P., & Shepherd, M. (1988). The development of a computerized assessment for minor psychiatric disorder. *Psychology Medicine*, *18*, 737–745.

Locke, S., Kowaloff, H., Hoff, R., Safran, C., Popovsky, M., Cotton, D., Finkelstein, D., Page, P., & Slack, W. (1992). Computer-based interview for screening blood donors for risk of HIV transmission. *Journal American Medical Association*, *268*, 1301–1305.

Lundsgaarde, H.P. (1987). Evaluating medical expert systems. *Social Science & Medicine*, *24*, 805–819.

Mackenzie, T., Popkin, M., & Callies, A. (1985). Pedagogic applications of a computerized data base. *General Hospital Psychiatry*, *7*, 125–127.

Mathisen, K., Evans, F., & Meyers, K. (1987). Evaluation of a computerized version of the Diagnostic Interview Schedule. *Hospital and Community Psychiatry*, *38*, 1311–1315.

Maurer, K., Biehl, K., Kuhner, C., & Loffler, W. (1989). On the way to expert systems. Comparing DSM-III computer diagnoses with CATEGO (ICD) diagnoses in depressive and schizophrenic patients. *European Archives of Psychiatry and Neurological Sciences, 239*, 127–132.

Miller, M. (1994). A critical review of principles involved in quality mental health software available from computer bulletin board systems (BBSs). *Psychiatric Annals*, *24*, 9–12.

Miller, M. (1987). A program for evaluating depression. *MD Computing*, *4*, 49–54, 63.

Miller, R. (1987). Computer-based diagnostic decisionmaking. *Medical Care*, *25*, S148–S152.

Molnar, G., & Feeney, M. (1985). Computer-assisted review of antipsychotics on acute care units. *QRB Quality Review Bulletin*, *11*, 271–274.

Morelli, R., Bronzino, J., & Goethe, J. (1987). Expert systems in psychiatry. A review. *Journal Medical Systems*, *11*, 157–168.

Moreno, H., & Plant, R. (1993). A prototype decision support system for diferential diagnosis of psychotic, mood, and organic mental disorders. *Medical Decision Making, 13*, 43–48.

Morss, S., Lenert, L., & Faustman, W. (1993). The side effects of antipsychotic drugs and patients' quality of life: Patient education and preference assessment with computers and multimedia. *Proceedings of the Annual Symposium on Computer Applications in Medical Care* (pp. 17–21).

Murphy, J.W., & Pardeck, J.T. (1988). Expert systems as an adjunct to clinical practice: A critique. *Child Psychiatry Quarterly*, *21*, 137–147.

Overby, M. (1987). Psyxpert: An expert system prototype for aiding psychiatrists in the diagnosis of psychotic disorders. *Computers in Biology and Medicine, 17*, 383–393.

Paperny, D., Aono, J., Lehman, R., Hammar, S., & Risser, J. (1990). Computer-assisted detection and intervention in adolescent high-risk health behaviors. *Journal of Pediatrics, 116*, 456–462.

Petty, L.C., Lynch, E.A., & Rosen, E.F. (1993). A ToolBook computer program to develop course objectives and assessment measures. *Behavior Research Methods, Instruments & Computers*, *25*.

Plugge, L., Verhey, F., & Jolles, J. (1990). A desktop expert system for the differential diagnosis of dementia. An evaluation study. *International Journal of Technology Assessment in Health Care*, *6*, 147–156.

Politser, P., Gastfriend, D., Bakin, D., & Nguyen, L. (1987). An intelligent display system for psychiatric education in primary care. *Medical Care, 25*, S123–S137.

Powsner, S., & Byck, R. (1989). The "Electric Resident," a computer system for training psychiatry residents. *Academic Medicine, 64*, 485.

Powsner, S., & Miller, P. (1992). Automated online transition from the medical record to the psychiatric literature. *Methods of Inference in Medicine, 31*, 169–174.

Safran, C., Porter, D., Rury, C., Herrmann, F., Lightfoot, J., Underhill, L., Bleich, H., & Slack, W. (1990). ClinQuery: Searching a large clinical database. *MD Computing, 7*, 144–153.

Safran, C., Slack, W., & Bleich, H. (1989). Role of computing in patient care in two hospitals. *MD Computing, 6*, 141–148.

Schneider, D.J., Taylor, E.L., Prater, L.M., & Wright, M.P. (1991). Risk assessment for HIV infection: Validation study of computer-assisted preliminary screen. *AIDS Education & Prevention, 3*.

Schwartz, M.D. (1986). Computers in psychiatric education. *Psychiatric Annals, 18*, 228–235.

Servan–Schreiber, D. (1986). Artificial intelligence and psychiatry. *Journal of Nervous and Mental Disorders, 174*, 191–202.

Sherman, P.S. (1989). A micro-based decision support system for managing aggressive case managment programs for treatment resistant clients. *Computers in Human Services, 4*, 181–190.

Slack, W. (1984). A history of computerized medical interviews. *MD Computing, 1*, 52–59, 68.

Slack, W., & Slack, C. (1972). Patient-computer-dialogue. *N England J Medicine, 286*, 1304–1309.

Slack, W., Hicks, G., Reed, C., & Van Cura, L. (1966). A computer-based medical history system. *N England J Medicine, 274*, 194–198.

Slack, W., Safran, C., Kowaloff, H., Pearce, J., & Delbanco, T. (1995). A computer-administered health screening interview for hospital personnel. *MD Computing, 12*, 25–30.

Stein, D. (1994). Expert systems for psychiatric pharmacotherapy. *Psychiatric Annals, 24*, 37–41.

Stout, C.E. (1988). Personal computer software for teaching differential psychodiagnostics. *Behavior Research Methods, Instruments, & Computers, 20*, 106–107.

Strain, J.J., Fulop, G., Strain, J.J., Hammer, J.S., et al. (1986). An approach to psychiatric teaching: The evaluation of a computer enhanced teaching program. *Journal of Psychiatric Education, 10*, 178–186.

Strain, J., Hammer, J., Lewin, C., Mayou, R., Huyse, F., Lyons, J., & Easton, M. (1990). The evolution of a literature search schema for consultation/liaison psychiatry: The database and its computerization. *General Hospital Psychiatry, 12*, 1–53.

Strain, J., Norvell, C., Strain, J., Mueenuddin, T., & Strain, J. (1985). A minicomputer approach to consultation-liaison data basing: Pedagog-Admin-CLINFO. *General Hospital Psychiatry, 7*, 113–118.

Werner, G. (1987). Methuselah—an expert system for diagnosis in geriatric psychiatry. *Computers in Biomedical Research, 20*, 477–488.

Wilkinson, G., & Markus, A. (1989a). PROQSY: A computerised technique for psychiatric case identification in general practice. *British Journal Psychiatry, 154*, 378–382.

Wilkinson, G., & Markus, A. (1989b). Validation of a computerized assessment (PROQSY) of minor psychological morbidity by relative operating characteristic analysis using a single GP's assessments as criterion measures. *Psychological Medicine*, *19*, 225–231.

Appendix

Table of Contents

This Appendix is organized as follows:

1. Introduction

This appendix was conceived as a thorough but rather specific listing of computer-based resources for those concerned with mental health education. These resources include multimedia programs available to individual users (generally on CD-ROM or videodisk), electronic references (bibliographic, pharmaceutical, medical, and various other assorted references), teaching software, Internet resources (electronic conferences, interest groups, data and software repositories), and printed directories or trade publications. This Appendix is not intended to be a comprehensive listing of all available resources, but rather is representative of those resources.

With regard to Internet listings, only those sites and resources deemed to offer a substantial number of relevant services of listings have been included, so that this Appendix might offer the reader fast and satisfying access to core resources. All of the Internet resources listed herein will also lead the interested reader to other useful sites. Because Internet addresses and offerings tend to change rapidly and without notice, many of the Internet resources listed in this Appendix refer instead to comprehensive on-line lists maintained dynamically by other experts. In this way, these Appendix entries will not become outdated as rapidly, because the addresses of the master lists should be more persistent than their contents.

These listings were accurate and verified as of February 1995. The authors have made reasonable efforts to provide correct information but cannot be responsible for the accuracy of the information presented.

1.1 Data Collection

This listing was compiled by searching through several published catalogs and directories of multimedia software, gleaning tidbits of information from specialized catalogs and periodicals, and by personally "surfing" the Internet via keywords and promising threads and links from particularly rich Internet sites, many of which are listed below as Major Sources of Information.

1.2 Major Sources of Information

The short list of resources that follows may also be particularly useful to the reader interested in doing his or her own research.

1.2.1 Major Printed Catalogs and Directories Used as Resources

- *SilverPlatter Directory, A Directory of Electronic Information Products*, published by SilverPlatter Information, Inc. SilverPlatter specializes in the sale of reference data bases on CD-ROM (1994)
- Scott Alan Stewart's *1994 Interactive Healthcare Directories* (1994)
- Health Sciences Consortium catalogs of health sciences educational media (1993–1995)

1.2.2 Major Internet Sites Providing Threads/Links

WWW Sites

- *http://kuhttp.cc.ukans.edu/cwis/units/medcntr/Lee/HOMEPAGE.HTML* — The Medical Matrix—Guide to Internet Medical Resources
- *http://www.ashe.miami.edu/ab/medweb.html* — MedWeb: Adam's Guide to Medical Resources on the Internet
- *http://www.cc.emory.edu/WHSCL/medweb.lists.html* — MedWeb: Biomedical Internet Resources
- *http://www.primenet.com/~gwa/med.ed* — The Medical Education Page
- *http://www.realtime.net/~mmjw/* — Specifica: An evolving resource of information and services for people in need

Gopher Sites

- *gopher://bubl.bath.ac.uk* Port 7070 — Bath University Bulletin Board for Libraries (BUBL)
- *gopher://ftp.gac.edu/1/pub/E-mail-archives/fam-med* Port 70 — FAM-MED

1.2.3 Major Resource Lists Found on the Internet

- Gary Malet and Lee Hancock's *The Medical List* (1994)
- J. Alvoeiro's *Subject Specific Resource List in Psychology* (1995)

1.2.4 Major Internet Directories (Sites Listed by Subject)

WWW Sites

- *http://www.ncsa.uiuc.edu/SDG/Software/Mosaic/MetaIndex.* — Internet Resources Meta-Index, from

html   National Center for
                                                  Supercomputing
                                                  Applications
                                                  (NCSA)

- *http://home.netscape.com/*   NetScape offers links to
  escapes/internet-directory.html   many major Web
                                                    directories

- *http://www.yahoo.com/*   Yahoo
- *http://galaxy.einet.net/*   EINet Galaxy
- *http://info.cern.ch/hypertext/*   WWW Virtual Library
  DataSources/bySubject/   Subject Catalog
  Overview.html
        <u>Gopher Sites</u>
- *gopher://riceinfo.rice.edu/*   RiceInfo, offers links
  1/Subject/MoreAbout   Port 70   to major gopher
                                                      directories

- *gopher://gopher.tamu.edu/1/.dir/*   TAMU
  subject.dir   Port 70
- *gopher://liberty.uc.wlu.edu/*   Washington and Lee
  1/internet   Port 70   University, offers
                                                     links to major subject
                                                     directories

**1.2.5 Major Internet Search Engines (Search Title and Content by
         Keywords)**

<u>WWW Sites</u>
- *http://home.netscape.com/*   NetScape offers links to
  escapes/internet-search.html   many Web search
                                                     engines

- *http://www.infoseek.com*   InfoSeek
- *http://lycos.cs.cmu.edu*   Lycos
- *http://www.webcrawler.com/*   WebCrawler
<u>Gopher Sites</u>
- *gopher://chico.rice.edu/1/*   RiceInfo, offers links to
  Subject   Port 70   major gopher search
                                                      engines

- *gopher://honor.uc.wlu.edu*   Jughead, Veronica
  Port 1020
<u>Anonymous FTP Sites</u>
- *gopher://liberty.uc.wlu.edu/1/*   Archie
  internet/hytelnet/sitesz/arcøøø
  Port 70
- *telnet://archie.sura.net*   Archie (log in as
                                                     archie)

Listservs, Phonebooks
- *gopher://honor.uc.wlu.edu*
  Port 1020

Washington & Lee
University, offers
links to search engines
for Listserv mailing
lists, institutional
telephone books,
E-mail addresses,
and more

1.3 Format of Internet Listings

When Internet resource addresses are given, they are listed in the Universal Resource Locator format: *method://site.name/filepath*. For example, *gopher://odie.niaid.nih.gov/1/aids* indicates that the site can be accessed via Gopher, the site address is *odie.niaid.nih.gov,* and the directory of interest is */1/aids*. Other access methods include FTP (ftp://), Telnet (telnet://) and WWW (World Wide Web, denoted as http://). E-mail addresses are listed in the standard format: *recipient@site.name* (note no end period). Subscription information for Usenet Newsgroups and Listservers is not listed here, but publications in which this information can be found are noted.

1.4 Terminology

Internet: Used in this context to refer to the global network of computers that provide information services.

E-mail: Electronic mail allows a person to send a private message (sometimes with an embedded file) to another person. Each person has a unique E-mail "address" that identifies the person and the computer at which the person can be found. Addresses are in the form *username@computer.site* and may be quite long, with lengthy multidotted descriptions of where to locate the user's computer.

Mailing List (Maintained by Listservers): Topical discussions are carried out via electronic mail (E-mail), with each person on the mailing list receiving a copy of each message as it is posted. One must specifically "subscribe" to a mailing list.

Usenet Newsgroups: These news groups are similar to mailing lists, but use special software (newsreaders) that keeps track of "threads," or conversational topics. One must specifically "subscribe" to a news group.

Electronic Conference: A real-time interactive dialog among many participants who are connected via the Internet. The conference generally centers around a predetermined topic and is often moderated, with one person granting "the floor" in turn to participants who indicate they have comments.

Forum: This can be a real-time interactive dialog among many participants who are connected via the Internet, or it can be analogous to passers-by writing comments on a posted sheet of paper: one can participate at any time, reading past comments, adding new ones, or replying to specific comments from others. Forums are most often in free-form, question-and-answer format. They are usually broadly topical, as for an interest group, and are wonderful repositories of expert opinions.

Telnet: A mechanism for connecting to another computer as if you were only on a dumb terminal and not really some fancy computer with its own cool icon-driven software. You must use whatever command language is present on that host (Unix, VMS, etc.) to navigate around that system.

Bulletin Board (BBS): A computer site that provides resources (software, forums, and other services) to the general public. Bulletin boards are traditionally accessible via direct dial-up by modem, but many are also available via telnet connections.

FTP: This is just what is name ("File Transfer Protocol") implies: an efficient way of transferring files between computers. Many sites have "Anonymous FTP" access, which means that certain files are available to the general public. FTP must be used for the file transfer on both your computer and at the remote site, and requires an Internet connection (some sites will optionally deliver these files by E-mail instead).

Gopher: A user-friendly, menu-driven (or icon-driven) way to explore the Internet. Certain sites will support Gopher connections that make file transfers and computer-hopping a breeze. Gopher does not display graphic files.

World Wide Web (WWW): Mosaic and Netscape are the best-known software tools for exploring WWW resources, but there are also other Web browsers. The attraction of WWW is its ability to present graphic information (The Rolling Stones gave a live concert over WWW), and to navigate the Internet using a point-and-click interface. While this is at the moment a fairly slow way to explore the Internet (due to the amount of information that must be transferred to your computer to support the interface), further development will ensure the supremacy of WWW.

2. Catalogs and Directories

These are general catalogs and directories that contain many listings for computer-based education and computerized resources for the mental health professional and patient.

<u>1994 Interactive Healthcare Directory: Healthcare CAI Directory</u>
<u>1994 Interactive Healthcare Directory: Healthcare CD-ROM/CD-i</u>
<u>Directory</u>

These are comprehensive catalogs of computer-assisted instruction and CD-ROMs that run on either IBM or Macintosh computers. Many of the listings in this Appendix were drawn from this directory.

Scott Alan Stewart, ED., Stewart Publishing, Inc., 6471 Merritt Court, Alexandria, VA 22312, 703-354-8155

<u>Health Sciences Consortium</u> (HSC)

HSC is a consortium of 1327 medical schols, nursing schools, hospitals, professional organizations, dental schools, and other organizations. Its goal is to share peer-reviewed instructional materials developed by faculty and professionals. Institutional members get a 30% discount on purchases and other benefits.

Consortium focus is on instructional material (videotape, computer-based programs, interactive videodisk, and traditional media) in medicine, nursing, allied health professions, dentistry, the behavioral sciences/psychology/counseling, patient education, and hospital personnel training. Catalogs of especial interest from the Consortium include: Medical, Nursing, Allied Health, Patient Education, and Computer-Based Education.

Health Sciences Consortium, 201 Silver Cedar Court, Chapel Hill, NC 27514-1517, 919-942-8731

Selected Items

<u>Computer-Aided Instruction</u>

AIDS Vignettes for Physicians

Decision-making situations, managing and coping with AIDS

AIDS Vignettes for Nurses

Decision-making situations, managing and coping with AIDS

Pharmacology

Drug interactions

MED-CAPS Manager (Medical Computer-Assisted Problem Solving)

Course manager for instructional modules, tracks student progress. Modules written by independent medical authors, and include Adolescent Medicine Problems, Psychiatry Problems, as well as modules in other medical specialties.

NURS-CAPS (Nursing Computer-Assisted Problem Solving)

Course manager for instructional modules, tracks student progress. Modules written by independent nursing authors. Sample modules include Alzheimer's Disease and the Family, Older Adults in Surgical Settings, and The Childbearing Family Experiencing Complications.

Medical Terminology Made Easy

Learn medical terminology, plus digitized pronunciation

Erectile Dysfunction Support System
Evaluation and treatment for impotence
Neuropathology Test and Review
Seven tests, each with 20 questions
Interactive Education for the Healthcare Professional
Three modules are available in this series: Human Diseases,
The Laboratory in Pharmacology, and Drug Interactions.
Interactive Videodisk (note that specific software and videodisk
hardware are required)
Difficult Diagnostic Decisions
Instruction and simulations with real patients
Psychiatric Interview Series
Instruction and simulation with real patient
*Developmental and Genetic Aspects of Clefting Disorders: A
Clinical Approach*
Includes information on genetic evaluation and counseling
Medi-Sim®/Williams & Wilkins Electronic Media
Software, video, and multimedia for healthcare education.
AWHONN, ONS, AACN, and ANA continuing education credit
available.
Medi-Sim®/Williams & Wilkins Electronic Media, 428 East Preston
Street, Baltimore, MD 21202-3993, 800-527-5597/410-528-4000
Selected Items
Mental Health Computer Aided Instruction
Clinical simulations in psychiatric and mental health nursing,
with interactive tutorials
Pain Management Computer-Aided Instruction
Oncology nursing
Pharmacology Computer-Aided Instruction
Clinical simulations in psychiatric nursing pharmacology
Reference
Medical terminology teaching programs
Stedman's Electronic Medical Dictionary
MedSpeak (medical dictionary with digitized pronunciation)

3. References

The following items should be of special use for either the mental health
professional or the graduate student. They include Internet sites and
listings of general interest to those in the mental health field, medical
software, electronic bibliographic resources, pharmaceutical references,
programs adaptable for patient education, traditional medical references
(Merck Manual, medical dictionaries) in electronic forms, and physician
directories.

3.1 Interent Resources

3.1.1 Conferences, Resource Lists

AIDS and HIV—Information and Resources

http://www.ircam.fr/solidarites/sida/index-e.html

Compilation of information from HIVNET Paris, CRIPS, INSERM, National Library of Medicine, and other sources, Includes calendars of conferences; lists of U.S. and French Internet resources, including links to NIH, WHO, CDC; prevention guides; news and information from organizations such as ACTUP, HIVNET, PWA; information and articles on nursing and available treatments; links to bibliographic data bases such as AIDSLINE, CRISP, MEDLINE, and TOXNET; and access to ArtAIDS, a digital art collaborative. Maintained by Michael Fingerhut (mf@ircam.fr) of the Centre Georges Pompidou, Paris.

AskERIC

gopher://ericir.syr.edu   Port: 70

Information about ERIC (Educational Resources Information Center), the largest education data base in the world containing more than 800,000 records of journal articles, research reports, curriculum and teaching guides, conference papers, and books. Each year, approximately 30,000 new records are added to this free, public-access data base sponsored by the Office of Educational Research and Improvement at the U.S. Department of Education.

Bath University Bulletin Board for Libraries (BUBL)

gopher://bubl.bath.ac.uk   Port: 7070

http://www.bubl.bath.ac.uk/BUBL/home.html

In the *Subject Tree* section at this site, there are sections for both *Psychology* and *Psychiatry*. The *Psychiatry* section (*/1/Link/Tree/Psychiatry*) and *Psychology* (*/1/Link/Tree/Psychology*) section have a wide selection of information.

Selected Items From Psychiatry:

- Psychiatry Software, primarily psychological testing, and assessment software
- PsyComNet Conference Transcripts, see InterPsych description elsewhere in this section
- InterPsych Newsletter, see InterPsych description elsewhere in this section
- Primer for Mental Health Professionals, an orientation guide to the Interent

Selected Items From Psychology:

- Subject Specific Resource List in Psychology
- Link to ERIC Clearinghouse for Testing and Assessment

- Psyc-couns, mailing list for students and researchers in counseling psychology
- PSYCGRAD project, forum for psychology graduate students

CANCERNET Information

gopher://gopher.nih.gov/1/clin/cancernet port 70

Includes access to CANCERLIT citations/abstracts, *Physician Data Query* (available also in Spanish) regarding current clinical information, information about rehabilitation, and other supportive care information.

College and University Home Pages—Alphabetical Listing

http://www.mit.edu:8001/people/cdemello/univ.html

List of 1,000 colleges and universities that have World Wide Web home pages that then give access to that university's phone books, departmental Web servers, and other resources. About 570 of the entries are United States, and the rest foreign. List maintained by Christina DeMello (cdemello@mit.edu).

FAM-MED

gopher://ftp.gac.edu/1/pub/E-mail-archives/fam-med
port 70

Lists of resources for computers in family medicine, with many items of interest to mental health professionals. Maintained by Paul Kleeberg, M.D. at Gustavus Adolphus College (Paul@GAC.edu).

Selected Items

- Lists of medically related electronic bulletin boards (*Black Bag Medical BBS* listing)
- Lists of Federal electronic bulletin boards
- Lists of Internet medical discussion lists
- Lists of clinical medicine Internet resources (*The Medical List*)
- Bibliographies of medical informatics, health policy, and medical education
- Windows hypertext program for browsing Internet health resources (*Healthmatrix*)
- Data base of conferences (postings from FPEN-C, Family Physicians/Electronic Network)
- Software reviews that appeared in *Journal of Family Practice*

GNN Medical Table of Contents

http://nearnet.gnn.com/wic/med.toc.html

WWW links to various Internet health resources. Includes sections on mental health, safer sex, and medical education, along with several news groups.

InterPsych

http://www.psych.med.umich.edu/web/intpsych/

Site is focused on interdisciplinary psychopathology, with 7,000 members in 40 countries from anthropology, computer science, neuroscience, nursing, pharmacology, philosophy, psychiatry, psychology, and sociology. A nonprofit, voluntary organization, it was founded in 1994 by Ian Pitchford at U. Sheffield, UK. *PsyComNet*, which hosts real-time conferences, was founded by Ivan Goldberg in 1985 and merged into *InterPsych* in 1994. For more information, contact Ivan Goldberg, M.D., at Columbia University College of Physicians and Surgeons (psydoc@netcom.com).

Conents of InterPsych:

Mailing Lists (some are limited to professionals)

- Attachment
- Child psychiatry
- Clinical psychophysiology
- Depression
- Emergency psychiatry
- Forensic psychiatry
- Helplessness
- Managed behavioral healthcare
- Psy-art
- Psy-language
- Psych current issues
- Psychiatry
- Psychiatry assessment
- Psychiatry resources
- Psychoanalysis
- Psychopharmacology
- Psychotherapy
- Rural care
- Transcultural psychology
- Traumatic stress

Real-Time Forums

Forums (electronic conferences and "Staff Lounge") take place once per week at designated time that maximizes international participation.

Electronic Conference

Published paper is selected and presented in abstract form. Conference is a moderated interactive discussion of paper and ideas derived from it.

Staff Lounge

Informal discussions about cases, particular problems Professional consultation resource.

InterPsych Virtual Campus

World Wide Web site for mental health education is under construction. Projected opening date mid-1995 to mid-1996. May offer CME credits.

Examples of Virtual Campus planned resources

- Data bases
- Electronic library
- Clinical and research section
- Patient and relatives support
- Book reviews
- Electronic conferences

InterPsych Newsletter

Monthly free publication to *InterPsych* members. Includes current events in mental health, new Internet mental health resources, list of conferences (physical and electronic), employment listings, updates from electronic conferences, and *InterPsych*. For more information contact Sean Sullivan, editor-in-chief (ssulliva@opal.tufts.edu).

Major Computing Services

Compuserve, Prodigy, and America On Line all have various health-related topics, both for dissemination of health-related information to professionals and the general public, as well as for support groups.

Selected Compuserve Items

- PsycINFO, access to Psychological Abstracts bibliographic data base
- PaperChase™, access to Medline bibliographic data base
- AMIA Medical Forum, American Medical Informatics Association
- Cancer Forum

Selected AOL Items

- Issues in Mental Health
- National Alliance for the Mentally Ill
- National Multiple Sclerosis Society
- Better Health and Medical Forum
- Several forums on specific mental disorders, medications, life stresses, abuse, etc. Software libraries provide information and suggest resources.

Selected Prodigy Items

- Health and Lifestyles Board: About painc attacks
- Health and Lifestyles Board: Antidepressants
- Medical Support Board: AIDS
- Medical Support Board: Cancer

MedWeb: Adam's Guide to Medical Resources on the Internet
http://www.ashe.miami.edu/ab/medweb.html

Comprehensive list that includes sections on medical education, informatics, patient education/support groups, Listservs, sites categorized by medical specialty, and links to
major government sites such as NIH, NLM, CDC. Maintained by Adam R. Block (Adam.R.Block@students.
miami.edu).

MedWeb: Biomedical Internet Resources
http://www.cc.emory.edu/WHSCL/medweb.lists.html

Extensive links to resources such as those in sections entitled
Medical Centers and Medical Schools; Mental Health,
Psychiatry, Psychology; and Lists of Internet Resources.
Also includes Listservs and special interest sections such
as AIDS and Alternative Medicine. Maintained by Steve
Foote (libsf@web.cc.emory.edu).

National Institutes of Health (NIH)
gopher://gopher.nih.gov   port 70
http://www.nih.gov

Mainly administrative information, including, grants, E-
mail and telephone directories, and links various NIH
institutions.

National Institute of Allergy and Infectious Disease (NIAID)
gopher://odie.niaid.nih.gov/1/aids   port 70

AIDS information from national organizations (government
and nongovernment) regarding statistics, clinical guidelines, general information, study recruitment, and links to
other resources. One sample item is *UCSF FOCUS: a
Guide to Research and Counseling*

National Institutes of Mental Health (NIMH)
gopher://gopher.nimh.nih.gov   port 70
ftp://ftp.nimh.nih.gov

Calendar of events, research reports, NIMH publications,
program announcements, other links.

National Library of Medicine (NLM)
gopher://gopher.nlm.nih.gov   port 70
http://www.nlm.nih.gov

Applications for and access to online data bases compiled by
NLM (in particular, *Medline*), along with *Grateful Med*
bibliographic software to search these data bases; lists
of journal titles indexed in *Index Medicus* and *Medline*;
HSTAT (Health Services/Technology Assessment Text), a
full-text data base of clinical practice guidelines, quick-
reference guides for clinicians, and consumer brochures

(also available via telnet and FTP); and various resource
lists and biblioigraphies, including a Health Hotline list of
800-numbers of organizations providing information and/
or support for health-related problems.

Natural Medicine, Complementary Health Care, and Alternative
Therapies

http:///WWW.teleport.com:80/~amrta

Sponsored by Alchemical Medicine Research and Teaching
Association, to provide information regarding various
forms of alternative medicine: mind/body therapy, chiro-
practic, homeopathy, acupuncture, Chinese herbal medicine, and more.

Selected Items

- PARACELSUS, a mailing list limited to health care professionals in both "conventional" and alternative
fields
- IBIS, "Interactive BodyMind Information System," a
sort of Merck Manual for alternative medicine
- Lists of Internet resources, newsgroups, and mailing lists

Psychology/Psychiatry Resources

gopher://una.hh.lib.umich.edu/1/inetdirsstacks   *port 70*

This is a list of electronic discussion lists, forums, journals,
newsletters, and Usenet newsgroups as of January 1994. It
was compiled by Paul Fehrmann and is part of the Directory
of Scholarly Electronic Conferences from Kent State
University Libraries.

Selected Items

- ADDICT-L, research and information on nondrug, non-
alcohol addictions
- APSSCNET, forum for American Psychological Society
Student Caucus
- BEHAVIOR, behavioral disorders
- DIV28, psychopharmacology
- FAMILYSCI, family studies
- MACPSYCH, discussion and software archive for psy-
chologists using the Macintosh in research and teaching
- PSYC, refereed electronic journal Psycholoquy spon-
sored by American Psychological Association
- PSYCGRAD, for psychology graduate students
- PSYCH-EXPTS, discussion and software for experiment
generation for teaching and research
- PSYCHIATRY, integrates biomedical and psychodyna-
mic approaches to psychiatry and abnormal psychology
- SCHIZ-L, schizophrenia research
- sci.med.psychobiology, psychiatry, and psychobiology

- SCR-L, study of cognitive rehabilitation from traumatic brain injuries
- SLFHLP-L, self-help/mutual aid discussion
- TIPS, teaching of psychology

Subject Specific Resource List in Psychology

gopher://bubl.bath.ac.uk/1/Link/Tree/Psychology *port 7070*

Large list of E-mail and discussion lists, Usenet newsgroups, Psychology libraries and departments offering Internet access, and lists of other interesting sites and resources, for example software archives, many government sites and national organizations, and Harvard University Press and Cambridge University Press. Compiled by J. Alvoeiro (J.Alvoeiro@psychology.hull.ac.uk).

Selected Items

- VIRTPSY, virtual reality psychology
- EUITLIST, educational uses of information technology
- SCR-L, study of cognitive rehabilitation
- ACSOFT-L, academic software development
- FAMCOMM, marital/family and relational communcation
- PSYCGRAD, psychology graduate students discussion group
- TECGRP, technology and social behavior group
- HYPERMED, biomedical hypermedia instructional design

The Medical List

gopher://una.hh.lib.umich.edu/1/inetdirsstacks *port 70*

This is a comprehensive list of Internet medical resources for both professionals and the general public. It includes lists of mailing lists, FTP, Gopher, WWW, and WAIS resources, Usenet newsgroups, BBSs, and electronic journals, as well as some institutional E-mail addresses. It is not limited to mental health, but has many items of interest to mental health professionals, and also includes detailed instructions on how to subscribe to mailing lists, access FTP sites, and other tidbits for the novice. It was compiled by Dr. Gary Malet and Lee Hancock of Healthtel Corp. Many sites listed elsewhere in this Appendix were drawn from this list.

Selected Items

- ADDICT-L, scholarly mailing list for discussions of non-alcohol/nondrug addiction (e.g., sexual, eating, etc.)
- BEHAVIOR, behavioral and emotional disorders in children
- HMATRIX-L, discussion list for on-line health resources

- INFO-AIDS, information and discussion about AIDS
- MEDFORUM, medical student forum
- PSYCHIATRY, unmoderated forum for psychiatry and abnormal psychology
- SCHIZOPH, unmoderated forum schizophrenia information exchange
- SNURSE-L, student nurse discussion list
- STUTT-L, research and clinical practice on stuttering
- TRNSPLNT, discussion list for organ transplant recipients
- Black Bag Medical BBS, list of over 400 medical, fire/ EMS psychology, science, recovery, AIDS, and disABILITY related bulletin board systems.

The Medical Matrix—Guide to Internet Medical Resources
http://kuhttp.cc.ukans.edu/cwis/units/medcntr/Lee/ HOMEPAGE.HTML

This is a WWW presentation of many of the sites and resources found in The Medical List, accessible via point-and-click interface. However, there are many offerings not found in The Medical List, for example sections on Medical Education, and Patient Education and Support. This is an excellent and comprehensive resource. Maintained by Gary Malet, Lee Hancock, and Robert King as a project of the Internet Working Group of the American Medical Informatics Association

U.S. Department of Education (DE)
gopher://gopher.ed.gov   port 70

The Office of Educational Research and Improvement provides *ERIC*, an educational data base of 800,000 citations that are managed via special-interest clearinghouses (e.g., higher education). See *AskERIC* listing in this Appendix for information specific to *ERIC*.

3.1.2 Medical Software

Macintosh Medical Software, U. Michigan
gopher://gopher.archive.umich.edu/1/mac/misc/medical port 7055

Variety of software, graphics, and courseware useful to medical professionals in all areas. List below only highlights selections of particular interest to mental health. Questions, problems, and comments regarding archive should be addressed to med.archivist@umich.edu.

Selected Items

- Fundamentals of pharmacology

- Alcohol Withdrawal Syndrome
- List of health science related resources, including DOS medical archives
- List of medical, fire/EMS, science, recovery, AIDS, and disABILITY related bulletin board systems (*Black Bag Medical BBS* list maintained by Dr. Delgrasso, 610-454-7396 (ed@blackbag.com).
- Templates for preparation of NIH grant applications
- Review questions for medical exams
- HIV and AIDS transmission and disease progression
- Photographic album of AIDS issues

Medical Education Software Repository

ftp://ftp.uci.edu/med-ed   anonymous FTP

Large resource for MS-DOS software (little Macintosh software), also includes health newsletters, information on Chronic Fatigue Syndrome and Multiple Sclerosis. Maintained by Steve Clancy, M.L.S. (slclany@uci.edu) and Albert Saisho, M.D. (saisho@uci.edu) at the University of California Irvine.

Selected Items

- APECS, demo of Advanced Patient Education Computer System, a patient-controlled graphical presentation of surgical procedures
- BRAINIAC, neuroanatomy atlas
- ESIE, Expert Systems Inference Engine, development tool for expert systems
- EXPERGEN, "learns" rules to generate expert systems
- LITEVAL, aid to critically evaluate statistical results in literature
- MD003I, undergraduate curriculum for teaching medical informatics to medical and nursing students
- MEDTUTOR, medical terminology
- MMGDEMO and MMGDEMO2, demos of graphical patient eduction program for back pain, carpal tunnel surgery, knee surgery
- PC-QUIZZER, development tool for computer-based training
- PSYCAL, PSYchiatry Computer-Assisted Learning, simulations of five psychiatric disorders
- PSYMED, quick-reference guide to psychotropic medicines
- QUIZMAKER, development tool for multimedia quizzes
- ZOOM, development tool for hypertext educational software

Mental Health Software, Indiana University–Purdue University
at Indianapolis (IUPUI)
  ftp://FTP.IUPUI.EDU/pub/psychiatry   *anonymous FTP*
  Large collection of software. Descriptions of software are
    listed in
  gopher://bubl.bath.ac.uk/1/Link/Tree/Psychiatry/PsychiGen
  Port: 7070
  Selected Items
  • Behavior Mod education
  • Computer-Assisted Learning about psychiatry
  • Psychotropic Drug Education
  • Description of Posttraumatic Stress Disorder
  • Suicide Prevention Triangle
  • Neuroanatomy Game
Collection maintained by Marvin Miller, M.D.

3.2 Bibliographic Resources

3.2.1 Publishers of Specialized Bibliographic Data Bases
  Certain vendors offer search engines and distributions on CD-
    ROM for IBM or Mac personal computers, or through
    dialup or network services
AIDS Compact Library
  Consolidates several authoritative resources around the
    world, including *Medline, AIDSLINE, AIDSDRUGS*, and
    Bureau of Hygiene and Tropical Diseases AIDS data base.
    Many full text articles. Also includes *AIDS Knowledgebase*
    from San Francisco General Hospital
  Publisher: Macmillan New Media, 124 Mount Auburn
    Street, Cambridge, MA 02138, 800-342-1338/617-661-2955,
    ×135
AIDSLINE
  AIDS literature (journal articles, government reports,
    letters, technical reports, meeting abstracts, monographs,
    dissertations, special publications), 1980–present
  Publisher: U.S. National Library of Medicine, MEDLARS
    Management Section, 8600 Rockville Pike, Bethesda, MD
    20894, 800-638-8480 (E-mail: mms@nlm.nih.gov)
CANCERLIT
  Cancer literature (journal articles, U.S. government reports,
    meeting abstracts, books, dissertations), most recent 5
    years
  Publisher: U.S. National Cancer Institute, International
    Cancer Information Center, Building 82, Room 111,
    Bethesda, MD 20892, 301-496-7406 (also in conjunction

with U.S. National Library of Medicine, MEDLARS
Management Section, 8600 Rockville Pike, Bethesda, MD
20894, 800-638-8480)

CINAHL

Cumulative Index to Nursing and Allied Health (journal
articles, 1983–present

Publisher: CINAHL Information Systems, 1509 Wilson
Terrace, PO Box 871, Glendale, CA 91209-0871, 800-959-
7167, 818-409-8005

ClinPSYC

A subset of *PsycINFO* tailored to clinicians

Publisher: American Psychological Association, PsycINFO
User Services, 750 First Street NE, Washington, DC
20002-4242,   800-374-2722/202-336-5650   (E-mail:
psychinfo@apa.org). Other information is available from
gopher://gopher.apa.org

Current Contents: Clinical Medicine

Weekly listings of tables of contents from 850 journals,
including those in psychiatry

Publisher: Institute for Scientific Information, 3501 Market
Street, Philadelphia, PA 19104, 800-336-4474/215-386-
0100, ×1449

Current Contents: Social & Behavioral Sciences

Weekly listings of tables of contents from 1300 behavioral
science journals

Publisher: Institute for Scientific Information, 3501 Market
Street, Philadelphia, PA 19104, 800-336-4474/215-386-
0100, x1449

Drug Information Full-Text: American Hospital Formulary
Service (AHFS) Drug Information

Commercially available and experimental drugs in the
United States (monographs)

Publisher: American Society of Hospital Pharmacists
(ASHP), 4630 Montgomery Avenue, Bethesda, MD
20814, 301-657-4383

EMBASE

Excerpta Medica

Publisher: Elsevier Science Publishers, PO Box 945, Madison
Square Station, New York, NY 10160

ERIC

Journals and research in education. *Resources in Education*
plus *Current Index to Journals in Education*. 1966–present.
Free public access via dialup or Internet, also available on
CD-ROM from several vendors. Sixteen clearinghouses
compile information pertinent to education, including

higher education, educational management, and the use of technologies in education

Publisher: US Educational Resources Information Center (U.S. Dept. of Education), ERIC Program, 202-219-2289, or the ERIC Clearinghouse on Information & Technology, 800-464-9107 (E-mail: askeric@ericir.syr.edu) or ACCESS ERIC, 800-LET-ERIC (E-mail: acceric@inet.ed.gov)

MEDLINE

Index Medicus, Index to Dental Literature, International Nursing Index (journal articles and monographs), 1966–present. This is probably the primary electronic resource for published medical literature

Information about gaining access to *Medline* (and other NLM data bases) directly from the National Library of Medicine can be obtained from the NLM gopher server (listed elsewhere in this Appendix), or by calling 800-638-8480. There is a charge for data base access. *Grateful Med* is software that helps automate searching on IBM and Macintosh computers and is also available from NLM

Many other third parties offer their own searching software and subscriptions to *Medline*

Publisher: U.S. National Library of Medicine, MEDLARS Management Section, 8600 Rockville Pike, Bethesda, MD 20894, 800-638-8480 (E-mail: mms@nlm.nih.gov)

PsycINFO

Psychology, psychiatry, sociology, anthropology, education, linguistics, and pharmacology (books, chapters, dissertations, journal articles, technical reports), 1967–present

Publisher: American Psychological Association, PsycINFO User Services, 750 First Street NE, Washington, DC 20002-4242, 800-374-2722/202-336-5650 (E-mail: psychinfo@apa.org); other information is available from gopher://gopher.apa.org

PsycLIT

Psychology, behavioral aspects of education, medicine, sociology, law, and management (journal articles since 1974, books and chapters since 1987)

Publisher: American Psychological Association, Psyc-INFO User Services, 750 First Street NE, Washington, DC 20002-4242, 800-374-2722/202-336-5650 (E-mail: psy-chinfo@apa.org); other information is available from gopher://gopher.apa.org

SEDBASE

Meyler's Side Effects of Drugs, full-text articles from *Meyler's Side Effects of Drugs* and *Side Effects of Drugs Annual*, (full-text articles)

Publisher: Elsevier Science Publishers, PO Box 945, Madison Square Station, New York, NY 10160

Social Works Abstracts Plus

Social Work Abstracts (450 journals) and *The Register of Clinical Social Workers* (directory of U.S. social workers, including name, address, education, employment history), 1997–present

Publisher: National Association of Social Workers, Suite 700, 750 First Street NE, Washington, DC 20002 800-638-8799

The Lancet

Complete text of *The Lancet* for the last 5 years, including citations back to 1966

Publisher: Macmillan New Media, 124 Mount Auburn Street, Cambridge, MA 02138, 800-342-1338/617-661-2955, ×135

The (Macmillan) New England Journal of Medicine

Complete text of *The New England Journal of Medicine* for the last 5 years, including citations back to 1966

Publisher: Macmillan New Media, 124 Mount Auburn Street, Cambridge, MA 02138, 800-342-1338/617-661-2955, ×135

3.2.2 Specialized Electronic Bibliographic Reviews

QuickScan Reviews, MedInfo Manager

Sponsored by Albert Einstein College of Medicine and Montefiore Medical Center, *QuickScan Reviews* is a subscription service in which 42 psychiatric and related journals are distilled by medical experts into 15–20 monthly reviews of the most important research in psychiatry. QuickScan Reviews also offers CME credits in AMA Category 1 or AOA Category 2-B

MedInfo Manager is a "databank" that organizes and searches the accumulation of reviews and allows the user to add notes, full text, or generate reprint requests

Publisher: Educational Reviews, Inc., 6801 Cahaba Valley Road, Birmingham, AL 35242-9988, 800-633-4743

3.3 Electronic References

3.3.1 Pharmaceutical Reference on CD-ROM

AskRx

Pharmaceutical reference, by drug or condition, includes prescription writer and patient data base

Publisher: Camdat Corporation, 1111 Bayhill Drive #465, San Bruno, CA 94066, 415-588-5409

DRUGDEX
Drug information
Publisher: MICROMEDEX INC., 600 Grant Street, Denver, CO 80203, 800-525-9083/303-831-1400

DRUG-REAX
Drug interactions
Publisher: MICROMEDEX INC., 600 Grant Street, Denver, CO 80203, 800-525-9083/303-831-1400

PDR Library on CD-ROM
Physician's Desk Reference (PDR); PDR for Nonprescription Drugs; PDR Guide to Drug Interactions, Side Effects, Indications
Available from American Medical Association, 515 North State Street, Chicago, IL 60610, 800-621-8335/312-464-5000

Prescription Drugs——A Pharmacist's Guide
Describes the most widely used prescription drugs, including interesting trivia
Publisher: Quanta Press Inc., 1313 Fifth Street #223A, Minneapolis, MN 55414, 612-379-3956

3.3.2 General Medical References and Directories on CD-ROM

BiblioMed Essential Medical Reference
Combines the *Merck Manual, Stedman's Medical Dictionary*, and *Physicians' GenRx*
Publisher: Healthcare Information Services Inc., 2335 American River Drive, Suite 307, Sacramento, CA 95825, 800-468-1128/916-648-8076

Directory of Physicians in the United States
Searchable full text of the *Directory of Physicians in the United States*
Publisher: American Medical Association, 515 North State Street, Chicago, IL 60610, 800-621-8335/312-464-5000

Electronic DSM-IV
Publisher: American Psychiatric Press, Inc., 1400 K Street, NW, Washington, DC 20005, 800-368-5777/202-682-6268

Health and Medical Care Directory
National Medical Yellow Pages of America, data on more than 1 million American health-related businesses
Publisher: Innotech Inc., 2001 Sheppard Avenue East #118, North York, ONT M2J 4Z7, Canada, 416-492-3838

Health and Psychosocial Instruments CD-ROM (HaPI-CD)
Data on measurement instruments (questionnaires, rating scales, etc.) abstracted from leading journals

Publisher: Behavioral Measurement Database Services, PO Box 110287, Pittsburgh, PA 15232, 412-687-6850

3.3.3 Pocket-Sized Information Managers

There are several pocket-sized information managers, which are calculator-sized computers available with PCMCIA modules (matchbook-sized insertable hardware and software modules) that offer various electronic versions of standard medical references (such as the *PDR*), as well as functionality that is not exclusively related to medical needs (e.g., address books, telecommunications, and many other applications). Some of these modules may be interchangeable between different brands of information managers

Franklin® Desktop Digital Book System

Pocket-sized information manager has matchbook-sized insertable (PCMCIA) "book" modules: *The Merck Manual, Pocket PDR^{TM}, The Medical Letter® Handbook of Adverse Drug Interactions, Harrison's Principles of Internal Medicine Companion Handbook, Washington University Manual of Medical Therapeutics.* Currently available in American Medical Association catalog, 515 North State Street, Chicago, IL 60610, 800-621-8335/312-464-5000

Franklin® MedSpell

Pocket-sized spelling checker. Includes terms from *Stedman's, USP Dictionary of Drug Names*, and *Merriam Webster Dictionary*. User can enter new words as well. Currently available in American Medical Association catalog, 515 North State Street, Chicago, IL 60610, 800-621-8335/312-464-5000

Hewlett–Packard HP 100LX and HP 200LX Palmtop PC

Hewlett–Packard Corporation, 1000 North East Circle Blvd., Corvallis, OR 97330, 503-715-2004

Sharp Wizard

Sharp Corporation, 600 International Parkway, Mount Olive, NJ 07828, 800-321-8877

3.3.4 Patient Education

These are primarily resources for the physician to generate printed take-home information for the patient

Electronic Drug Reference Version 5.0

Drug information from 6 major references, includes information in lay language that can be printed and distributed to patients

Publisher: Clinical Reference Systems Ltd., 7100 E. Belleview Ave #208, Greenwood Village, CO 80111, 800-237-8401/303-220-1661

FYI: Information Printouts for Patients
> Prints out information for patients to take home, including a bibliography and list of national support organizations when applicable
>
> Publisher: p.r.n. medical software, 755 New York Avenue #210, Huntington, NY 11743, 516-424-7777

MedTeach
> Contains ASHP's *Medication Teaching Manual*, plus program to access and author monographs, that can be modified for patient education
>
> Publisher: American Society of Hospital Pharmacists, 4630 Montgomery Avenue, Bethesda, MD 20814, 301-657-4383

4. Educational Resources

These items are of especial interest to the graduate student and mental health professional responsible for or seeking training. They include graduate school, fellowship, and residency data bases; clinical tutorials and simulations; medical terminology tutorials; examination aids; and systems for tracking student progress

4.1 Graduate/Postgraduate Programs

AMA Fellowship & Residency Electronic Interactive Database Access System 1993 (AMA/FREIDA)
> Companion to the printed book *Directory of Graduate Medical Education* to customize search for ideal residency
>
> Publisher: American Medical Association, 515 North State Street, Chicago, IL 60610, 800-621-8335/312-464-5000

Peterson's GRADLINE
> Data base of 28,000 graduate and professional programs in 300 academic disciplines in 1500 colleges and universities in North America, including faculty information
>
> Publisher: Peterson's Publishing Group, PO Box 2123, 202 Carnegie Center, Princeton, NJ 08543, 609-243-9111

The medical Education Page
> *http://www.primenet.com/~gwa/med.ed*
>
> A site of especial interest to medical students, with resources such as AMA Medical Student Section, Erick's Guide to Medical School Admissions, The Princeton Review guide to medical schools, and 1995 ratings for medical schools; however, there are also resources of general professional interest, including links to medical schools, medical centers, and departments, as well as WWW multimedia "medical courses" in many specialties, offering audio, video, and still photography to illustrate diagnostic concepts. Maintained by Gregory Allen at Loma Linda University

4.2 Topical Tutorials

CYBERLOG: Anxiety Disorders
  Tutorial on neurophysiology, clinical picture, and treatment of anxiety
  Publisher: Cardinal Health Systems Inc., 4600 West 77th Street Suite 150, Edina, MN 55435, 800-328-0180/612-835-6941
Death: A Personal Encounter
  To aid in effective counseling, promotes self-awareness about death and one's own personal death
  Publisher: American Journal of Nursing, 555 West 57th Street, New York, NY 10019, 800-223-2282/212-582-8820, ×551
Meeting the Psychological Needs of Critically Ill Clients
  Addresses psychosocial problems of critical care patients
  Publisher: Computerized Educational Systems, PO Box 536905, Orlando, FL 32853, 800-275-1474/407-841-6230
Pharmacology TextStack
  Electronic text of *Pharmacology*, problems and reviews written by Theoharis C. Theoharides of Tufts University
  Publisher: Keyboard Publishing Inc., 482 Norristown Road, Suite 111, Blue Bell, PA 19422, 800-945-4551/610-832-0945
Protecting Patient/Resident Rights
  Game-type format to review patient rights
  Publisher: Computerized Educational Systems, PO Box 536905, Orlando, FL 32853, 800-275-1474/407-841-6230
Therapeutic Patient Communications I and II
  Basics of therapeutic communication techniques, includes simulation
  Publisher: Computerized Educational Systems, PO Box 536905, Orlando, FL 32853, 800-275-1474/407-841-6230
The Therapeutic Counseling Session
  Builds on *Therapeutic Patient Communications I* and *II*, includes simulation
  Publisher: Computerized Educational Systems, PO Box 536905, Orlando, FL 32853, 800-275-1474/407-841-6230
Therapeutic Communication With the Chemically Dependent Client
  Specific techniques to deal with defense mechanisms
  Publisher: Computerized Educational Systems, PO Box 536905, Orlando, FL 32853, 800-275-1474/407-841-6230

4.3 Medical Terminology

Elements of Medical Terminology
  Teaches derivations (roots, prefix, suffix) of medical terminology
  Publisher: Applied MicroSystems Inc., PO Box 832, Roswell, GA 30077, 404-552-9000

Exploring Medical Language: A Student Directed Approach
  Student-directed approach to teaching medical language
  Publisher: NIMCO, 117 Hwy 815–POB 9, Calhoun, KY 42327,
    800-962-6662/502-273-5050
MEDiLEX: A Guide to the Language of Medicine
  Derivations, etymologies, historical context, diagrams
  Publisher: Chariot Software Group, 3659 India St., San Diego, CA
    92103, 800-242-7468/619-298-0202

4.4 Medical Education Support

Education Tracking System
  Maintains continuing medical education information for personnel
  Publisher: Reliant Software Corporation, 2080-B Walsh Avenue,
    Santa Clara, CA 95050, 408-988-0891
METS: Medical Education Tracking System
  Tracks medical student, intern, and resident clinical and nonclinical
    activities
  Publisher: NEAR Computer Systems Inc., 836 Cattell Street,
    Easton, PA 18042, 215-253-0103
Mount Sinai School of Medicine Self-Testing System Version 3.20
  Over 20,000 timed exam questions in the National Board format,
    general and 100 specialties
  Publisher: ILOC Inc., PO Box 232, Granville, OH, 43023, 614-
    587-2658

5. Resources for the Mental Health Patient

The following are items of special interest to mental health patients. They
include listings of support groups, computerized interactive informed
consent, informational guides, and family health publications

5.1 Support Groups

Emotional Support on the Internet
  gopher://bubl.bath.ac.uk/1/Link/Tree/Psychiatry/PsychiGen
  Port: 7070
  http://www.bubl.bath.ac.uk/BUBL/home.html
  This document can be retrieved from the *Psychiatry* data base in
    the Subject Tree of Bath University Bulletin Board for Libraries
    (BUBL)
  This is a list of support groups, not informational repositories, on
    over 150 topics, from sexual addiction to panic, depression,
    infertility, phobias, and trigeminal neuralgia. Compiled by Steve
    Harris (steveha@cix.compulink.co.uk)

Emotional Support: Physical Loss, Chronic Illness, and Bereavement:
A Guide to Internet Resources

gopher://una.hh.lib.umich.edu/1/inetdirsstacks   *port70*
http://asa.ugl.lib.umich.edu/chdocs/support/emotion.html

List of support resources for people with chronic illness, who have
lost a loved one, or who have suffered amputations or other
physical losses. Compiled by Joanne Juhnke and Chris Powell

5.2 Interactive Informed Consent

Shared Decision-Making Programs™

Interactive multimedia videodisk programs for the clinical setting.
Includes general information about particular medical conditions,
with descriptions of the risks and benefits of alternative treat-
ments. Available disks include: *Treating Your Breast Cancer:
The Surgery Decision; Benign Prostatic Hypertrophy: Choosing
Surgical or Nonsurgical Treatment; Treating Your Breast Cancer:
Adjuvant Therapy; Treatment Choices for Low Back Pain;
Treatment Choices for Mild Hypertension; Treatment Choices for
Prostate Cancer; Treatment Choices for Ischemic Heart Disease.*

The Foundation for Informed Medical Decision Making, Inc., P.O.
Box 5457, Hanover, NH 03755, 603-650-1180

RSVP MED Clinical Information Center

Customized computerized patient education and informed consent.
Multimedia presentation incorporates on-screen presentations by
individual institution's physicians and staff members. System will
track a patient's progress through the instructional presentation
and record answers to interactive questions.

RSVP Information, Inc., 14 Story Street, Cambridge, MA 02138,
617-354-6066

5.3 Family Health Publications

While not specific to mental health, these may be useful in educating
those patients with medical-related anxiety or hypochondria; health
and fitness computer programs may be helpful as means of stress
reduction and preventative medicine. For more information about
many of these products, see recent review in *CD-ROM Today*
(Gregor, 1994).

5.3.1 General Health References

Dr. Schueler's Home Medical Advisor Pro

Special features include detailed graphic information of
medical procedures and disease symptoms, with censor
button for the squeamish.

Publisher: Pixel Perfect, 10460 South Tropical Trail, Merritt
Island, FL 32952, 800-788-2099/407-777-5353

Mayo Clinic CD series (Family Health Book, Pharmacist, The
Total Heart, Sports Health and Fitness)
   Publisher: IVI Publishing, 7500 Flying Cloud Drive, Suite
      400, Minneapolis, MN 55344-3739, 800-432-1332/612-996-
      6000
The Family Doctor
   Special features include prescription drug reference guide,
      lists of support groups, and health-related organizations
   Publisher: Creative Multimedia Corporation, 514 NW 11th
      Ave., Suite 203, Portland OR 800-262-7668/503-241-
      4351
Total Health: Body and Mind
   Special feature includes wellness program that assesses level
      of health, including stress management, and recommends
      diet and fitness program. *PharmAssist: The Family Guide
      to Health and Medicine* (see description below) is also
      included, along with *Bodyworks 3.0* (anatomical program),
      and *MasterCook II* (recipe and nutrition manager).
   Publisher: ICS Learning Systems, Scranton, PA, 800-233-
      4191
Health Today
   Includes information on stress, drugs, AIDS, cancer, birth
      defects, depression, suicide, and more
   Publisher: Queue Inc., 338 Commerce Drive, Fairfield, CT
      06430, 800-232-2224/203-335-0906

5.3.2 Pharmaceutical References

Most of the following are illustrated pharmacopoeia that include
   information about class of drug, brand names, generic equi-
   valents, interactions, and side effects.
HealthSoft Complete Guide to Prescription and Non-
Prescription Drugs
   Also includes photographs of drugs for identification
   Publisher: Great Bear Technology, Morago, CA, 800-795-
      4325
Mayo Clinic Family Pharmacist
   Can search to identify drug by color, shape, drug ID number,
      and size
   Publisher: IVI Publishing, 7500 Flying Cloud Drive, Suite
      400, Minneapolis, MN 55344-3739, 800-432-1332/612-996-
      6000
PharmAssist: The Family Guide to Health and Medicine
   Also includes what to do about missed doses
   Publisher: Softkey International, Inc., 1 Athenaeum St.,
      Cambridge, MA 02142 800-227-5609

The Pill Book
Can search for drug information by article, idea, or illustration
Publisher: Compton's NewMedia, 2320 Camino Vida Roble, Carlsbad, CA, 92009 800-216-6116/619-929-2500

5.4 Specific Psychiatric Problems

Specifica: An Evolving Resource of Information and Services for People in Need
http://www.realtime.net/~mmjw/
Particular strength in areas of specific problems in mental health (addiction, Alzheimer's disease, OCD, ADD, bipolar disorder, eating disorders, mood disorders, sexual assault, and others), providing information regarding the problems, support groups, pharmaceutical information, reference citations, data base access, electronic conferences, and information on related disorders. Also offers a section on other medical problems, including AIDS/HIV and Cancer, and descriptions of university programs, electronic journals, and self-help programs. Maintained by Jeanine Wade, Ph.D. (mmjw@bga.com).

Stress Management
Learning to identify causes of stress and to manage it
Publisher: Psychological Psoftware Company, 11127 Carlota Street, San Diego, CA 92129, 619-627-1631

Suicide and Depression
For grades 7–12, discusses adolescent depression and suicide, presents resources for help
Publisher: NIMCO, 117 Hwy 815, POB 9, Calhoun, KY 42327, 800-962-6662/502-273-5050

Weight Control and Eating Disorders: Anorexia and Bulimia
For grades 7–12, describes eating disorders, ways to manage them, and the importance of doing so
Publisher: NIMCO, 117 Hwy 815, POB 9, Calhoun, KY 42327, 800-962-6662/502-273-5050

5.5 Bibliographic Medical References for the Layperson

MDX Health Digest
Consumer health data base in lay terms (magazines, newsletters, newspapers, medical journals)
Publisher: Medical Data Exchange

6. Publications

The following are general (nonmedical, nonelectronic) publications that may be useful resources in researching multimedia hardware and software. Many of them may be available on newsstands.

6.1 Multimedia/CD Magazines

CD-ROM Today
> GP Publications, Inc. 1350 Old Bayshore Highway, Suite 210, Burlingame, CA 94010, 415-696-1661

CD-ROM World
> Meckler Corporation, 11 Ferry Lane West, Westport, CT 06880, 203-226-6967

Instruction Delivery Systems
> Society for Applied Learning Technology, 50 Culpeper Street, Warrenton, VA 22186, 703-347-0055
>
> Bimonthly magazine concerned with the use of technology in education, training, and job performance; good buyer's guide

Inter@ctive Week
> Inter@active Enterprises, 100 Quentin Roosevelt Blvd., Garden City, NY 11530, 516-229-3700
>
> Free publication for qualified applicants

Microsoft Multimedium!
> Affinity Publishing division of Penn Well Publishing Company, PO Box 1950, Tulsa, OK 74101, 918-831-9405

Multimedia Today
> Redgate Communications Corp., 800-779-2062

MULTIMEDIA WORLD
> PC World Communications, Inc., 501 Second St. #600, San Francisco, CA 94107
>
> Subscription Dept. PO Box 58690, Boulder, CO 80323-8690

New Media
> HyperMedia Communications, Inc., PO Box 1771, Riverton, NJ 08077-7371, 609-786-4430

New Media News
> Boston Computer Society, Hypermedia/Optical Disk Publishing Special Interest Group, Building 1400, One Kendall Square, Cambridge, MA 02139, 617-252-0600

6.2 Health and Computing

Healthcare Informatics
> Health Data Analysis, Inc., Box 2830, 2902 Evergreen Parkway, Ste. 100, Evergreen CO 80439, 303-674-2774

InfoCare (Information Strategies for Healthcare Networks)
> Health Data Analysis, Inc., Box 2830, 2902 Evergreen Parkway, Ste. 100, Evergreen CO 80439, 303-674-2774
>
> A regular *Healthcare Informatics* supplement

7. Other Resources

American Medical Informatics Association (AMIA)

This national organization is concerned with computer applications in medicine. A member may be able to offer further assistance with specific questions.

Send mail to amia@camis.stanford.edu

References

SilverPlatter Information, Inc. (1994). *SilverPlatter directory*. Norwood, MA.

Stewart, S.A. (Ed.). (1994). *1994 Interactive healthcare directory: Healthcare CD-ROM/CD-i directory*. Alexandria, VA: Stewart Publishing, Inc.

Stewart, S.A. (Ed.). (1994). *1994 Interactive healthcare directory: Healthcare CAI directory*. Alexandria, VA: Stewart Publishing, Inc.

Health Sciences Consortium. (1993–1995). *Health sciences consortium catalogs (1993–94 medical, 1994–95 nursing, 1993 allied health, patient education, 1995 computer-based education)*.

Malet, G., & Hancock, L. (1994). *The medical list*. Healthtel Corp. (From gopher://una.hh.lib.umich.edu).

Alvoeiro, J. (1995). *Subject specific resource list in psychology*. Kent OH: Kent, State University Libraries. (From gopher://bubl.bath.ac.uk).

Gregor, A. (1994). Rx for home: Personal health and fitness on CD-ROM. *CD-ROM Today*, December, 66–72.

19
Systems for Accessing Knowledge at Point of Care
Kenric W. Hammond

Knowledge Is Vital to Patient Care

High quality, state of the art patient care depends on a host of factors, but an irreplaceable one is assurance that the clinician's storehouse of learning and judgment is continuously refreshed with new knowledge. Knowledge is necessary cognitive "fuel" for clinical decisions, but is perishable once tapped, and has a limited shelf life when stored. The new discoveries and insights that augment established truth require lifelong learning if caregivers are to their serve patients in the best possible way. For optimal benefit, knowledge needs to be present during the patient care encounter. Lack of critical knowledge can stymie the seasoned practitioner and novice alike.

Patient-specific information must accompany domain knowledge in the care setting, and progress in computer-based record systems has been substantial. Likewise, important advances have occurred in storing and managing published clinical knowledge. Integration of these information streams in the clinical information processing environment remains incomplete. To understand the barriers and opportunities involved it will be useful to examine knowledge sources that are potentially valuable in patient care settings and identify ways to integrate them in the task of managing patient care information.

Traditional Approaches to Knowledgeable Patient Care

Health care organizations recognize the value of clinical knowledge in their hiring, credentialing, and continuing education and training programs. Academic medical centers possess extensive libraries and teaching opportunities, and most hospitals provide at least a small medical library and staff support. Nonacademic organizations, outpatient clinics, community mental health centers, and private offices can be relatively know-ledgepoor environments. For them, the chief organizational investment in knowledge maintenance may consist of educational leave and tuition grants to skilled employees, and in-service training for the less specialized. Beyond meeting minimum continuing education hourly requirements, specifics of staying current are pretty much left to practitioners and may only erratically eliminate knowledge gaps. Great variability exists among the strategies practitioners use to find knowledge during patient care encounters. Improving access, and possibly reducing the variation in how knowledge is obtained could have a favorable impact on quality of care. Before discussing technologic advances that may help, let us briefly review typical clinical knowledge management tasks and the tools used to accomplish them.

Fact Finding With Standard References

Looking up a fact is the most frequent clinical knowledge acquisition chore. For this, standard works such as a medical dictionary, the Physician's Desk Reference (PDR) (Arky & Greenberg, 1994), the latest Diagnostic and Statistical Manual of Mental Disorders (DSM) (American Psychiatric Association, 1994), and fact repositories published by the parent health care organization, such as formularies, guidelines for laboratory testing, and policy and procedure manuals, are quite satis-factory and usually near at hand. Often these references are found in common areas set up to serve office clusters. Sharing in this way is economical, but not infrequently the best books have a distressing habit of disappearing unless they are literally chained down. Many clinicians purchase their own reference materials for rapid access in their offices, but at any given time a fair number of these works are likely to be outdated. Finding a fact in a good dictionary is fast, but locating drug information in the PDR can be tedious.

Reviewing Knowledge With Textbooks

Most practitioners keep a standard textbook or two from their field, and possibly a guidebook such as the Washington Manual of Psychiatry (Shader, 1994) to refresh previous learning and to review rarely visited subjects. These sources may provide useful guidance for treatment plan-ning, but retrieving knowledge from texts is slower than with a dictionary, because relevant information is scattered about, necessitating several lookups from an index.

Staying Current With Periodicals

Scholarly and trade journals usually share space with textbooks on the shelf. Periodicals are indispensible sources of new knowledge, but furnish it in smaller portions than textbooks. To supplement current issues clinicians keep photocopies of review articles; but once collected, the material quickly goes out of date. Retrieving knowledge from this reservoir can be a random exercise in associative memory. Alternatives include keeping several years of journals on shelves and developing a reprint filing system. Incompleteness and erratic cataloging plague all but the most assiduous reprint collectors.

Exploring Knowledge in the Library

When it is acceptable to defer finding a fact, a good medical library is an excellent place to browse current literature and explore conceptual connections. This is a luxury. Most clinicians are too busy taking care of patients to conduct knowledge exploration in the workplace, let alone go to a library as often as they would like, especially when the library is located elsewhere. This is frustrating because patients often present situations where exploration of the literature could enrich a clinical decision.

Knowledge Access Via Clinical Information Systems

Contemporary patient care information systems provide limited access to clinical knowledge, but this situation changes rapidly. The first generation of health care information systems consisted of financial applications running on costly mainframe systems. Successive waves of development saw growth in departmental systems to support key functions such as lab and pharmacy, followed by progressively integrated facility-based patient tracking systems, and the beginnings of computer-based patient records. Each phase of growth has brought more computer terminals into the workplace and involved more users. Decreasing costs of computer equipment and recognition of efficiencies gained from computerization have steadily propelled development of patient care information systems. Advances in high speed data networks and user interfaces capable of integrating information from multiple sources together have increased the power of clinical information to support decision making, and currently put clinical computing on the threshold of explosive growth in data access and connectivity. Growing awareness that practicing in information-rich environments pays dividends in quality of care sets the stage for realizing that *knowledge-rich* computing will confer similar clinical benefits.

Building Knowledge-Rich Clinical Microenvironments

This section will review several information technology solutions to the office dilemma outlined above, focusing on technology available to "average" readers equipped with today's "average" 1995 home computer.

These machines, equipped with 486, Pentium, or RISC processors; 4 to 20 MB of RAM; several hundred megabytes of disk storage; 14.4 kbaud modems; and CD-ROM drives are available at discount stores for under $2,000 and are more than adequate for the applications described. Attention will focus on the practical applicability, *at the point of care*, of current computer-assisted approaches to the principal knowledge retrieval tasks: fact-finding, focused subject matter review, acquistion of new knowledge, and knowledge exploration.

Basic Strategies for Retrieving Knowledge With Computers

To begin it will help to discuss standard strategies for finding specific knowledge "needles" in information "haystacks". "Where do you want to look" and "What do you want to know?" are the first essential questions in a knowledge search. "Where do you want to look?" depends on the array of knowledge sources available, and the scope of the request. When the objective is to retrieve a quick fact or definition, a dictionary or a glossary is appropriate. When richer detail is desired, textbooks or similar reference works are preferred. Reviewing a discrete topic in the current literature may lead the seeker to a narrow set of periodicals; but when the question spans several disciplines or the seeker is uncertain where the best information resides, a broad net must be cast, equivalent to a trip to the library. Once the knowledge source is targeted a request can be formulated via the computer program's human interface, using one or more of the techniques described below.

Word and Phrase Lookups. Finding a definition is reasonably simple, but even a simple lookup benefits from considerate human engineering. Most systems allow users to type in a word that is then looked up, usually with a satisfactory result. Correctly spelled user input is expected, though, and many systems do not forgive misspellings. Lookup methods usually attempt to match input with the initial portions of target words, and display a list of matching "hits" for selection, meaning that a very short or very common input string can produce a long pick list for the user to resolve. Systems that limit users to entering single input words are quite restrictive when the target concept is a phrase (e.g., major depression, recurrent). Systems that permit entering *several* short fragments of a phrase minimize typing, reduce misspellings, and yield smaller hit lists. Glossaries, dictionaries, and other references that organize returned information around a single concept work well with single phrase lookup techniques.

Browsing. An approach that resembles browsing a table of contents is often available as an alternative to word or phrase input. In a typical example, the user selects a topic from a list that exposes successive subsidiary lists of narrower topics until the desired term is found. Browsing is not very efficient for finding specific terms, but is useful when one has a general idea of the target and wishes to explore it. When using an automated version of the PDR, for example, a word-based search is good for looking up information on a specific drug, but a topical browse beginning with a drug class is better for identifying treatment alternatives.

Indexed Searching. Indexes, familiar to all readers of texts, permit recovery of units of information that are indexed by one or more terms. Glossaries and dictionaries index each *entry* with a unique term and work well with a single phrase lookup technique. Other units of information can be indexed as well, and it is important to remember the *type* of unit one is seeking in a particular search. In bibliographic systems the unit is almost always a single article, indexed by key words. Page references found in book indexes refer to variable units judged important by the author. Topics that occur frequently in a volume may be subdivided. Building indexes is labor intensive and requires the indexer to make relevance judgments. Size constraints of paper-based indexing systems limit citations to important concept occurrences, but automated full-text storage systems permit finding a target phrase anywhere in a text.

Full-Text Searching. When complete documents are available on-line, some systems will locate and highlight search words in the text, much as a word processor does. Once a knowledge unit (which could be a definition, an abstract, an article, or a chapter) is located, it is often useful to scan the returned unit with a word search. Some systems, such as SilverPlatter's Medline data base on CD-ROM, automatically highlight search terms in the retrieved abstracts. Word finding locates desired information in the knowledge source and is a useful way to refine a search. Systems implement this capability differently. Some highlight target words and make it easy to issue a "find again" command. Others move the cursor to the found word without offering the find again capability, necessitating repeated string input. When one must quickly navigate through multiple occurrences of a target word, prominent highlighting and single-keystroke find again are very helpful.

Combinatorial Searching. When a reference volume is richly indexed, in the extreme case tagging every meaningful phrase, looking up a single phrase can return an unusably large number of hits. Here it is almost always better to request results tagged by more than one term. Because beginners often encounter difficulty with this powerful technique, it is important to explain what actually occurs in searches that combine two or more terms. Almost always the search begins with specifying the *units of information* to be searched for occurrence of index terms. Medline indexes, for instance, point to key words associated with individual articles.

Medline searches return reference citations and, optionally, abstracts. Many full-text storage systems permit specifying articles or chapters, or smaller components, such as sections, paragraphs, or sentences, as units to be searched. These systems may also support specifying how many words apart the target terms can fall. An inappropriate searching unit can result in retrieving too few or too many hits. Users unaware of how to refine search criteria by manipulating search terms and searched units may abort prematurely.

Figure 1a illustrates applying combinatorial logic in a Medline search to retrieve journal articles indexed by keywords. In the example, the seeker wants information relating the drug clonazepam and the illness

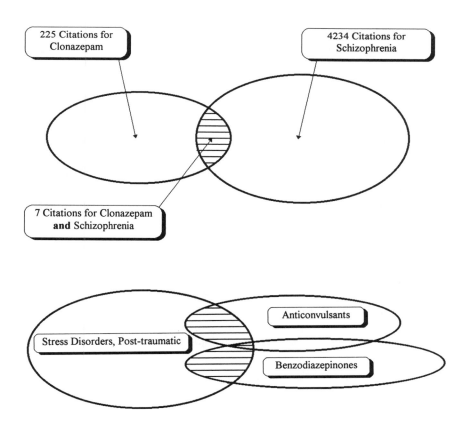

Figure 1. Combinatorial Search Logic. (a) Finding citations indexed by the terms schizophrenia AND clonazepam together. (b) Finding citations indexed by stress disorders, posttraumatic, AND *either* of benzodiazepinones OR anticonvulsants.

schizophrenia. Logically, this is expressed by the statement: "find articles indexed by the term 'schizophrenia' AND by the term 'clonazepam'." Four thousand two hundred thirty-four citations are indexed by the term schizophrenia, 225 by the term clonazepam, and 7 are indexed by both terms at once. As shown, combining terms quickly leads the searcher to a small group of information units containing the desired information. Most systems permit combining up to four concepts. Users of this technique need to remember that each additional search term significantly *narrows* the scope of a search, and in most cases, combining more than two components is unhelpful. In some situations it can be very useful to review citations when *either* of two different terms combines with a third. In this case, the first component consists of two terms joined by a logical OR, either of which may co-occur with a third term. Figure 1b illustrates a request for citations indexed by Stress Disorders, Posttraumatic, together with *either* of the topics benzodiazepinones or anticonvulsants.

Controlled Vocabularies. The somewhat peculiar form of the search terms in the above examples illustrates another important feature in some bibliographic systems: use of a "controlled" vocabulary. Compound expressions, particularly complex combinations of lengthy terms, are quite vulnerable to performance degradation introduced by spelling errors, variant spellings, and synonyms. Controlling the spelling and form of a search concept reduces this source of error. The United States National Library of Medicine (NLM) Medical Subject Heading (MeSH) vocabulary, which provides the sample terms above, enjoys standard usage in bio-medical knowledge retrieval systems, and formulating a search with any of its 16,000-odd terms eliminates noise introduced by misspelling and synonymy. MeSH brings its own complications to be sure: One must find the proper MeSH term and spell it correctly. MeSH resembles, but does not exactly match, the clinical vernacular. Searchers who have not memorized MeSH terms must look them up somewhere, but most systems using MeSH furnish term-finding assistance. Because NLM indexers apply MeSH in a consistent fashion, search performance is predictable. MeSH concepts are organized hierarchically, and a search that fails because it has been too narrowly or broadly focused can be easily reformulated using a related MeSH from higher or lower in the hierarchy of specificity.

Computer-Assisted Knowledge Sources Available in 1995

Knowledge Media

Table 1 presents a rough comparison of salient characteristics of media that deliver clinical knowledge. "Annual" cost is used to permit comparison between per-use subscription services and resources distributed

Table 1. Overview of Computer-Assisted Knowledge Sources

Medium	Annual User Cost/Knowledge Units Stored	Accessibility and Portability	Response Time	Currency	Storage Capacity
Silicon chip	++++	++++	++++	+++	+
Floppy disk	+++	++	++	+++	+
Fixed disk	+++	++	++++	++	++
CD-ROM	++	+	++	+++	+++
Network	+	+	++	++++	Unlimited

on readable media. "Network" refers to accession of knowledge sources via telephonic, local, or wide area networks.

More important than the media involved are the real-world considerations of cost, usability, accessibility, response time, and currency that distinguish practical tools from conversation pieces. Keeping this in mind, we can now review a number of contemporary computer-assisted knowledge resources, grouped by knowledge task: fact-finding, reviewing knowledge, acquiring new knowledge, and knowledge exploration.

Fact Finders

Medical dictionaries and the PDR are fact containers. Dictionaries store many static facts, and accrue new entires slowly enough that new editions are needed only every half-decade or so. PDR is published annually on paper, and has aggressively entered the electronic media market with a pocket PDR on a chip. Annual updates cost about $200. This medium also offers the Washington Manual of Medicine and the Harriet Lane Handbook of Pediatrics, each costing about $150 per module. The hand-held display of 48 columns by 8 rows is small, but portability is excellent. PDR is also published on compact disk. Site licenses are available that permit installation on a local area network. Organizations that have made the necessary investment in LAN hardware and multiplatter CD players may find this mode of distribution more economical than the paper product. CD-ROM lookups are slow with standard drives, and slowness is compounded if the CD must be mounted before it can be read. Quad-speed drives are better, and are recommended to individual users contemplating a CD-ROM library. Topic lookup speed is comparable to using a paper dictionary, but ability to search the fine print of a PDR listing for a word occurrence is a distinct advantage of electronic fact-retrieval systems.

Reviewing Knowledge With Textbooks

Medical and behavioral texts aim to provide their readers with current authoritative knowledge. Reference texts tend to be very complete, but the pace of scientific discovery produces rapid obsolescence of content, posing a perennial problem for publishers of expensive technical texts. In 1978 Scientific American Medicine, a modular textbook assembled in a loose leaf binder made its debut, providing its "subscribers" with regular chapter updates and a new index every month (Dale & Federman, 1978–1995). Since 1990 Scientific American Medicine has been distributed in CD-ROM form, at about three times the price of the paper version. Multiuse licenses to install CD-ROM publications reduce the cost per user to about $100 (excluding equipment cost). The true value of on-line texts remains to be established. Texts on compact disks save shelf space, permit rapid searching of their contents, and in contrast to fact finders and dictionaries, return many pages of information, and can include images and sound. Texts can be difficult to read on low-resolution displays, and slower CD-ROM drives produce delays. On the other hand, rapid access to textbook information in clinical environments could far outweigh such disadvantages. CD-ROM deserves consideration when a network is available.

Acquiring New Knowledge in Electronic Periodicals

For a decade now, almost all major journals have been composed digitally and are transferable to computer media. Currently CD-ROM is the dominant electronic format for distribution of biomedical periodicals and every year more journals are available on CD. Although CD-ROM has been available since the mid-1980s, its growth as a viable publishing medium accelerated rapidly in 1992, in parallel with steep drops in the price of multimedia computers targeted at the home market. CDs able to store thousands of pages of text are not ideal for distributing single periodicals. A solution adopted by the American Psychiatric Press and several other publishers has been to bundle several years' worth of several journals with reference texts and to provide periodic update releases.

The American Psychiatric Press Electronic Library (APEL) introduced in 1992, costs single users about $800 for four quarterly updates. It includes 3 years' worth of the *American Journal of Psychiatry*, *Hospital and Community Psychiatry*, the *American Journal of Neuropsychiatry*, a number of annual review volumes and the DSM-IV. Update releases have been delayed several times, at no penalty to subscribers. I have used it since May 1994 and find the system to be a mixture of pros and cons. Its compactness liberates at least 6 feet of shelf space. Ability to search the full text of books and journals is quite powerful and hits are very rapidly found, but retrieving the text of citations thus located is slow with a single-speed CD-ROM drive. The search engine permits restricting searches to books or periodicals, and allows specifying how many words apart co-occurring target terms are allowed to fall, and whether to restrict the search to titles, authors, text, or reference sections. Lack of support for a controlled vocabulary, such as MeSH, to index articles and chapters limits ability to refine the scope of a search statement, and renders Medline search skills acquired elsewhere irrelevant. Unlike Medline, which returns reference citations suitable for inclusion in bibliographies, APEL only inconsistently returns suitable reference citations. APEL yields page numbers for articles from the *American Journal of Psychiatry,* but not *Hospital and Community Psychiatry* or textbooks. On the other hand, the full text includes authors' reference sections, providing another way to locate useful citations. APEL's price does not exceed the cost of purchasing its component publications separately, but $800 per year is expensive for individuals who do not need the whole collection. The product is suitable for library usage and network installation, at a premium price based on the number of users.

From the perspective of a serious researcher, the chief limitation of APEL, as with any limited selection of journals or texts, is incomplete coverage of the world literature on a subject. Eventually, libraries offering electronic access to full texts of most major journals will be the norm, and scholarly work will be transformed. Before this potential is realized fully, however, CD systems must provide better support for the MeSH controlled vocabulary and separate the knowledge they store from the proprietary search interfaces they support, so they can respond to standard queries issued by a search interface of the user's choosing. Greater demand for controlled vocabulary support will influence electronic publishers to perform more extensive indexing prior to electronic distribution.

A number of CD-ROM publishers distribute full-text journal sets along with Medline subsets, combining the advantages of MeSH-based searching and full-text retrieval. Annual cost per single user for a 1 year subscription is about $600, but network licensing arrangements can reduce costs per user by up to 80%.

Knowledge Exploration Tools. Bibliographic systems that index large numbers of publications and return abstracts rather than full text exhibit strengths and weaknesses that are complementary to electronic publications on CD-ROM. The prototype, Medline, has had an enormous impact on improving access to medical literature. Supported by NLM since 1971, Medline has been a vital driving force in medical research. Its key components are:

1. Citation and abstract listings accessible over telephone lines,
2. The MeSH indexing system,
3. A standard search language (MEDLARS), and
4. Frequent updates.

Medline's original market targeted medical libraries, but the familiar trends of personal computing (small size, low cost, and better performance) have contributed to revolutionary broadening of its availability. In 1971, equipment and telephone costs and the specialized MEDLARS search language restricted Medline's power to trained library staff, requiring nonexperts to submit written requests and wait for printouts of citations. The ability of Medline to meet immediate clinical knowledge needs was limited until advances in personal computing technology put the librarian's tools into the hands of caregivers. Today, several options to access Medline exist, and some of them are extremely economical.

Medline Options

Grateful Med was developed by NLM for lay searchers using personal computers. A "front-end," Grateful Med insulates users from MEDLARS search language and eases establishing a telephonic connection. A simple electronic form lets users compose search statements. Software translates the search specifications into MEDLARS commands prior to connecting to Medline. Once connected, Grateful Med accesses the requested data base, runs the search, and captures results on the user's disk. The batch operation minimizes connect and on-line costs, but allows a leisurely browse of the results. Search results can be printed or stored, and search logic can be stored for future reuse. Grateful Med can be configured to access several health sciences data bases besides Medline, including TOXNET and AIDSLINE.

Most searches conclude in a few minutes, and the average cost per search is less than a dollar. Since Grateful Med was introduced in the early 1980s, costs per search have steadily dropped, yet usage and response times have improved. The advent of packet-switch networks such as Compuserve and Tymenet has eliminated long distance telephone costs, and recently, access over Internet connections using the Telecommunications Protocol/Interconnect Protocol (TCP/IP) and Telnet protocol has permitted even more rapid, and less costly searches.

As with most computer systems, the chief barrier to using Grateful Med is learning how to use it effectively. McKibbon and Haynes studied this in detail and concluded that 2 hours of hands-on tutorial was the minimum training required to achieve proficiency (McKibbon, Haynes, Johnston, & Walker, 1991). Grateful Med's screens are text based, but can be configured to work with a mouse. Although straightforward and flexible, limitations exist: Grateful Med does not retrieve full texts of articles. Many abstracts are available, but requesting them by default costs considerably more than retrieving citations alone. When citations of interest are retrieved, it is relatively awkward to instruct Grateful Med to request abstracts for specific articles. Use of the MeSH controlled indexing vocabulary improves search returns, but selecting a MeSH term requires several steps. Grateful Med provides limited access to the MeSH hierarchy, making it somewhat difficult to rapidly "re-scope" a search. Figure 2 illustrates formulation of a Grateful Med search and an example of a returned citation.

The trial and error required to develop a feel for designing productive searches with Grateful Med can create anxiety over accrued search costs and may discourage beginners from getting sufficient practice with the system. A new NLM pricing policy that offers flat annual fees to institutions connecting to Medline via an Internet connection should change this perception. The number of Medline subscribers grew from 21 in 1971 to over 100,000 in 1994, and continued growth is certain.

CD-ROM Systems for Knowledge Exploration

In 1994 CD-ROM versions of Medline were very popular, and as noted, some products combine Medline features and full-text retrieval. Libraries in particular find the unlimited searching permitted with a local CD-ROM system to be a cost-effective alternative to accruing per-search charges. Multiuser installations require a local area network and concurrent mounting of many disks so the overhead cost of equipment enters the equation as well. Library reference sections often include on-line text-books and other reference materials in addition to MEDLINE. Specialized data bases such as PsychLit are available on CD-ROM, and many of these allow searching and retrieval of full article texts.

Embedding Knowledge Access in Clinical Systems

The flexibility and portability of electronic data open up the possibility of integrating patient record applications and knowledge access within the electronic workspace. Depending on the equipment and software, pro-gressively sophisticated levels of integration are possible. Examples of very simple setups include on-line access to hospital policies, formularies, and patient medication instructions, where information resides on the same media that store clinical data. While simple, this information can have a noticeable impact on practice. Slightly more complex is establishing a gateway to a knowledge resource stored on CD-ROM, such as the Medline. With appropriate networking technology, this capability can be implemented on the "dumbest" text-based terminals. Substituting a per-sonal computer for a terminal increases the options, and depending on the workstation's operating system, may permit concurrent access to patient information via a data port and telephonic access to a bibliographic

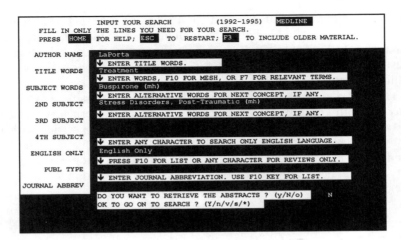

Figure 2a. Composing a Grateful Med Medline search.
Grateful Med users fill in as many blanks as needed. Searchers may combine up
to four subject words. Author and title specification may help locate specific
articles. Pressing F10 instead of <enter> after typing text in a subject field opens
a dictionary of MeSH terms, denoted by the suffix (mh). Searches can be
restricted to English, to reviews only, or to specific journals, and abstracts may be
requested.

```
2
UI  - 92242543
AU  - LaPorta LD
AU  - Ware MR
TI  - Buspirone in the treatment of posttraumatic stress
      disorder
      [letter] [see comments]
CM  - Comment in: J Clin Psychopharmacol 1994 Feb;14(1):79-81
PT  - LETTER
LA  - Eng
SO  - J Clin Psychopharmacol 1992 Apr;12(2):133-4
```

Figure 2b. A Medline citation.
Citations returned by Grateful Med have a unique identifier (UI) whose first two
digits indicate the year of publication, and indicate the authors (AU), title (TI),
comments (CM), publication type (PT), language (LA) and source (SO).

resource. When the workstation supports a networking protocol, such as
TCP/IP, concurrent access to patient information, local knowledge sources
on CD-ROM, and remote knowledge sources is possible with a single
port. The broadest application of this concept is the unlimited potential to
link to remote computers via the World Wide Web over the Internet.

So far though, the methods for accessing knowledge described involve switching *between* clinical and knowledge-seeking sessions. More intriguing is the possibility of accessing knowledge while *inside* a clinical information processing task. For example, it is easy to imagine the benefits of access to an electronic PDR while ordering or reviewing drug therapy, or to APA's Electronic DSM-IV, when recording a diagnosis. Unfortunately, most available knowledge sources do not yet respond to queries issued by another computer program, but when this happens, embedded queries will be feasible. Several promising experiments in this area have been conducted. In the Medline Button System, prototyped by Cimino at Columbia–Presbyterian Medical Center, the clinical workspace provides such a knowledge gateway (Cimino, Johnson, Aguirre, Roderer, & Clayton, 1992). At any point in clinical processing information, users may click a button and conduct a literature search. The system anticipates topics and search strategies for drug interactions and therapeutic guidelines, making knowledge acquisition rapid, and bringing it directly to bear on clinical decisions. Nielson has described a system based on the Microsoft Windows Help program, that offers on-line access to compiled bibliographic resources (Nielson, Smith, Lee, & Wang, 1994).

At the American Lake VA medical center I developed a comparable system, Clinical Library Assistant. Implemented in a multitasking environment under Microsoft Windows, Assistant extracts data from computer-based patient records and allows users to use them to specify and execute a Medline search. Patient-specific terms from the clinical system such as diagnoses and drug names are translated to the MeSH controlled vocabulary via tables derived from the NLM's Unified Medical Language System (UMLS). UMLS is a superset of standard controlled vocabularies that interrelates MeSH, International Classification of Diseases-9th ed. (ICD-9), DSM-III-R, and about a dozen other well-established terminology systems (Lindberg, Humphreys, & McCray, 1993). The Clinical Library Assistant enables users to:

1. Perform Medline searches at clinical workstations;
2. Employ MeSH terms that correspond to patient data;
3. Refine and rerun searches against older data bases;
4. Obtain on-line abstracts from selected references; and
5. Transfer search results to electronic mail for storage, printing, or forwarding.

Inspiration for the Assistant came from an impression that serious errors in care can stem from lack of key medical knowledge at a crucial decision point. When a knowledge gap is narrowly circumscribed or obscure, precisely targeted Medline searches are often more useful than standard references, and provide very current information. Ready access to MeSH was judged important because searches using the controlled vocabulary perform better than searches based on free text (Lowe &

Barnett, 1994). User-typed input can also be converted to MeSH, and MeSH terms may be manipulated to yield broader and narrower concepts within the MeSH hierarchy. Once search terms are selected, the user sets up search conditions using a simplified version of the Grateful Med screen shown in Figure 2, and executes the search over a telephone line. Figure 3 presents an overview of the program flow. In the first 6 months after installing both Grateful Med and Clinical Library Assistant in four clinical locations, approximately 40 staff used these tools to conduct 1,000 searches at an average cost of 50 cents per search, retrieving 10,000 references. Recent acquistion of Internet connect capability at VA Medical Centers has eliminated the need for analogue telephone lines and modems to support the system, and permits installation at any data terminal location.

A Knowledge Layer in Patient Information Systems

One conclusion to be drawn from experiments like the Medline Button and Clinical Library Assistant is that it makes no sense to segregate

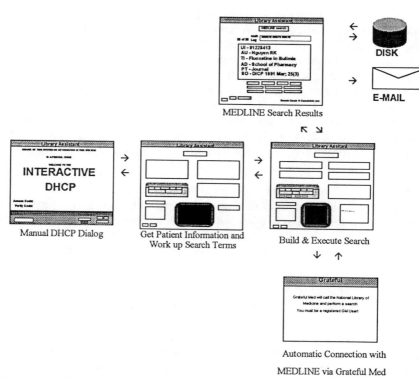

Figure 3. Clinical Library Assistant Program Flow.

patient information processing and knowledge accession, when both can be concurrently supported on the same inexpensive machines. Currently available electronic knowledge resources are powerful, but the extreme diversity of their user interfaces, query techniques, and output makes integrating them with patient care computing difficult. To overcome such obstacles, designers and purchasers of patient care and knowledge access systems need to begin thinking about a new element in clinical information architecture: a knowledge layer. In information systems layers are logical strata of functionality that operate concurrently to support the computational process. They include communications and networking protocols, operating systems, computer languages, applications, data, and the human–machine interface. Layers exchange messages, and when they are properly coordinated, only the topmost layer is visible to end users. Characteristics of an effective knowledge layer might include:

1. Ability to respond with suitably formatted knowledge at any point in clinical processing;
2. Sensitivity to the processing context;
3. Support of standard queries for different knowledge needs (e.g., definitions, facts, explanations, explorations);
4. Ability to locate and link to appropriate knowledge sources; and
5. Support for saving, applying, and communicating knowledge.

With a standard knowledge interface, we can expect rapid progress in the embedding of knowledge services in patient care systems. The data transport capacity of the Internet and robustness of the TCP/IP protocol will accelerate convergence of patient care and knowledge systems. To prepare for these changes, systems planners will do well to acquire support for internal and external TCP/IP connections and plan ample local and wide-area network capacity.

Dilemmas Facing Current Knowledge Vendors

Knowledge publishers will face crucial and possibly perilous strategic decisions about supporting the knowledge layer in clinical systems. CD-ROM vendors have not been shy to suggest that their products will help patient care, but such claims are weakened by their failure to furnish resources able to respond to queries issued by clinical applications. Furthermore, the rapidly increasing capacity of the Internet casts doubt as to whether CD-ROM sources will remain competitive with high-speed data networks. Today, data transfer rates for networked CD-ROM systems compare to a typical Internet-mediated knowledge resource, but pricing policies differ. For either a flat annual fee or per-search charge Medline subscribers can access the most current bibliographic information. CD-ROM users must buy update disks to stay current, and continually invest in platter-spinning capacity to support access to older material. If Medline connect fees continue to fall, and performance continues to improve, it is hard to see the more limited CD products thriving solely on the basis of their Medline services, that, after all, are no more than remarketed public domain data. CD-ROM vendors currently compete on the bases of price, value of the full-text sources they offer, and utility of their searching software. Their reluctance to support a standard query interface capable of serving clinical knowledge needs is understandable given the pressure this would create to "unbundle" search software from data resources, favoring the lowest cost vendor of each, thereby reducing profit.

CD systems continue to hold an advantage over Internet connections for full-text searching, but this advantage will decrease as Internet bandwidth increases. When that happens, we can expect publishers of journals and books to begin offering access to full texts over the Internet, eliminating middlemen. CDs will survive as excellent media for *archival knowledge storage*, replacing microfilm, but their importance for periodical distribution will lessen. Competitive pressures now discourage different publishers of original material from pooling products on single CDs (advantageous for libraries) because high-volume periodicals would lose their market edge. Servicing the knowledge layer through direct publishing over the Internet affords an interesting opportunity to publishers, especially when standard query and retrieval methods emerge. The impact on publishing economics (advertising and royalties, for example) is unclear, but we guess that the emerging knowledge market will be driven by the value health care providers find in point of care knowledge access. Initial experiments suggest that this value is substantial, and will increase when standard interfaces and high-speed data networks allow interchange between clinical systems and knowledge repositories. We make the following recommendations to planners of point of care knowledge systems:

1. Invest cautiously in distributable media technologies;
2. Link clinical workstations in high-speed local area networks; and
3. Furnish clinical networks with high-speed Internet connections.

References

American Psychiatric Association. (1994). *Diagnostic and statistical manual of mental disorders, Fourth Edition*. Washington, DC: American Psychiatric Press, Inc.

Cimino, J.J., Johnson, S.B., Aguirre, A., Roderer, N., & Clayton, P. (1992). The medline button. In *Proceedings of the Sixteenth Annual Symposium on Computer Applications in Medical Care* (pp. 81–85). American Medical Informatics Association. New York: McGraw–Hill.

Dale, D.C., & Federman, D.D., (Eds.). (1978–1995). *Scientific American medicine*. New York: Scientific American, Inc.

Lindberg, D.A.B., Humphreys, B.L., & McCray, A.T. (1993). The unified medical language system. *Methods of Information in Medicine, 32*, 281–291.

Lowe, H.J., & Barnett, G.O. (1994). Understanding and using the medical subject headings (MeSH) vocabulary to perform literature searches. *Journal of the American Medical Association*, *271*, 1103–1108.

McKibbon, K.A., Haynes, R.B., Johnston, M.E., & Walker, C.J. (1991). A study to enhance clinical end-user Medline search skills: Design and baseline findings. In *Proceedings of the Fifteenth Annual Symposium on Computer Applications in Medical Care* (pp. 73–77). American Medical Informatics Association. New York: McGraw–Hill.

Nielson, C., Smith, C.S., Lee, D., & Wang, M. (1994). Implementation of a relational patient record with integration of educational and reference information. *Journal of the American Medical Informatics Association Symposium Supplement: Proceedings, Eighteenth Annual Symposium on Computer Applications in Medical Care* (pp. 125–129). Philadelphia, PA: Hanley and Belfus, Inc.

Shader, R. (Ed.). (1994). *Manual of psychiatric therapeutics*. Boston: Little, Brown and Co.

Zurich, D.B., et al. (1995). *Physician's desk reference* (49th ed.). Montvale, NJ: Medical Economics Data, Inc.

20
Tools for Developing Multimedia in Psychiatry
Milton P. Huang and Norman E. Alessi

Multimedia refers to the use of graphics, sound, animation, and video in the transmission of information. By accessing several sensory modalities instead of only one, multimedia allows greater communication than simple text or simple speech. Creating a message with visual and auditory elements increases the density of information sent and permits greater impact. Furthermore, the term multimedia has also come to suggest a media that allows interactivity. Unlike a movie that must be seen from beginning to end in a fixed sequence, multimedia productions directly elicit information from the audience and alter themselves accordingly. Although present and utilized within medicine and psychiatry for over 20 years (Baskett, 1978; Miller, 1972), recent advances in computer technology have propelled multimedia to a new prominence. Increases in central processor speed and storage capacity have enabled the rise of digital media where text, music, and video are created and distributed with the use of computers. With the help of computer tools, the technical expertise required to develop media is more easily mastered and dispersed. Previously, artisans and artists spent their lives dedicated to a single realm such as printing, photography, etc. Now, anyone can produce professional results with the help of a desktop system. These effects are becoming evident in almost all areas of communication, entertainment, and education. The "digital revolution" is leading the way for what is thought of as the most significant advance since the development of the printing press.

Several areas within medicine have taken advantage of the potential of multimedia, although none have begun to realize the full impact that lies ahead. Radiology is one area that has demonstrated the development of multimedia applications for a number of uses. In clinical care situations, actual images and dictated reports can be made available from hospital workstations (Lemke, Faulkner, & Krauss, 1994; Huang et al., 1994; McGarty, 1991; Bélanger, 1990) or incorporated into an electronic

322

medical record (Ratib, 1994; Kitanosono et al., 1992). These images can also be sent to distant hospitals for consultation (Franken et al., 1992; Kagetsu & Ablow, 1992) or placed in teaching files on the Internet for community access (Galvin, D'Alessandro, Erkonen, Lacey, & Santer, 1994). Multimedia educational applications are being developed at several teaching institutions in multiple areas (Frisse, 1990) and studies have been done comparing its efficacy to that of standard lectures (D'Allesandro, Galvin, Erkonen, Albanese et al., 1993). Educational applications have been described in the literature of radiology (D'Allesandro, Galvin, Erkonen, Santer et al., 1993), pathology (Levy & Thursh, 1989), plastic surgery (Webber, Summers, & Rinehart, 1994), and psychiatry (Hyler & Bujold, 1994).

The continuing advances in digital technology will make multimedia production easier and such applications more common. With its increasing presence and a vast potential to improve communications in all areas of medicine and psychiatry, it is imperative for an informed physician to be familiar with multimedia. The goal of this chapter is to describe multimedia and discuss the tools and the issues involved in its production. The chapter is divided into three sections. The first section describes the components of multimedia. The second section provides an overview of the issues involved in the construction and presentation of multimedia, including a description of "authoring" software. The final section discusses the legal implications of copyright law as it pertains to multimedia.

Components of Multimedia

Multimedia is divided into the component media types of text, sound, graphics, animation, and video (Fig. 1). For each of these media types, we will describe how the media is used in computers as well as explain some of the technical jargon.

Text

Although text is a traditional media for communication, the digital revolution has transformed its use. From the early development of printing, text was laid out in "type." Each character was individually shaped to attain the appropriate audience response. Typography explores the ways in which type can influence expression within text (Baudin, 1988). Publishers now use sets of standardized typefaces, where a typeface is a defined set of aesthetically related characters. The text you are reading now is a particular typeface, chosen for readability and a professional feel. Many other typefaces exist, each with a different aesthetic sense or tone and consequent expressivity (Fig. 2). Individual typefaces are also referred to as fonts (Fenton, 1991).

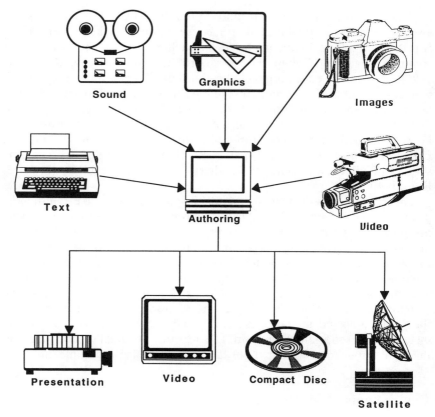

Figure 1. The components of multimedia.

The conversion of typefaces to computer form has allowed the creation of computer tools that simplify the choice and manipulation of type appearance. For example, the same typeface can be scaled to different sizes. These sizes are measured in "points," with approximately 72 points

Font Name	Example
New Century Schoolbook	Fonts and text
Clearface Gothic Monotype Bold	**Fonts and text**
Mecurius Bold Script Monotype	*Fonts and text*
Old English Text	𝔉onts and text
New Berolina Monotype	*Fonts and text*

Figure 2. Examples of fonts.

in an inch. Usual text is 10 to 12 point, but it can be scaled down to as little as 2 or up into the hundreds to obtain different effects. A particular typeface can also be altered in style or face, including **boldface**, *italic*, or underline. Some styles can be obtained by using a different face from the same typeface family. Thus, Times Roman font appears bold through the use of Times Roman Bold or italic through using Times Roman Italic or Oblique. Alteration in styles may also be generated by the computer. In such cases, underlining or boldfacing is extrapolated from an original font through calculation. Because they are created by the computer, these extrapolations can be combined so it would be possible to create bold words that are also underlined.

There are two major ways in which typefaces are converted into a form used by computers, creating either bitmapped or outline (or scalable) fonts. Bitmapped characters are represented by a grid of small squares that are either black or white (bits). All characters on a computer monitor are bitmapped because the screen is divided into pixels. One problem of using bitmaps occurs in scaling fonts to different sizes. A character that is bitmapped will have jagged edges (jaggies) that become more noticeable when enlarged because of the square edges of the component bits. Outline fonts such as PostScript and TrueType are now more commonly used. These fonts have characters that are drawn from cubic or quadratic formulas, allowing the calculation of a smooth curve at all point sizes.

Fonts are usually purchased as families. These families are available on disks, CD-ROMs, or from commercial electronic bulletin board services. There are also programs that allow you to create your own fonts or modify previously existing ones. Perhaps the most striking way of modifying fonts is to make them three dimensional (3-D). Such effects can be accomplished by many 3-D software packages (see Graphics section), although there are also programs that specifically specialize in creating "dimensional type."

Sound

The changes that have occurred in the recording and storage of sound provide a clear example of how media are affected by digital technology. Older storage mediums like tapes or vinyl records were analog. In other words, the sounds were translated into measures that could assume any value in a continuous range. In contrast, digital recordings store noncontinuous, discrete numbers. Fixing measurements as numbers makes them accessible to computers. This process of digitization is accomplished by a special board, a digital analog converter (DAC). In the case of sound, this board samples a microphone (analog) signal at regular intervals, measuring the volume and frequency as numbers, and storing these digital values. The input may be music, human speech, or any other sound. This technology is used in making the compact disk (CD) that has almost replaced older analog mediums because of the greater ease of making machines that process digital signals.

The quality of digital sound is controlled by the sampling rate and sampling size or resolution. The sampling rate is the measure of how often the analog input is sampled in 1 second. The higher the rate, the closer the recording can match the original sound. The sampling resolution is the stored size of the samples that is indicative of the range of values available to represent the magnitude of the sound. "8-Bit audio" uses 8-bit samples that can only be one of 256 values. 16-Bit audio samples can be one of 65,536 values, increasing the range of the recording. CD-quality audio specifies a sampling rate of 44.1 kHz or 44,100 samples per second with a sample resolution of 16 bits. Often, slower sampling rates (22 kHz) are used for sounds like human speech that may not need such high quality.

The advantage of converting sounds into digital form is the ability to apply digital (computer) tools. Because the information is stored as numbers, there is no loss of information when a sound is rerecorded, or copied. Computer programs can be written to create many different effects by rearranging the digital information or processing it through various equations. Sound editing software provide a range of editing abilities such as fading in or out, cutting and pasting, or changing the signal gain (volume). More advanced effects include adding echo, reverberation, or applying digital filters to equalize or eliminate particular frequency bands.

Although an entire musical piece can be stored as digital samples as described above, some computer systems use a different method of representing musical information. In wavetable synthesis, a digital sample of each musical instrument is stored instead of an entire piece. When an instrument needs to play, the computer looks up that sample in the table and plays back at different speeds to get different notes. This technique saves space because music files only need to save the instrument type, the notes played, and the timing of the notes. The file information is fed to the synthesizer chip to create the actual sounds. Such files are saved with the WAV extension. This wavetable setup is conducive to the use of MIDI (Musical Instrument Digital Interface). MIDI is a communication protocol for electronic instruments that uses similar information about note length and duration. It is a music industry standard and a necessary adjunct for using the computer for composition. MIDI was incorporated into the original multimedia PC (MPC) standard created for IBM compatible systems. Microsoft Windows has a built in ability to play MIDI files, and in 1994, MIDI was added to Apple's QuickTime standard (version 2.0) so that MIDI files can now be converted to QuickTime soundtracks.

Music and sound effects for computers can be purchased on disk or CD-ROM in standard audio or MIDI formats. Audio files are also available over electronic bulletin boards and the Internet. Having a digitizer board will allow direct capture of sounds through a microphone, or in some cases music directly from a music CD played in the computer's CD-ROM drive. Amateur musicians can create MIDI-based music with a keyboard, MIDI interface, and appropriate software.

Graphics

The term graphics can refer to many things. In this section, we include any still image as being a graphic. Therefore graphics will include simple drawings as well as photographic images. As graphic images vary greatly in their native state, so does their translation into a digital form. Simple black and white drawings were some of the first images converted for computer use. Like fonts, these were bitmapped, divided into an array of small bits or pixels that are either on or off. Shades of gray could be simulated by a process referred to as "dithering." This worked by alternating white and black dots in a checkerboard pattern that blends into a gray appearance from a distance. The sharpness of such images is determined by the resolution or number of pixels per inch. Higher resolutions allow for smoother appearing lines without jaggies. Just as for fonts, some graphics avoid this problem by storing shapes as equations or vector graphics instead of bitmaps. The most common standards for this mode of graphic storage are EPS (encapsulated PostScript) format or WMF (Windows Metafile) format.

The availability of greater storage and computational power has allowed computer graphics to move beyond black and white images to a wider use of color. Quality of color graphics is determined not only by resolution, but also by the color depth. The depth is the number of computer bits that each pixel in a graphic can represent. Thus, with 8-bit color each pixel on the screen can be one of 2^8 or 256 different colors. Human ability to perceive variations in color reaches a limit at 24 bits (about 16.7 million colors). Of course, the memory required to store these pictures increases proportionally with the depth. The standard monitor size is 640 × 480 pixels. An image this size (full screen), would take up 38 K (kilobytes) in black and white, but 307 K in 8-bit color. 16-Bit color would take up twice that (there are 8 bits in each computer storage byte).

Because of these large file sizes, compression algorithms are often used. These are mathematical routines that are applied to the digital data to remove redundant information. In such cases, decompression routines can retrieve the original data exactly. Other algorithms do not allow full retrieval of the original information. These "lossy" techniques like JPEG (Joint Photographic Experts Group) eliminate data that appears unnecessary, such as color changes that are too subtle to be detected by the human eye. Other common standards used with color images are PICT (picture), GIF (graphics interchange format), TGA (Targa),

TIFF (Tag Image File Format), or Kodak Photo-CD (see Appendix for details). In addition to storage, large image sizes make demands of the computer processing power as well. The number of calculations needed to decode file information and transfer it to the monitor often calls for dedicated video boards to perform these tasks.

Perhaps the most spectacular and computationally intensive graphics are those created by 3-D graphics programs. These sophisticated photographlike images are built up through the use of a series of computer tools. Modeling programs first allow the creation of 3-D geometric objects, shaping them through extruding, lathing, or other functions. Such objects are represented by a wire-frame outline. Once an object is defined in the right shape, a surface or texture is mapped onto it. Thus a cylinder becomes either a marble column or a wood post. The final step is "rendering," where an image is created by arranging the designed objects in an imaginary space, specifying particular views and types of illumination for the scene. Several levels of quality exist depending on whether the rendering program is adjusting for shadows, multiple lights, reflective surfaces, or refractive objects. The complexity can reach the point that even the fastest machine can take hours to days to create a single scene. On the other hand, such techniques can be used with high-powered computers to create a virtual reality where a person can "walk" through the space they designed while the computer continuously rerenders the image to account for the ongoing change in perspective.

Like other computer medias, graphics can be purchased on disk, CD-ROM, or obtained through a network. Collections of small images are usually referred to as clip art for the way they can be cut and pasted into document and presentation layout. Such simple images can be edited or created de novo using a drawing program. These programs create graphic objects in different layers that can be separately manipulated or joined. This is ideal for working with the vector graphic (EPS) type pictures or designing logos where it is desirable to shift objects around with respect to one another. In contrast, photographic images cannot be created de novo, but must be purchased or directly digitized. The most common means of digitizing is scanning. Like a photocopy machine, the scanner runs a light bar and capture device over the target image. The quality of the image is determined by resolution and color depth. Newer digitizing options include the digital camera that captures an entire scene in digital form, like a still from a video camera. Whether purchased or captured, the digital nature of these images allows the computer to perform calculations that result in changing colors, adding shadows, duplicating elements, and other types of image retouching.

Animation

The illusion of motion is created using graphics through the process of animation. Graphics images appear to move by redrawing the graphic slightly differently, several times per second. When these are shown in rapid enough sequence, the brain perceives a single object moving instead of two separate objects. Humans perceive motion when an object appears to change at a rate of approximately 5 to 10 frames per second (fps). For professional quality animations, higher frame rates are used and thousands of separate frames may be needed for a few minutes of animation.

Computer programs can simplify this creation process by generating frames automatically. Such programs allow users to create 2-D or 3-D objects and describe a path for moving them across an imaginary stage. The computer then creates the necessary images. Many of the programs that generate the complex 3-D images described above are also able to change the positions of objects or lights and generate another frame for animation.

Animations require large amounts of disk space. As calculated above, the size of a full screen image in 8-bit color is 307 K. A minute of animation played at 30 fps would then occupy over 550 MB (megabytes). As most frames of animation are very similar to one another, animation files can be compressed by saving only the changes that occur between frames. An animation of a person swallowing a pill would only need to redraw the moving pill between frames and does not need to alter the drawing of the person or the background behind them. Space is saved because the full screen 8-bit color image does not have to be rerecorded each frame. This technique is used to create the Flick (FLI) animation files used on IBM compatibles. PICS was the most common animation format on the Mac until the advent of QuickTime.

Digital Video

Like the process described under Graphics, digital video involves capturing a photographlike image and digitizing it into a computer compatible form. The difference is that several captures must be done every second. Quality is determined by resolution, color depth, and number of frames per second. Standard video in the United States (National Television Standards Committee video) plays at an image size of about 640 × 480 with 16-bit color and 30 fps. Using the same calculations from the animation section, this would result in a file size of 1 GB (gigabyte) to store a minute of video without compression and ignoring the need to store audio. Furthermore, most computer storage devices cannot move data to the computer at that speed (18 MB/second). For this reason, many applications show only small video windows on the screen (320 × 240 or 160 × 120 pixels) and all use compression. Video compression requires compression of the graphic image, the accompanying sound, and information used to synchronize the two signals. One common standard for the compression of such information is MPEG (Motion Picture Experts Group). Use of this standard can compress full screen, full motion video to the point where it can be played off a device with the speed of a CD-

ROM. Compressed data is taken from CD-ROM at its slow data rate. The data is fed to the faster computer processing chips for rapid decompression and display on screen. IBM and Mac systems currently do not have a fast enough processor and require a specialized MPEG playback card to perform this task.

Although clips of videos can be purchased, undoubtedly the most clinically relevant video will be digitized from videotape. Video enters the computer from an external source, usually a VCR. The video source is connected to the computer via a video digitizer board. This board captures video frames of a specified size at some maximal rate, sending the images to the computer. Depending on the particular board, there will be a trade-off between the two variables of size and rate. For example, a chosen board might offer the option of capturing a frame size of 160 × 120 pixels at 30 fps versus capturing a 640 × 480 pixel frame at 5 fps. As described above, compression of this raw information is important. Some of the more expensive boards include chips to perform hardware compression while the video is being captured. Others rely on software compression, using the computer's CPU to perform the work. In this case, "postcompression" is used. The raw information is temporarily stored until the capture period is complete. Then during the "post" phase, the computer goes through the computations for compressing this data. The final results of video digitization are stored as QuickTime or AVI files. These digital files can be manipulated by video editing programs that allow users to take these files and cut, copy, or paste them. More sophisticated programs allow the addition of complex transitions between film clips or special effect filters.

Construction of Multimedia

Although familiarity with the components of multimedia is a necessary foundation, they are only components. In this section, we will discuss the issues that the multimedia author faces in combining these different medias into a coherent and communicative whole. We divide these issues into three subsections. First will be issues of authoring design. This explores how multimedia are implemented as an effective communication tool. Second will be a detailed review of the steps in the authoring process with a review of authoring software and its use. The third topic is that of the authoring environment. This includes details specifying the hardware and software the author needs to have available to be able to create.

Authoring Design

An essential part of multimedia is interactivity. Multimedia technology not only uses multiple media paths to reach audiences, but also provides a medium that can change and adjust to the unique responses of that audience. This option of interactivity enhances the learning process, increasing how engaged the user becomes. Part of the challenge in creating multimedia is to craft a series of experiences that provide and organize information, engage the audience around that information, and finally distill the information into the specific message to be conveyed. Within this context there are several areas of interest. These include the user interface, the structure of information presentation, and the degree of interactivity possible.

The user interface of a computer is the mechanism through which the computer communicates with the user. This interface needs to be easy to use, intuitive, and flexible to avoid user frustration. The rapid spread of the graphical user interface (GUI) among personal computers is testimony to the importance of these qualities. A GUI provides instructions to a computer by use of graphic images instead of text commands. In 1984, Apple's Macintosh computer helped introduce the use of a GUI through their metaphor of a desktop. Icons of documents on the desktop could be grabbed and moved into icons of folders. Because this metaphor is intuitive, it is quickly grasped and employed by the computer user, giving them a sense of understanding and control. In designing multimedia productions, appropriate use of metaphor will give users a sense of familiarity and direction that should be exploited. Many presentations, for example, use the graphic of a push button with the familiar forward, reverse, and stop symbols from VCRs and tape decks. Although nothing is really being pushed, the user immediately knows to click their mouse in the appropriate area. A poorly designed interface will have the opposite effect, leaving the audience uncertain as to where they are and where they need to go.

Beyond the issues of interface, it is important to control the structure of the interaction with the user appropriately. The simplest structure is that of a slide show. A slide show is a linear structure where each screen is displayed in sequence, approaching the intended denouement. Screens can contain buttons or controls that allow the viewer to move among screens at a self-chosen pace. A slide show metaphor usually also allows a reverse in the direction of the presentation so that the user can review any point. More complex, nonlinear structures are built through "hypertext" or "hyperlinks." Hyperlinks are connections made to text or graphics that allow the user to leave the previous track they were on and explore a new track related to the chosen text or graphic. These links can facilitate involvement with the experience by freeing the user to pursue their learning in an active mode, rather than passively accepting a linear structure. The multimedia author needs to use an appropriate balance of linear and nonlinear structures to guide the audience to the desired teaching point while at the same time maximizing their native enthusiasm and desire to explore.

With an appropriately designed interface and structure, the degree of interactivity becomes limited by computing power and imagination. The highest level of interactivity is the simulation. This creates interactivity by placing the user in an imaginary situation where they can alter variables and receive auditory and visual feedback about the results. To design a presentation teaching the use of an ECT machine, one could create a visual representation of the machine controls. A simulated case history could be presented on the screen and the user could visually set the controls using a mouse. A resultant EEG strip and patient response could be generated to give feedback. Such a presentation would be much more effective than simply displaying text and photographs in a linear sequence.

Authoring Process

The process of multimedia production will be briefly reviewed here with an emphasis on authoring software. More in-depth books on production and production values are available (Wolfgram, 1994). If preproduction steps are complete (including determining the message to be communicated, analysis of the audience, analysis of delivery constraints, and the final creation of the idea), the next step is to convert the idea into an actual production. This task is accomplished with authoring software. These applications range in complexity and the amount of control the author has over creating effects for the audience. Some specialize in simple linear slide presentations, while others are used to create the types of complicated simulations described above.

Basic presentation software packages provide a wide range of tools for multimedia production. First, they have tools for structuring the presentation. This is usually in the form of an outliner. Another part of the program is used for the construction of slides that illustrate points of the outline. Sounds, movie clips, animated charts, etc. can be included by importing the files or using included media manipulation tools. Different presentation programs have different strengths, such as tools to create graphs or animation. Other features may include ability to work with spreadsheets, painting tools, animation tools, sound recording and editing capabilities, and digital video support. Many of these programs support the ability to link slides using on-screen buttons, promoting interactivity.

Using more advanced authoring programs allows more options in promoting interactivity, but also requires a greater understanding of how computers are programmed. The above slide show programs involve little control of computer functions. Greater control would allow an author such options as writing files to disk, making mathematical calculations based on user input, or controlling external devices like a laserdisc player. Such control is obtained by using a programming language. Some authoring programs use traditional high-level programming languages like Visual BASIC or C++. These languages have the advantage of being widely taught in computer programming classes, but are not specific to multimedia design and can be clumsy in how they work with medias. Other authoring programs therefore use proprietary scripting languages. These languages give the author similar control abilities as the high-level programming languages, but are specifically designed for authoring. The main drawback to these languages is that they can only be used with the particular authoring program in which they are included.

Most authoring programs combine the functions of the presentation program and a programming language. They use icons to represent screens or component media. The author arranges these icons along a graphic time line or a flowchart, and augments this structure with instructions from the scripting language. Examples of such instructions might be: "turn on the buzzer sound if the user does nothing for 30 seconds" or "if the user clicks on the second curve in the patient course plot, then display the 'manic episode' message ."

Authoring Environment

In this section we will review the hardware and software components of the authoring environment. Although an authoring package is essential, it is important to also have a media library, a development platform, and a display system.

Media Library. Authors need to build and organize a library of media. Each moment in a multimedia production requires appropriate images, sounds, and text. To be free to create these moments, authors need to have a large set of media at their fingertips. The fastest way to build such a library is to purchase clip media. This suffices for generic images and sounds, but may not be adequate for covering specialized topics within psychiatry. Someone interested in the automatisms of autism, for example, may need to capture many such examples on videotape, creating a library of analog media that will act as a source for digitization. Such media is not available through any other means.

In addition to having a sufficient quantity of material, a media library needs a system of organization. This permits rapid access to whatever images, sounds, etc. that are pertinent to a production under construction. Organizing large numbers of images, sounds, and video clips is simplified through the use of a multimedia database program. These programs create a collection of small thumbnail images that can be organized and quickly searched or browsed to help find the location of the desired image. Icon representations of sounds and thumbnails of video images complete the database index.

Development Platform. Any development platform for multimedia requires at minimum a computer of sufficient power, a mass storage device, and sufficient hardware for digitally capturing desired media.

Computer. To create simple multimedia presentations, an extremely powerful computer is not usually necessary. The Multimedia PC (MPC) standard was established in 1991 to specify the minimum components of a machine that can run multimedia applications. It lists a 386SX machine, 2 MB random access memory (RAM), 30 MB hard drive, 8-bit color, a sound board that is Sound Blaster compatible with 8-bit audio and sampling at 22.05 and 11.025 kHz rates, music synthesizer, and single speed CD-ROM. It was rapidly replaced by a newer MPC level 2 specification (see Appendix), and more specifications may arise as computers continue to become more powerful. The main consideration for a system is to have sufficient RAM and hard disk space. More powerful systems are only needed for more intensive graphics or video editing because of the computational demands of these tasks.

Storage. Besides the basic computer hardware and CD-ROM, a multimedia developer should strongly consider acquiring a mass storage device. These devices are slower than a hard disk, but have removable media that can be used to backup data and guard against the possibility of a hard disk crash and consequent loss of information. DAT (digital audio tape) drives are a commonly used backup device. These store 1 to 10 GB on a 4 millimeter wide tape, depending on the drive and compression technology. Magnetic QIC data cartridges are an alternative that store from 40 MB to 2.5 GB with faster access speeds. The ability to transfer large files to other machines is sometimes a consideration beyond the function of simple backup. Removable drives are a widely used format in publishing houses. These cartridges store 44 to 270 MB. Magneto-optical or MO drives are an extremely versatile media that range in size from 3.5 or 5.25 inch disks and store 128 MB to 1.3 GB.

Digitization Boards. To round out a development platform requires appropriate digitizing hardware. The particulars will vary with the individual author's needs. Almost all developers require a sound board for digitization of audio. This is included in the MPC configuration. The need for the addition of a scanner, digital camera, or VCR and video digitizer board are more variable.

Display System. The final component that is important to multimedia development is the system used for presentation. To give a computer-based presentation, it is necessary to display a computer screen so that a large group of people can see it. There are three basic ways of achieving this: a large screen (27–40 inch) monitor, a liquid crystal display (LCD) projector system, or a LCD panel. LCD panels are small units that work in conjunction with a standard overhead projector. Combined with a notebook computer, they create a portable presentation system.

Copyright Law and Multimedia

In this section we discuss some of the legal considerations that affect all multimedia authors as part of copyright law. Multimedia is a new and growing field, and many details of what is or is not covered by copyright have not been tested in the court system. This discussion will cover what is protected by copyright, what rights copyright provides, and what rights are important in using copyrighted media.

Copyright protects "original works of authorship fixed in any tangible medium of expression, now known or later developed, from which they can be perceived, reproduced, or otherwise communicated either directly or with the aid of a machine or device" (U.S.C. 17, section 102). A multimedia production, and all the component media that compose it, fall in this category. This protection exists as soon as the presentation is "fixed" in the computer. Examples of "fixation" include loading onto disk, placing into RAM, or displaying on a monitor. No copyright notice or copyright registration is necessary to secure these rights, although these help clarify ownership.

The rights protected by the copyright act of 1976 are described in U.S.C. 17, section 106. It states:

The owner of copyright under this title has the exclusive rights to do and to authorize any of the following:

(1) to reproduce the copyrighted work in copies or phonorecords;
(2) to prepare derivative works based upon the copyrighted work;
(3) to distribute copies or phonorecords of the copyrighted work to the public by sale or other transfer of ownership, or by rental, lease, or lending;
(4) in the case of literary, musical, dramatic, and choreographic works, pantomimes, and motion pictures and other audiovisual works, to perform the copyrighted work publicly; and
(5) in the case of literary, musical, dramatic, and choreographic works, pantomimes, and pictorial, graphic, or sculptural works, including the individual images of a motion picture or other audiovisual work, to display the copyrighted work publicly.

These rights are broad and complex. To illustrate them in the case of a videotape clip, the law states the copyright owner has the exclusive right to make a copies of the tape. No one else can distribute copies or play the tape to any group of people "outside of a normal circle of a family and its social acquaintances," unless granted permission by the owner. The owner also has the sole rights to prepare a derivative work, that is any work that is based on the tape. Thus no one else could create a new version of the tape by enhancing the sound track or converting the images to black and white.

The issues are further complicated by the fact that these different rights may be owned by different parties. The music rights may belong to the music composer, the choreographic rights to the choreographer, etc. The actors may have rights to their own images, and the studio may own the rights to broadcast and distribute the film. To use a videotape clip in a multimedia production, a license for use would need to be obtained from all of these parties. Because of the difficulty of obtaining all of these rights, many multimedia producers only work with media they develop themselves and therefore have complete rights to. Another way of avoid copyright problems is to use media for which the copyright has expired and that therefore falls into the public domain. This occurs 50 years after the death of the author (U.S.C. 17, section 302).

The exclusive rights of the authors are limited by the fair use provisions (U.S.C. 17, section 107). This states:

> ... the fair use of a copyrighted work, including such use by reproduction in copies or phonorecords or by any other means specified by that section, for purposes such as criticism, comment, news reporting, teaching (including multiple copies for classroom use), scholarship, or research, is not an infringement of copyright. In determining whether the use made of a work in any particular case is a fair use the factors to be considered shall include—
>
> (1) the purpose and character of the use, including whether such use is of a commercial nature or is for nonprofit educational purposes;
> (2) the nature of the copyrighted work;
> (3) the amount and substantiality of the portion used in relation to the copyrighted work as a whole; and
> (4) the effect of the use upon the potential market for or value of the copyrighted work.

Thus a multimedia production that copies a videotape could claim their use was fair if they copied an insubstantial part of it for nonprofit educational purposes for use only at a specific educational institution. The restricted distribution of the production provides evidence that the effect on the tape's potential market is small. (Samuelson, 1994).

Summary

Multimedia technology is rapidly developing. Its potential application in psychiatry is profound because it will allow the demonstration of patients and mental status findings to others for purposes of communications and education. In order for a psychiatrist to use it, a significant effort is needed to understand the components, tools, and legal issues involved. With time, multimedia will become easier to use, and a grasp of the essential tools of multimedia will prepare psychiatrists for the advances of this technology and the changes it will bring.

References

Baskett, S.J. (1978). Teaching psychiatry in a new medical school: A multimedia approach. *Southern Medical Journal, 71*, 1507–1510.

Baudin, F. (1988). *How typography works (and why it is important)*. New York: Design Press.

Bélanger, G. (1990). The missing link: Multimedia communications. *Dimensions in Health Service, 67*, 18–21.

D'Allesandro, M.P., Galvin, J.R., Erkonen, W.E., Santer, D.M., Huntley. J.S., McBurney, R.M., & Easley, G. (1993). An approach to the creation of multimedia textbooks for radiology instruction. *American Journal of Radiology, 161*, 187–191.

D'Allesandro, M.P., Galvin, J.R., Erkonen, W.E., Albanese, M.A., Michaelsen, V.E., Huntley, J.S., McBurney, R.M., & Easley, G. (1993). The instructional effectiveness of a radiology multimedia textbook (HyperLung) versus a standard lecture. *Investigative Radiology, 28*, 643–648.

Fenton, E. (1991). *The Macintosh font book* (2nd ed.). Berkeley, CA: Peachpit Press.

Franken, E.A., Berbaum, K.S., Smith, W.L., Chang, P., Driscoll, C., & Bergus, G. (1992). Teleradiology for consultation between practitioners and radiologists. *Annals of the New York Academy of Sciences, 670*, 277–280.

Frisse, M.E. (1990). The case for hypermedia. *Academic Medicine, 65*, 17–19.

Galvin, J.R., D'Alessandro, M.P., Erkonen, W.E., Lacey, D.L., & Santer, D.M. (1994). The virtual hospital: A link between academia and practitioners. *Academic Medicine, 69*, 130.

Huang, H.K., Arenson, R.L., Lou, S.-L., Wong, A.W.K., Andriole, K.P., Bazzill, T.M., & Avrin, D. (1994). Multimedia in the radiology environment: Current concept. *Computerized Medical Imaging and Graphics, 18*, 1–10.

Hyler, S., & Bujold, A. (1994). Computers and psychiatric education: The "Taxi Driver" mental status examination. *Psychiatric Annals, 24*, 13–19.

Kagetsu, N.J., & Ablow, R.C. (1992). Teleradiology for the emergency room. *Annals of the New York Academy of Sciences, 670*, 293–297.

Kitanosono, T., Kurashita, Y., Honda, M., Hishida, T., Konishi, H., Mizuno, M., & Anzai, M. (1992). The use of multimedia in patient care. *Computer Methods and Programs in Biomedicine, 37*, 259–263.

Lemke, H.U., Faulkner, G., & Krauss, M. (1994). Development towards multimedia medical workstations. *Computerized Medical Imaging and Graphics, 18*, 67–71.

Levy, A.H., & Thrursh, D.R. (1989). The implementation of a knowledge–based pathology hypertext under HyperCard. *Journal of Medical Systems, 13*, 321–329.

McGarty, T.P. (1991). Multimedia communications technology in diagnostic imaging. *Investigative Radiology, 26*, 377–381.

Miller, M. (1972). Multimedia teaching of introductory psychiatry. *American Journal of Psychiatry, 128*, 1219–1223.

Ratib, O. (1994). From Multimodality Digital Imaging to Multimedia Patient Record. *Computerized Medical Imaging and Graphics, 18*, 59–65.

Samuelson, Pamela (1994). Copyright's Fair Use Doctrine and Digital Data. *Communications of the ACM, 37*, 21–27.

Webber, W.B., Summers, A.N., & Rinehart, G.C. (1994). Computer–based multimedia in plastic surgery education. *Plastic and Reconstructive Surgery*, *93*, 1290–1300.

Wolfgram, D.E. (1994). *Creating multimedia presentations*. Indianapolis, IN: QUE.

Appendix

The following is a list of commonly used terms in multimedia. Each term is followed by a definition or explanation of its area of concern.

AIFF (audio interchange file format): File format for audio files developed by Apple Computer.

Authoring: The process of creating multimedia applications.

AVI (audio video interleaved): File format for Windows machines for storing audio and video information.

BMP (BitMaP): File format for IBM compatibles for storing bitmapped images.

CD-ROM (compact disc—read only memory): An optically based storage medium that computers can read from, but not write to. A 4.75 inch disk can contain up to about 650 MB.

Color Depth: The number of bits used to store color information, for example 8-bit color uses 8-bit numbers (ranging from 0 to 255) to represent different colors, 16-bit color has 65,536 colors, and 24-bit color has approximately 16.8 million colors.

DAC (digital analog converter): Any device that converts a signal between digital and analog forms.

Digitization: The process of converting an analog signal to a digital one.

Dithering: The technique of interspersing small dots of different colors to give the appearance of a new color.

DXF (Drawing Interchange Format): A file format that stores descriptions of 3-D objects, originally designed for AutoCAD.

EPS (encapsulated PostScript): File format for text, graphics, and images that are described by Adobe PostScript language (see PostScript).

FLI: A file format for IBM compatibles to store animation, developed for Autodesk Animator. Saves 8-bit color in a 320 × 200 pixel frame.

Font: A typeface or set of characters of related appearance.

GB or gigabyte: 1024 MB.

GIF (graphics interchange format): An efficient file format for compressing 8-bit color graphics, originally created for the Compuserve on-line service.

GUI (graphical user interface): An interface or means of interacting with the computer that uses pictorial (graphical) metaphors to let the user know the status of the machine and change that status.

Interlacing: Technique by which two fields compose a video frame. The first field is a scan of odd numbered horizontal lines from left to right. The second field is the set of even lines. The two fields are interlaced for a video frame, thus 30 frames per second = 60 fields per second.

Jaggies: Jagged edges that result from the use of bitmapped displays instead of smooth, calculated lines.

JPEG (Joint Photographic Experts Group): An image compression standard developed by the committee of the same name designed to compress natural (photographic) images in 24-bit color.

LCD (liquid crystal display): Electronic device that can display information using crystals suspended in a liquid.

MIDI (Musical Instrument Digital Interface): A standard for communication between electronic instruments that sends a device number (instrument to be played), signal to start playing, what note (pitch) to play, and how loud (velocity).

Modeling: The process of creating a 3-D object.

MPC 1 (Multimedia PC level 1): Specification designed by the Multimedia PC Marketing Council for standardizing the components of a multimedia machine. It specifies a 16 MHz 386SX with 2 MB RAM, 30 MB hard drive, single speed CD-ROM drive, 8-bit digital sound, 8-note polyphony, MIDI playback, MIDI input/output (I/O), joystick, and 640 × 480 video display with 8-bit (256) colors.

MPC 2 (Multimedia PC level 2): Newer specification designed by the Multimedia PC Marketing Council (see MPC 1). It specifies a 25 MHz 486SX with 4 MB RAM, 160 MB hard drive, double speed CD-ROM drive, 16-bit digital sound, 8-note polyphony, MIDI playback, MIDI I/O, joystick, and 640 × 480 video display with 16-bit (65,536) colors.

MPEG (Motion Picture Experts Group): Group that meets under the ISO (International Standards Organization) to generate standards for audio and video compression. MPEG 1 and MPEG 2 are standards they have released that are used to compress digital video in computer systems.

Multitrack: A recording that runs in parallel channels, such as stereo sound. Video and audio editing programs need this capability for mixing simultaneous signals from different sources.

NTSC (National Television Standards Committee): Refers to the type of video signal used for broadcast, tape, etc. in the United States, Japan, and Latin America (see also PAL, SECAM).

PAL (Phase Alternate Line): Refers to the type of video signal used for broadcast, tape, etc. in much of Europe (see also NTSC, SECAM).

PCX: Color bitmap file format used on IBM compatibles, developed for PC Paintbrush.

PICS: A Macintosh animation file format based on storing a series of PICTs.

PICT and PICT2: Macintosh (PICTure) file format. Used to store graphics as a set of Macintosh QuickDraw instructions. PICT2 was developed for Color QuickDraw.

PostScript: A language for describing scalable fonts and graphics, designed by Adobe systems. This language is used by computers to communicate instructions to PostScript printers.

QuickTime: Standard created by Apple Computer for storing and playing video.

Rendering: The process of creating a 3-D image after the different elements (objects, textures, orientation, lighting, etc.) have been specified.

RTF (rich text format): A text format that stores text as well as formatting information about point size, style (such as bold or italic), etc.

SECAM (Séquence Couleur à Mémoire): Refers to the type of video signal used for broadcast, tape, etc. in France and much of Eastern Europe (c.f. NTSC, PAL).

SMPTE (Society of Motion Picture and Television Engineers): This organization established the SMPTE time code standard (hr:min: sec:frame) used to identify video frames, as well as standards for synchronizing audio and video.

S-VHS (super VHS): An enhanced version of VHS that uses higher quality tape, can only be recorded and played on S-VHS tape decks; not the same as S-video although many mix the terms.

S-Video: Also know as Y-C. This is the transmission of a video signal in two separate components, lumina (brightness) and chroma (color). It requires two wires and the use of special S-video connectors.

Sample Resolution: The number of bits used to store sampled data. Thus, 8-bit data would be able to store numbers ranging from 1 to 256.

Sampling Rate: The frequency with which an analog signal is sampled in the process of digitization (see Digitization). Usually measured in samples per second.

TGA: A file format used on IBM compatibles for storing 16- or 24-bit color images, named for Truevision's Targa (TarGA) board.

TIFF (Tag Image File Format): An image file format developed by Aldus and Microsoft that was designed to carry image data flexibly. TIFF files are able to contain multiple objects as well as instructions on the handling of those objects.

TrueType: A type of scalable font, designed by Microsoft. These are stored in both Macintosh and IBM compatible files, but the two formats are not directly interchangeable.

Video for Windows: Microsoft's extension to its Windows operating system that allows storing and playing video.

VRAM (video random access memory): RAM that is dedicated to storing video images while the computer sends the image to the screen. More VRAM is needed for larger screens, higher resolution, and greater color depth.

WAV or RIFF WAVE: An audio file format developed by Microsoft and IBM, now a part of Windows. Stores wavetable information.

Wavetable Synthesis: A method for playing sounds that stores short patches or samples of instruments in a table. Musical notes are synthesized from the table.

Windows: A GUI interface designed by Microsoft to be used on IBM compatible machines. Uses a desktop metaphor.

WMF (Windows MetaFile): A graphic format used by Windows machines that stores graphics as a set of colored objects instead of a set of colored pixels.

21
Hypertext Access to Psychiatric Information
Neil Alex

What Is Hypertext?

The term hypertext, coined by Theodore Nelson in 1965, refers to linked, nonsequential information processing using a computer (Seyer, 1991). He could have been speaking of psychiatric record keeping when he stated "Everything is deeply intertwingled" (Horn, 1989, p. 259). It was Vannevar Bush, however, who first described a hypertextlike device he termed the MEMEX in an *Atlantic Monthly* article "As We May Think" in 1945. Bush saw this device as an extension of the human memory, and many of his concepts antedated the hardware developments that made them practical today (mass storage devices, scanners, modems). It was Douglas Englebart who first implemented such a system in 1962. Englebart also developed fundamentals of computing today such as the mouse and outline processing (Horn, 1989).

Hypertext appears to have special relevance to psychiatry, because much of the psychiatric record is not formatted for inclusion in the traditional structures associated with a data base. Hypertext does not require a priori decision making about the length or format of information to be entered. It allows the designer and/or user of the system to add information by the creation of linkages. A linkage is simply a jump to another topic relevant to the current topic. Unlike a text index, hypertext links allow the user to explore relevant data, and keep track of location in the system. The user can easily retrace steps or return to the initial starting point.

A hypertext system does not require costly maintenance personnel, because the system consists of simple ASCII text files, graphics files in standard formats, and sound files. Any of these can be linked to any of the others, allowing complicated topics to be explained with voice or graphic annotation or both.

Links tend to be associated with different patterns of thinking. They can be divided into hierarchical, structural, and associative types. The hierarchical link is characterized by passage down a decision tree structure with branching. It is a manner of thinking that in medicine is often associated with internists. Structural thinking, in which hierarchical thinking is combined with visualization of physical structure, is often considered to be characteristic of neurologists. Associative thinking, in which elements may not have simple hierarchical or spatial relationships, is often used by the psychiatric practitioner. The conflicts associated with implementing computer modeling of each of these representational structures has been a barrier to information exchange among medical specialists. The hierarchical thinker finds the associative thinker unscientific, while the associative and structural thinkers find the hierarchical thinker excessively rigid and missing subtleties of patient data.

Most attempts at encoding patient information have attempted to use data bases to store and represent their patient models. This has had somewhat limited success, because data bases have had difficulty showing relationships in the data set, and tend to be rigid, requiring entry of information in specific forms and sizes. Data base programs are often quite demanding of computer resources, and require sophisticated programming for automation of access to data and control of data entry. The learning curve for a neophyte data base user is often a steep one. Data bases are, however, the best choice for information in which the required output is a listing of data elements sorted on a specific criterion.

Associative and structural thinkers have tended to find the data base model too encumbering to represent such complex elements as a process description of a family interaction or the interactive elements in a focal neurological lesion. Some attempts have been made to use the word processor as an information storage engine. Because these programs continue to rely on the file model (in which discrete data elements are stored in separate files), it is often difficult to show structural relationships. Tools for searching for information are often rudimentary, and most word processors offer no tools for automation of creation of data links. They can also have a steep learning curve, and may be slow in multifile access.

Hypertext is, like the term spreadsheet, a class of programs rather than a specific program. It provides a number of benefits for the storage and retrieval of psychiatric information. First, it is extremely easy to use with minimal training time. Many hypertext programs for the IBM computer require only knowledge of the F1 key (for help) and the Up and Down arrow keys for moving up or down the page within a topic and the Right and Left arrow keys for moving deeper or shallower in the hypertext data system. Unlike most data base and word processing programs (spreadsheets are simply flat data bases in which a record is a line of data), hypertext systems track the user's path and allow retracing or returning to the starting point with a keystroke. In addition, linkages educate the user about the associations and interrelationships in the data.

The end user of a hypertext system is easily able to extend the system, and can equally easily link it to another user's hypertext system. It is this ease of extensibility and association of different structures that makes hypertext so powerful in a psychiatric context.

Making Hypertext

The construction of a hypertext system can be as simple as writing a few files using an ASCII editor, or as complex as linking thousands of graphics, sounds, and text files on a CD-ROM. Unlike most forms of computer software, the hypertext program is easily scaled from the smallest handheld computers to the largest personal computer systems.

The initial element in hypertext construction is determination of the domain of discussion. The system that was presented at the October 1993 Computer Application in Mental Health conference was a hypertext version of the Diagnostic and Statistical Manual of Mental Disorders-III-Revised (DSM-III-R), with release from the American Psychiatric Association for the use of the DSM-III-R for academic presentation (APA, 1987). An outline was created, using a series of "views of the data" as headings. These included diagnoses, decision trees, symptoms, and locally relevant practice data (such as hospital admission formats). The data from the DSM-III-R was typed into the appropriate headings, but could have been linked directly if a computer readable format was available or could have been scanned and read with optical character recognition software. The software, which is produced by Maxthink, permits cross referencing of topics automatically, indexing each word as it is entered. Software tools are available to produce jumps to any selected word or element, such as links to all references to depression. Software is also available to create a glossary that allows the user to understand areas with which they may be unfamiliar and to find related topics easily. The creation of the DSM-III-R hypertext software presented took approximately 60 hours, the bulk of which consisted of data entry time. The system runs on any IBM compatible computer, but was presented on an HP 100 palmtop computer, which runs on AA batteries and weighs 11 ounces.

If this volume were organized in hypertext, the reader would be able to choose from a series of links (buttons, words, or pictures) that would bring together related concepts in the diverse articles present and jump among them, while keeping track of the reader's position. This feature is particularly useful in allowing disparate parts of large organizations to maintain information in their own manner, yet link all areas and keep all information accessible to the entire work group.

Data Reuse: A Major Benefit

One of the major benefits of the hypertext approach is the "reuse" of data. Unlike a data base system, in which the same information may be entered many times in a variety of records, a hypertext system makes a linkage to a piece of data and allows multiple locations to access that link. The information on Imipramine, for instance, may be germane to discussion of ADHD, depression, pain management, and enuresis. The pharmacological data need be entered only once, and can be accessed by a simple link under each of these topics. It is also possible to make customized handouts or summaries of data for patients or referral sources simply by using the clip and print function of the hypertext system.

Linking Information Systems With Hypertext

The recent expansion of Internet access and the use of World Wide Web navigation tools, such as Mosaic and Cello, are beginning to give a glimpse of the full potential of a hypertext-linked information system. One can imagine the efficiencies to be gained if hospital requirements or governmental regulations were available at a keystroke, clinical records accessible (with appropriate security control) in an instant, and decision support tools were available just as easily. The psychiatrist could easily access the expertise and thought sequences of the neurologist or internist (or attorney), and only need a formal consultation for situations of unusual complexity. The potential cost savings are significant. This is particularly evident in large medical organizations, such as HMOs, where minimization of unnecessary referrals means both dollars saved and improved access for those patients for whom consultation is truly needed.

Problems With Hypertext

Unlike traditional word processing documents, hypertext documents require careful thought to the "chunking" of the data, as it is not possible to assume that the reader came upon the information in a specific sequence. Unlike the assumption of the book reader that "you start at the beginning and read through to the end," the hypertext reader is encouraged to browse related information using links encountered in the exploration of the hypertext system. It is extremely useful to the reader if the author of the system is consistent in the use of structures for the presentation of data, using the concepts of Information Mapping developed by Robert Horn et al. (Horn, 1989). In this system, the physical structure of the data presented gives specific indications of where specific information can be found. He presents four principles (chunking, labeling, relevance, and consistency) that encourage authors to limit information to small, easily handled chunks, consistently presented, relevant to the topic, and labeled with a heading separate from the body of the text or picture.

Without a good index or a strong search tool, hypertext can be a confusing web of data that does not convey meaning or show relationships. Too many World Wide Web linkages on the Internet give no hint of the relationship of the data linked to the data viewed. This is confusing to the user and can even be disorienting. Although not an issue for personal systems created by the individual who will use them, it is a significant issue in organizational systems in which the author and the user have no relationship beyond organizational membership.

Confidentiality of hypertext documents is a major concern, and solutions are gradually becoming available. These range from the use of public key software encryption tools to the use of encoded "smartcards" for data access. Each has a cost, either in terms of time to retrieve the data (which must be decrypted) or in terms of ease of data access (when you must put in a card and have it verified by the system). No solution is fully satisfactory at present, and all solutions remain susceptible to normal human carelessness. The doctor who leaves the computer logged on with his or her access code is likely to be a greater risk to confidentiality than the computer hacker. This issue is also present with nonhypertext patient data bases, where access to the computer can give access to hundreds of confidential records.

Hypertext has several political issues associated with it that can be barriers to implementation of hypertext systems. By the nature of the medium, hypertext systems tend to ignore traditional organizational boundaries and permit much more open access to information than is traditional in many organizations. This leads to anxiety in individuals with a high need for control of their environment. This is, of course, the trade-off for the time saved in not having to organize all data at the level of the minimum data set on which the organization can agree.

Working in the Hypertext Environment

In daily practice, it is fully possible to work entirely within a hypertext environment, calling up specific subprograms (telecommunications, spreadsheets, etc.) when they are needed. Using automation tools (macros) built into many of these programs, it is possible to edit a picture, make a spreadsheet, or download a Medline search and include any or all of these directly into a hypertext linkage, accessible to the entire system. Fax documents, which are easily converted to standard PC graphics formats, can be included as well. What develops is an information system in which the associations and uses of data become obvious to the user. This conveys information and insight in ways often not provided by a data base structure (Alex, 1989). Hypertext is a relatively new form of software tool that offers many benefits for dealing with the often unstructured, multifaceted, changing needs of the psychiatric information system. It helps reduce complexity without reducing information, permits graphic and sound annotation without large investments in PC hardware, and provides speed often factors of 10 greater than other forms of multimedia information retrieval.

References

Alex, N. (1989). Hypertext decision support for psychiatry. In B. Barber, D. Cao, D. Qin, & G. Wagner (Eds.), *MedInfo 89* (pp. 266–268), New York: Elsevier Science Publishing.

American Psychiatric Association. (1987). *Diagnostic and statistical manual of mental disorders, third edition, revised*. Washington, DC: American Psychiatric Association.

Horn, R.E. (1989). *Mapping hypertext: Analysis, linkage, and display of knowledge for the next generation of on-line text and graphics* (pp. 252–253, 258–259). Lexington, MA: The Lexington Institute.

Seyer, P. (1991). *Understanding hypertext concepts and applications* (pp. 4, 5). Blue Ridge Summit, PA: Tab Books.

22
Knowledge Coupling: Support for Psychiatric Decision Making

Willie Kai Yee

The human mind has a limited capacity for retaining and processing knowledge. Memory is imperfect, and some problems are too complex to be solved by an individual brain. The implications of these for psychiatric practice are largely ignored. Recognizing and addressing these facts as they affect the process of medical decision making is critical if health care is to be delivered more effectively.

Decision making as discussed here refers to the clinical process of making diagnoses and selecting treatments based on that diagnosis. Psychiatric decision making is subject to the same constraints as medical decision making in general, and in addition must deal with: difficulties inherent in the state of psychiatric knowledge, as reflected in the literature; the subjective, cultural, and individual nature of psychosocial problems; ideological conflicts within the field; and the context of psychiatric treatment and evaluation that may involve the exploration of private and sensitive matters.

Knowledge Losses in Decision-Making

Medical-psychiatric decision making is a heterogeneous process. It may involve a spectrum of strategies ranging from the "hunch" of the clinician, to variably grounded and integrated clinical experience, to logical deduction based on a thorough review of the best available scientific data. Most clinicians will employ a variety of methods depending on the clinical situation and the information that is available to them.

There are severe limitations to this process. First, the decision process may involve multiple variables. The limitations of the human mind in this regard are well documented. Studies have shown that in a variety of areas, clinical judgment, the evaluation of multiple variables by the unaided human mind, is inferior to actuarial decision making, where evidence is combined and evaluated according to known rules and established statistical methods (Dawes, Fust, & Meehl, 1989).

Second, the recall of data is subject to numerous errors as applied to clinical situations. It begins with the data obtained in a study. The data is filtered as it is put into publication, and some of what may have been learned as clinically useful may not be included in the publication for various reasons. As the information is applied to the clinical situation, its relevance may be in question: The population in the study may not reflect the characteristics of the patient. For example, patients selected for an antidepressant medication trial may exclude those with a concurrent personality disorder. In clinical practice, however, depression and personality disorder frequently present together. Thus what was learned from the drug trial may not be applicable to the individual patient.

Further knowledge loss occurs as the information is reproduced in publications or presentations. The summarization procedure will inevitably leave out some material from the original publication. In some cases, what is selected will be that which is relevant to the clinical case. In others, material left out may be deemed to be irrelevant to the purposes of a review or presentation, but may turn out to be essential to a particular patient.

Overall losses in knowledge occur because access to the information varies: Information in papers or books that the practitioner has not read is not available to the decision-making progress (Huth, 1989). In this case, the information simply does not exist. If the practitioner has read or heard the material, errors of comprehension may enter: The material or its significance may be misunderstood (Evidence-Based Medicine Working Group, 1991). Finally, in the actual clinical situation, recall of the material is entirely dependent on the memory of the clinician. This is inconsistent at best, and may be decreased due to overwork, stress, or preoccupation.

Once information is imparted to a patient, as in a recommendation or a prescription, additional knowledge losses occur. The patient may not be presented with all the information that is relevant to the situation, may not hear or understand all that is presented, may not remember what was understood, and may not be motivated to follow what is remembered.

When viewed in toto, even small knowledge losses at each step add up to a potentially frightening degree of misinformation at the time that a treatment is administered.

Solutions: Philosophy and Technology

The means to address these matters discussed above already exist. They involve the use of a new philosophy and appropriate technology brought to the process of clinical decision making.

Knowledge Couplers: Technology to Aid Clinical Decision Making

Problem Knowledge Couplers (PKCs) are computer programs developed specifically to aid clinicians in the process of making accurate clinical diagnostic and treatment decisions. Each coupler covers a clinical problem as presented by the patient: either a symptom to be diagnosed or managed, or a known condition that requires management.

The coupler begins with a series of questions that are answered by the clinician, or when practicable, by the patient. Without further effort such as writing or dictation, a click of a button creates a record of the findings for that patient. The list of findings is used by the program to vote for various diagnostic and management options. Both the findings and the options are presented with appropriate comments that may be printed out and presented to the patient.

A detailed description of the Problem Knowledge Coupler system is provided in the Appendix to this chapter.

Principles of Rational Decision Making in Health Care

The elements of a required philosophy have been described by Lawrence L. Weed, M.D. (1991).

1. Provide the best information tools available.
2. Maximize the contribution of every provider.
3. Couple knowledge to action on the patient's behalf.
4. Put the patient at the center of the health care process.
5. Provide real means for the continuous improvement of quality.
6. Remove the risks associated with variation among providers.
7. Deliver precisely and ethically the necessary and sufficient care each patient requires.

Each of these has relevance to mental health care, and raise issues particular to psychiatry.

Provide Best Information Tools Available. Few tools have been generally available to aid psychiatric decision making, although these have been under development at various institutions. These tools vary widely in their scope, reflecting their origins. Some that have developed out of academic institutions use search and retrieval or artificial intelligence strategies. Others have developed from diagnostic classifications, especially the Driagnostic and Statistical Manual of Mental Disorders (DSM), and from structured diagnostic interviews. The PKC system was developed for use in medical settings after an examination of the decision-making process itself, and a determination of the types of information access that would be most clinically useful. Using the principles and tools of the PKC system, it has been possible to develop programs that address common psychiatric problems such as depression, anxiety, and psychosis.

Evaluation of the PKC system, or any other knowledge tool, raises complex issues. The clinical interview is not an acceptable "gold standard." The variability in unstructured clinical evaluations is the very problem that knowledge couplers are trying to address. Allowing a wide variety of procedures as the input into a research project cannot produce meaningful results. The question of evaluation must be framed in light of decades of research demonstrating the limitations of unaided human decision making. Because of demonstrated deficiencies and an insoluble research design dilemma, a different approach is needed. It is as though cardiologists asked for double-blind studies on the superiority of the stethoscope before using it. The question should be settled on the basis of actual familiarity and usage of the tools in question.

Maximize the Contribution of Every Provider. Present day medicine has developed multiple roles in addition to physicians (primary and specialty), for the provision of health care in specialty/technical areas (e.g., radiology technicians or ICU nurses) and in primary care (nurse practitioners and physician assistants). A shared knowledge base and a shared set of standards, terminology, and conventions reflected in the medical record are essential to consistent and rational administration of health care by multiple providers, whether organized as a team or not.

"Support providers" are used widely, especially in hospital and community psychiatry, and include psychologists, social workers, occupational and recreational therapists, psychiatric nurses, community mental health workers, and others. Although they may use a common medical record, and may participate in regular interdisciplinary treatment planning meetings, disparities in treatment philosophies, ideologies, and the arena of contact with the patients may lead to varying and conflicting views of the patient and his or her problems.

Problem Knowledge Couplers address these conflicts by providing a common framework for evaluating a patient, and providing a problem list shared by all providers. Couplers are able to integrate knowledge from multiple disciplines, so that all providers have relevant information from other disciplines as diagnostic and treatment decisions are made. A means of including input from all providers allows the coupler to become a mechanism for the cumulative and cooperative acquisition of knowledge across professional boundaries.

Couple Knowledge to Action on Patient's Behalf. All clinical decision making involves the retrieval of information from a base of knowledge, and selecting and combining the information relevant to the clinical problem. Computer tools can extract knowledge that is relevant to the situation. Proper program design means that the clinician will not have to depend on memory or wade through a textbook, library, or computer data base to have access to the most appropriate material.

In addition to remembering a base of technical knowledge, applying it to a clinical problem involves the correlation of multiple variables of the clinical situation (history findings, symptoms, physical examination, mental status, and laboratory results) with the variables presented in the literature. A given problem may involve dozens of diagnostic possibilities, each with several findings, many of which overlap. The number of combinations exceeds the capacity of the human mind to carry out a complete correlation. Mental strategies used in such situations inevitably involve simplifications, abstractions, and other methods that omit information, and carry the risk of introducing error into the decision-making process.

Accurately correlating multiple variables is something that computers can do well. Although much research and discussion has gone into discussing the representations of knowledge (algorithms) that are best used, it has been shown that even the simplest models (linear models or simple but accurate lists) can aid accurate clinical decision making (Dawes & Corrigan, 1974).

As psychiatric knowledge expands and is put on a more scientific basis, the application of that knowledge remains in a centuries-old mode. The number of effective interventions that have been demonstrated continues to increase. For example, the number of antidepressants presently available on the market is close to 20, with a half-dozen classes of augmenting or alternative agents, and many medications that may be used for comorbid conditions. Although all are effective against depression, the literature lists a number of demonstrated indications and contraindications for each agent and class of agent. Published guidelines may attempt to rationalize the selection of medication, but these omit details that may be relevant to an individual patient, and again rely on the memory and processing capability of the clinician to implement them.

Knowledge couplers written for psychiatric problems are able to create the relevant links between the ever-expanding psychiatric literature and the unique presentation of the individual patient. Beginning by asking those questions that should be asked for every problem, a coupler is able to produce the links to all relevant knowledge from the literature, including the rare illness, the disorder that is the province of another medical specialty, and the multiple causes that may be present in a complex case.

Put the Patient at the Center of the Health Care Process. Discussions of health care reform largely proceed on the assumptions that patients are passive recipients of health services, and that the provider is at the center of the process. True reform must recognize the patient as the final arbiter of health care actions, and must recognize patients as active participants. When patients themselves are seen as the primary providers of health care, and information access is restructured to facilitate that process, compliance increases, prevention is emphasized, and health care costs are brought down in numerous ways (Ferguson, 1987). Similarly, the recognition of families as a health care delivery system has a demonstrated impact on the course of psychiatric illness, as shown by the abundant literature on the psychoeducational family treatment of schizophrenia.

Psychiatric implementation of this involves an educational component that helps to relieve stigma, utilize resources, such as self-help groups, that lie outside the province of formal psychiatric care. Respect is maintained for the patient's ability to determine the combination of symptom severity, disability, side effects, risks, benefits, and costs with which he or she wishes to live.

Knowledge couplers provide a key link in transforming the center of health care decision making. Their use in the earliest phases of evaluation, and the provision of information that has been selected to be specifically applicable to the problem at hand insures that the importance of the consumer is recognized. As the patient reviews the coupler output with the provider, a collaborative rather than passive and dependent relationship is established.

Provide Real Means for Continuous Improvement of Quality. The vast amount of information available is both a blessing and a curse. From a scientific and clinical point of view, this is a wonderful time to be in the field of psychiatry. New medications, greater understanding of brain function, and the establishment of a firm research foundation for various psychosocial treatments make psychiatry an exciting and challenging field. The difficulty here, as in all rapidly advancing fields, is that the explosive growth of knowledge makes it impossible to keep abreast of all significant information, especially while engaged in a busy practice. Even if one is able to keep up to date, the knowledge losses described above render the application of knowledge to the clinical situation a haphazard process.

Computer systems have the ability to track large amounts of information, and to provide for regular updating of that information. Implementation of the PKC system includes regular updating of information as it is reviewed in the literature by coupler authors and as suggested by users of the PKC system.

Remove Risks Associated With Variation Among Providers. Psychiatry is making progress in establishing a consistent language for diagnosis (the DSM) and standards for the treatment of psychiatric disorders (practice guidelines). The actual implementation of these at the level of the practitioner still remains a haphazard process. The training, philosophies, and literature bases of various disciplines result in additional variation in case evaluation and management between providers of different disciplines. However, knowledge couplers, based on the problem-oriented approach, insure that relevant knowledge from all disciplines is available to all providers.

Consistent input is applied to every case, regardless of the practitioner's specialty, discipline, training, orientation, or practice setting. Although diagnostic classifications, clinical guidelines, and computer-based knowledge systems cannot reduce the variation associated with individual patients, consistent input can be used to ensure that all providers are working from the same data base of information about the patient, and from the same base of knowledge derived from the literature. Interventions, when chosen from recommendations coupled to the findings for a patient, may be more rationally selected. When interventions are not selected from these recommendations, the variation is clear. In either case, the consistency of input means that outcomes can now be meaningfully assessed.

Deliver Precisely and Ethically the Necessary and Sufficient Care Each Patient Requires. Health care reform has involved a discussion of the financing of health care. Insurance schemes, mandatory coverage, caps on services, and public financing (i.e., taxes) are the language of such reform. Managed care attempts to control costs by limiting care on the basis of utilization statistics of populations of patients. The characteristics of individual cases that may justify care may be overlooked in the routine processing of requests for authorization or the often strained negotiation between authorizers and providers of care.

Limiting costs in this context involves limiting services in some way, either directly through caps on services, or indirectly by limiting fees or taxing benefits. Little discussion is given to the role of preventive care, other than in a few areas such as prenatal care, where a clear cost benefit advantage has been shown. Although there is discussion of the role of guidelines to limit the inappropriate use of expensive technology, there is no discussion about how guidelines or any other relevant medical information is actually used in the patient–physician interaction (Weed & Weed, 1994). Indeed, the topic of the patient–physician interaction is seen as a taboo subject, and the role of information technologies in this interaction is a matter left to a few specialists.

Computer software can be used to select treatment that is appropriate by matching the characteristics of the individual patient to those that have been shown to identify safe and effective treatments. Superficially, this may appear to be the same process as that utilized by managed care. The difference is that the coupling of information takes place as part of the process of clinical diagnosis and treatment, rather than an additional procedure that is imposed upon it. For example, cognitive therapy may be a recommended treatment for some depressions. If some other form of therapy were being practiced by the therapist, the recommendation for cognitive therapy by a managed care representative may be seen as an invasion into the therapeutic process. If this recommendation appeared at the time that the treatment was planned, it could be reviewed as an option by provider and patient together, taking into account the provider's skills and patient preference.

Utilizing continuously updated software provides a way of rationally integrating newer treatments into clinical practice. Techniques that the clinician may not have learned during professional training can be brought to the clinician's attention at the time when it is most appropriate to consider them for application, rather than at a distant time that may be convenient to the schedule of the clinician or the presenters of the information. It also allows newer treatments to be evaluated appropriately in the context of information about established treatments, with both risks and benefits available. The overprescription of newer medications because of pharmaceutical company marketing efforts, and their underutilization, due to reluctance to employ unfamiliar treatments and lack of adequate information, can be overcome by software that can provide the precise amount of information that the situation requires.

Health Care Reform

By ignoring issues that would improve health, make better clinical decisions, and better utilize existing services and technologies, the focus on economics will paradoxically result in poorer overall health of the people and greater cost of health care. Only by redirecting the goal of reform from how to pay for health insurance to how to improve the health of the citizenry can true cost control be achieved.

Knowledge Coupling in Clinical Practice

Problem Knowledge Couplers have been used for several years in a variety of psychiatric settings. The experience of users indicates fewer problems with acceptance than anticipated, and unexpected benefits.

Patient Acceptance of Computer Usage

Patients generally accept the use of the computer as part of a psychiatric evaluation. Except for paranoid patients, discussed below, I have never had a patient object to the use of the computer during an evaluation. Most patients react to the computer positively. They feel they are being evaluated with state-of-the-art methods, and that the physician is being thorough. Some patients have stated that the computer evaluation is evidence of care that is both personal and state-of-the-art. This is particularly true if they are given a printout for their own use either during or after the session.

Dealing With the Paranoid Patient

Paranoid patients may object to the use of the computer. I have handled this simply by asking the patient to sit by my side where he/she can see the screen while I run the program. Paranoid patients are usually quite curious, and will take the opportunity to see what is happening. Once they have accepted this offer, they have now become allies with me against a new "adversary"—the computer. After several minutes using the PKC system, I have found most paranoid patients lose interest, probably because screen after screen of text lacks the appeal of video games and other computer graphic displays that they may have been exposed to. At this point, however, the mistrust of the computer is no longer an issue.

Paranoid patients may object to or falsely answer some questions in the coupler "Psychotic-like Behavior, Thinking, and Speech," the one that is most likely to be used in their cases. This can be overcome by running a coupler that is more neutral for them, such as Anxiety or Depression, first. The patient may then lose interest in specific questions before the coupler for psychosis is run.

Psychiatrist Resistance

Resistance, usually passive, to the use of the computer in clinical settings is more likely to come from the psychiatrist than the patient. Patients may pick up the psychiatrist's discomfort with the situation, and may then express the discomfort as their own.

Use in Clinical Practice

One user said of the PKC system "It's like having a friendly consultant at your side." For practitioners in solo practice, or working in isolated areas, the PKC system can be a valuable resource in maintaining and augmenting their own clinical skills.

To serve its function, the PKC system should be used on a regular basis. I routinely do the appropriate couplers on all evaluations. Occasionally, on what appears to be a clear cut case, I will omit doing the coupler. Within a few weeks, I usually regret the decision, and do the coupler at that point. In short, actual experience with couplers shows that they can become integrated into psychiatric practice. After using them regularly, and having the comprehensive, relevant, and reliable data base available for each patient, it is difficult to conceive of practice without such a system.

Mr. A., a 42-year-old engineer, consulted me several years ago for mild depression, marital conflicts, and difficulty getting his life in order. After several months of psychotherapy, he felt he had made sufficient progress to discontinue therapy. He returned a few years later, and as part of his reevaluation, the couplers Psychiatric Screening and Depression and Loss of Interest were run. In addition to major depression, four out of nine possible findings indicating Attention Deficit Disorder (ADD) were present. A more thorough evaluation of this confirmed the presence of ADD, and a trial of stimulants was begun. The results were dramatic, with both remission of all depressive symptoms and an enormous improvement in organizational ability and productivity at work that has been sustained for a year.

This case illustrates the critical issues concerning the use of couplers. I might well have picked up the presence of ADD in this patient without the coupler had I been more aware of it as an issue. On the other hand, I might not have, and did not on the first encounter of this patient. With the use of coupler, my awareness of the prevalence of ADD and of the need to explore the findings of ADD in this patient were not required to properly evaluate and manage this case. The steps in the evaluation are documented, consistent, and justified.

Integration of Couplers Into Psychiatric Evaluation

There are several approaches to utilizing couplers in the actual clinical situation of evaluating and treating patients. The three that follow discuss the various points in the evaluation at which the couplers may be run, along with the pros and cons of each approach.

After Clinical Evaluation. The coupler appropriate to the patient's problems may be run after completing the clinical evaluation and allowing the patient to leave the office. This has several advantages. If the clinician is just becoming familiar with the PKC system, this will allow time to study all the aspects of the coupler, and to become more adept at handing the mechanics of navigating the coupler system.

One disadvantage of this method is that the user will inevitably find a few questions that were not asked during the interview. Because the use of a coupler requires that the user answer all questions, the accuracy of the data generated will be compromised. One of the reasons that couplers were developed was to be certain that all pertinent questions were asked, and this method is likely to defeat that purpose.

Another difficulty is that the results of the coupler are not available at the time decisions are made. For a diagnosis, this may just mean adding a chart entry; but if it affects treatment, the patient may be unavailable or confused by an alteration of treatment plan at this point.

In short, running a coupler after a clinical evaluation should be done only as a training exercise, or in those rare occasions in which the coupler session for some reason cannot be completed in the patient's presence.

Toward the End of Interview. The clinician may conduct the interview as he or she usually does, and run the coupler just before presenting the assessment and treatment plan to the patient. The coupler may be introduced by a comment such as "I would like to enter some information into the computer to make sure I do not forget anything." As the clinician selects the appropriate responses in the coupler, she may ask the patient to answer any questions that were not asked during the earlier part of the interview. After coupling, the results may then be discussed with the patient. This allows the clinician to evaluate the patient with little disruption of his or her usual style, and still allows access to the results of coupling as treatment decisions are made. This also allows the clinician who may not entirely trust or understand the coupling process to form her own clinical opinion, against which the coupler-generated options may be compared.

Patients may sometimes feel that the clinician is involved in some secretive process from which he or she is being excluded. This may be handled by inviting the patient to observe the computer screen as the data is entered. This procedure also allows the patient to confirm the accuracy of responses as they are selected.

During Evaluation of Present Illness. The coupler may be run as soon as the main problem has been determined, near the beginning of the clinical interview. This allows the integration of the information gathering process for the coupler into the clinical interview. The running of the coupler becomes part of obtaining the history of the present illness and stresses its importance to both patient and practitioner. The clinician asks questions relevant to the patient's complaint at the time the patient presents the problem, and establishes the use of the computer as a natural part of the evaluation process.

Running the coupler early in the interview may mean that the evaluation process may be limited to the evaluation of the presenting problem. In an emergency, this may be acceptable, and may allow for prompt evaluation and initiation of treatment. There is, however, a risk that the evaluation may end here, and that other essential tasks such as obtaining a complete problem list or a thorough past history may be ignored.

Before the Interview. Another procedure that may be employed in clinic settings is to have a skilled interviewer, for example, a psychiatric social worker, nurse, or other trained interviewer, run the coupler before the evaluation. This makes the coupler results available at the time of the evaluation. None of the physician's time is used to enter data into the computer, and the interview may proceed as usual.

The discussion of coupler results may not take place immediately after the coupler is run because some of the content of the coupler may be considered beyond the knowledge level of the nonphysician interviewer. In a mental health setting, medical issues are more likely to be beyond the scope of a mental health worker, and in medical settings, psycho-therapeutic issues may be unfamiliar to medical personnel.

Although this may be a more efficient use of the psychiatrist's time, this procedure risks minimizing the importance of the coupling process, and the coupler results could even conceivably be ignored, just as critical laboratory reports may be overlooked.

Time Required

After becoming familiar with the structure of a coupler, it takes about 10 minutes to ask all the questions contained in a coupler. Most of these are questions that should be asked in the evaluation of the problem anyway, and answers are keyed in by pressing single number keys (i.e., no typing is involved). The actual amount of time that it adds to the evaluation is minimal.

If the patient presents with multiple complaints, more than one coupler may need to be run. I have found that two couplers can be run without interfering with the evaluation process. If an evaluation requires more than two couplers, it is best to schedule them over more than one session. Again, there is probably no additional increase in time involved, because these are cases that require a longer evaluation anyway.

The Personality Disorder Coupler is the only psychiatric coupler that may take more than 10 minutes to run, because it contains questions for each of the individual criteria of all the DSM-IV personality disorders. Because of this, a self-assessing questionnaire, the PsyComNet Self-Assessing Personality Disorders Inventory by Ivan Goldberg, M.D., has been adapted for use with the PKC System. The patient completes the questionnaire, and a clerical person can enter the data directly into the Personality Disorder Coupler using the Add to the List of Findings command from the Other Functions screen. This process takes about 10 minutes of clerical time, not counting time to print out the report. The results of the questionnaire, as with all self-assessing instruments in personality disorders, must be interpreted with caution (Hyler et al., 1989).

Conclusion

Unaided psychiatric decision making depends on processes that have limitations that have been defined by cognitive science, and that are becoming inadequate to handle the volume and complexity of psychiatric knowledge. Tools, such as Problem Knowledge Couplers directly address these limitations. Clinical experience has shown that the use of these knowledge tools in psychiatric practice is beneficial and acceptable to both practitioner and patient.

Appendix: Working With Problem Knowledge Couplers

PKCs are Windows™-based point-of-care information tools for identifying patient problems and risk factors, eliciting and recording patient findings, and considering and refining diagnostic and management strategies.[1]

Couplers are defined in three ways:

1. As screening tools to identify problems and risk factors that may require attention;
2. For problems presented at the level of a present illness, such as vomiting or headache, requiring diagnosis and management; and
3. For problems with known diagnosis, such as hypertension or diabetes, requiring management.

Many couplers provide both diagnostic and management information.

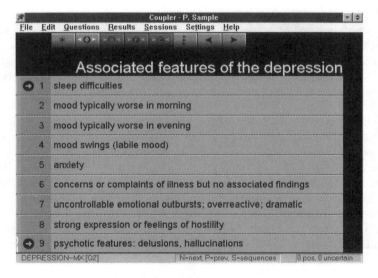

Positive (observed) findings for the patient are elicited and recorded through the use of sequences of findings displays. The provider and patient respond to a series of questions or statements, each corresponding to or qualifying a finding that may or may not be present in the patient. A finding is set to positive by clicking on it with the mouse, or by entering its number via the keyboard. Repeating this action will set the finding to "uncertain"; a third click will reset it to negative.

By clicking on toolbar icons or selecting pull-down menu choices, positive findings for the patient may be coupled with a medical knowledge base parsed from core and specialty medical literature and texts, kept current through periodic updates, to produce:

---

[1] Adapted and used with permission from the literature of PKC Corporation, One Mill St., Burlington, VT 05401.

1. An annotated summary of findings;
2. An index of possible causes or relevant management options;
3. An index of secondary options that may be pursued to further characterize the problem or initiate management; and
4. Information detail displays for each specific cause, management option, or secondary option.

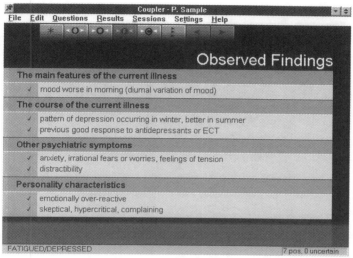

The Findings Summary includes all positive and uncertain findings entered for the patient. Positive findings are distinguished by check marks ($\sqrt{}$), uncertain findings by question marks (?). Findings are listed in broad groupings specific to each coupler. Comments directly relate each finding to one or more possible causes of the problem being defined, or give information for monitoring or further investigating the problem. One or more medical literature citations are associated with each comment.

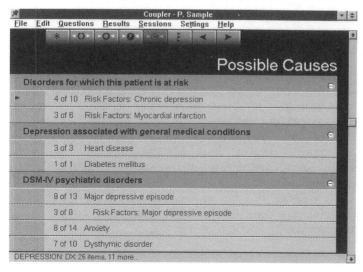

When all findings have been entered and reviewed via the Findings Summary, a list of possible causes or relevant management options for the problem as it is currently characterized may be generated.

The numbers at left for each cause indicate the number of positive (observed) findings for the patient, followed by the total number of possible findings in the coupler, indicating the cause may be present.

By clicking on any cause on this index, you may view all findings in the coupler that may indicate the presence of that cause.

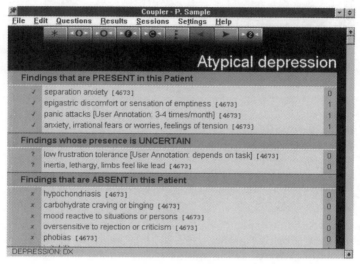

Findings that may indicate a specific cause are grouped into:

findings that are PRESENT in this patient;
findings that are UNCERTAIN in this patient;
findings that are ABSENT in this patient; and
other considerations.

PRESENT and UNCERTAIN findings are those previously entered for the patient. ABSENT findings are other findings that may have indicated the cause had they been present.

Other considerations are relevant texts pulled from the coupler's knowledge base that may have a bearing on the consideration of the cause, but that are not specific to any single finding.

The number in the right-hand column for each finding is the number of other causes in the coupler's knowledge base indicated by that finding.

Menus of secondary options to pursue to further characterize the problem or to rule in or rule out a specific possible cause or management option are available for some causes and options. Procedural and informational details are presented for each option as it relates to the cause or management strategy under consideration.

Storing and Retrieving Coupler Results

The set of positive and uncertain findings collected during a coupler session for a patient can be saved in an electronic file for later recall and modification, or printed to give to the patient or to include in a paper record. There is no need for transcription: The printed text is a complete, structured record of the encounter.

Each session is identified with patient ID, provider ID, date/time stamp, and an optional free-text comment. You can retrieve any stored session at any time to review the data or to add or delete findings. If you elect to restore after modifying findings, the old session will not be overwritten: The modified session will be assigned a new date/time and stored as a separate session. You therefore maintain a complete audit trail.

Patient and coupler session information is saved in dBASE compatible files using FoxPro indexing. (Please call PKC for information about dBASE III Plus, dBASE IV, and Clipper compatible index files.) If you are using couplers on a network, a dBASE compatible file is created for each client station for each session.

System Requirements

1. IBM-compatible PC with Intel 386 CPU (minimum) and one 3.5 inch disk drive
2. Microsoft Windows™ 3.1 or later
3. 20 MB available hard disk space
4. 4 MB main memory
5. 16 color EGA monitor or laptop monochrome (minimum)
6. Highly recommended: 256 color monitor

To realize maximum benefit, PKC also highly recommends a mouse and laser printer.

References

Dawes, R.M., & Corrigan. (1974). Linear models in decision making. *Psychological Bulletin, 81*, 95–106.

Dawes, R.M., Fust, D., & Meehl, P.E. (1989). Clinical versus actuarial judgment. *Science, 243*, 1668–1673.

Ferguson, T. (1987). Health in the information age: Sharing the uncertainty. *Whole Earth Review, 57*, 130–133.

Huth, E.J. (1989). The underused medical literature. *Annals of Internal Medicine, 110*, 99–100.

Hyler, S.E., Rieder, R.O., Williams, J.B., Spitzer, R.L., Lyons, M., & Hendler, J. (1989). A comparison of clinical and self-report diagnoses of DSM-III personality disorders in 552 patients. *Comprehensive Psychiatry, 30*, 170–178.

Evidence-Based Working Group (1992). Evidence-based medicine: A new approach to teaching the practice of medicine. *Journal of the American Medical Association, 268*, 2420–2425.

Weed, L.L., & Weed, L. (1994). Reengineering medicine. *Federation Bulletin: Journal of Medical Licensure and Discipline, 81*, 149–183.

Weed, L.L. (1991). *Knowledge coupling: New premises & new tools for medical care and education*, New York: Springer–Verlag.

23
Neural Network Models in Psychiatry

Satish S. Nair, John C. Reid, and Javad H. Kashani

Neural networks represent one of the most promising artificial intelligence tools at the present time, with successful application to a broad range of modeling problems. Neural networks are currently used in psychiatry in two widely different areas. The first one is the rapidly growing field of cognitive neuroscience (also referred as neuropsychology, behavioral neurology, or computational neuroscience) formed by the merger of the disciplines of cognitive science (psychology) and neuroscience (biological psychiatry). The second area uses advanced modeling and analysis techniques to study human behavior by scales and interviews. Both these areas are described in the foregoing with emphasis being primarily on the latter.

Cognitive neuroscience and its potential for studying psychiatric behavior are briefly described. Subsequently the other area of using artificial intelligence for advanced modeling and analysis techniques is described, starting with statistical approaches and leading to the promising neural network framework. The subsequent sections then deal primarily with these techniques for decision making. A novel sensitivity method using neural networks developed by the authors to ascertain quantitatively the importance of the causative factors (inputs) on the output(s) for such studies is described. Following that, two case studies in psychiatry illustrate the techniques described. The first case study investigates the relationship of personality, parental bonding, social support, and Diagnostic Interview for Children and Adolescents (DICA) variables to adolescent hopelessness using a data set gathered from 150 high school students. The second case study uses similar modeling and analysis techniques for determining the effectiveness of stages of change and a drug in panic disorder. The last section discusses the implications of the

This study was supported in part by the University of Missouri Research Board grant #94-013 and by National Science Foundation grant NSF CMS 9411866.

methodologies and their utility to psychiatry followed by some of the current research directions being pursued by the modeling and artificial intelligence community.

Cognitive Sciences and Biological Psychiatry

The area of cognitive neuroscience has emerged due to increasing awareness in the separate disciplines of cognitive science and neuroscience that adequate explanations of human behavior require both high-level (cognitive) and fine-grained (neuroscience) descriptions simultaneously. The high-level description of cognitive science attempts to understand human cognition in symbolic and abstract terms without reference to the brain mechanisms used to carry them out. This approach has successfully characterized important aspects of high-level cognition, such as multidigit arithmetic and problem solving, and many advances in artificial intelligence have been based on this premise. However the high-level approach has been less successful for problems in human cognition such as visual pattern recognition and language processing (Cohen & Servan–Schreiber, 1992). This has spurred research at the fine-grained level (neuroscience) wherein the functioning of the brain itself is being studied in an attempt to explain poorly understood phenomena in cognition. In psychiatry this approach, classified as biological psychiatry, has been dominant over the past 30 years, and represents a bottom-up attempt to gather as much basic neurobiological data as possible, and use this to build upward to understand behavior. Although such a fine-grained approach has resulted in increasing our understanding of basic brain mechanisms, it has not helped significantly to unravel how brain mechanisms result in behavior for psychiatric applications (Cohen & Servan–Schreiber, 1992). Also, psychopharmacologic therapy still relies on empirical trials rather than on causal understanding of the interactions between drugs and brain mechanisms.

The limited success of both the disciplines of cognitive science and neuroscience individually has motivated researchers to unify both these fields to create the area of cognitive neuroscience. Progress in cognitive neuroscience has resulted so far from new methods for simultaneously studying brain function and behavior, including neuroimaging techniques (such as positron emission tomography [PET] and magnetic resonance imaging [MRI]) and electrophysiological techniques (such as event-related potentials) that can be used in humans, as well as more detailed methods in animal studies (such as single-cell recording and microdialysis). Some examples of such studies are a neural model of the physiological effects of catecholamines to explain cognitive deficits in schizophrenia (Servan–Schreiber & Cohen, 1992), modeling schizophrenia (Hoffman & McGlashan, 1993), modeling the characteristics of Alzheimer's disease

(Kippenhan, Barker, Pascal, Nage, & Duara, 1992), and humans under central nervous system (CNS) stimulants (Cohen & Servan–Schreiber, 1992). The challenge for the new area is to complement the empirical techniques such as PET and MRI with a broad enough theoretical framework. Such a theoretical framework has begun to emerge from artificial neural network modeling, also called connectionism or parallel distributed processing. Neural network models mimic the brain structure with its parallel computation, massive interconnections between the basic units that have stochastic firing properties, distributed representation of information, and incremental learning. These issues and properties of neural networks will be discussed in more detail.

The area of cognitive neuroscience, as mentioned, is growing rapidly as evident from the popularity of the 6-year-old *Journal of Cognitive Neuroscience* and the formation of the new Cognitive Neuroscience Society (Waldrop, 1993). The examples just cited probably represent a minuscule portion of the research being performed in the area. The interested reader is referred to the new journal and the literature for further information related to the area. The purpose of this chapter is to present another promising area, that of diagnosis and decision making using new artificial intelligence modeling and analysis techniques. Such techniques hold considerable potential for application to psychiatry as we illustrate using two case studies later in this chapter.

Diagnosis and Decision Making

Several researchers infer characteristics of human behavior by using scales and interviews. These two tools, although used in conjunction at times, are fundamentally different with scales being quantitative and interviews being qualitative. By this we mean that scales are collected from a large sample of subjects and using appropriate mathematical and statistical techniques, the trends of interest in the population are determined. On the other hand, a psychiatric expert interviews one patient at a time, and, using the qualitative information from the interview and his/her knowledge base, arrives at an appropriate diagnosis. Few tools exist currently to capture such expert knowledge bases but several exist for analyzing data sets collected using scales. Statistical modeling, which is a large area in itself, is briefly reviewed next followed by neural network modeling, the main focus of this chapter, and then the utility of them both for a problem is presented.

Statistical Approaches

Statistical approaches include decision trees with various loss functions at each node in the tree, Bayesian analyses, sequential analyses where decisions are made after processing some of the data, and linear models, to name a few. All of these techniques have been incorporated into various algorithms and computer programs to help health professionals make decisions. However, these techniques are often time consuming to use and few have enjoyed wide popularity. Probably the most common are classical statistical techniques such as analysis of variance and linear models that are typically used to make decisions about a set of data. If the underlying structure of the data are complex, however, the statistical models can be difficult to interpret. The interested reader is referred to Kirk (1982) and Neter, Wasserman, and Kutner (1989) for more details regarding statistical techniques.

Neural Networks and Learning

Neural networks can quantify complex mapping characteristics in a compact and elegant manner. Neural networks have been successful in several areas including economic analysis, pattern recognition, speech recognition and synthesis, medical diagnosis, seismic signal recognition, and control systems (McCord–Nelson & Illingworth, 1991). The massive interconnections of rather simple neurons that make up the human brain provided the original motivation for the neural network models. The terms artificial neural network and connectionist models distinguish them from the biological networks of neurons in living organisms. Interest in neural networks is due, in part, to powerful new neural models, the multilayer perceptron, the feedback model of Hopfield, and to learning methods such as backpropagation (Rumelhart & McClelland, 1987). It is also due to the rapid recent developments in hardware design that have brought within reach the realization of neural networks with a large number of nodes.

In a neural network, a multilayered architecture is interposed between inputs and outputs (Fig. 1a). Elements of these interposed layers are called neurons. Each element, or neuron, of the interposed layer has weights and biases. Changing the weights and biases of a neuron alters its output, and, ultimately, the output of the entire network. The goal is to choose the weights and biases of the neurons to make a mathematical model that will map the inputs to the outputs. The neural network is initialized with random weights and biases that are adjusted based on an error minimization criteria called "training" the network. Training (or learning) is accomplished by adjusting these weights iteratively (typically, to minimize some objective function) when input/output pairs are repeatedly presented to the network. When the network has analyzed all the patterns once, it has trained for one epoch. These weights and biases provide the necessary memory for the learning process. A two-layer neural network with an arbitrarily large number of neurons in the interposed layer can approximate a continuous function over a compact set

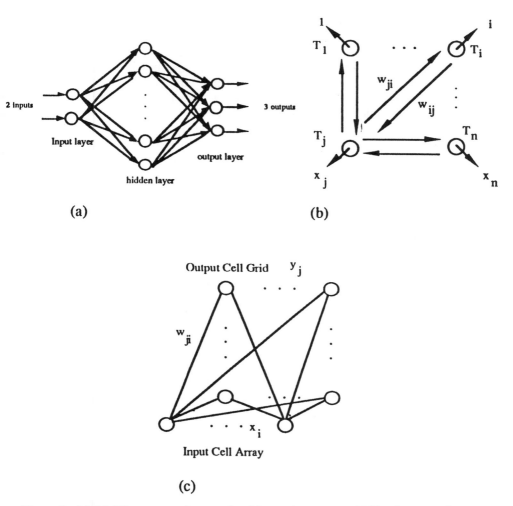

Figure 1. (a) Multilayer neural network with two inputs, one hidden layer, and three outputs; (b) Hopfield network; and (c) self-organizing feature map.

(Hornik, Stinchcombe, & White, 1990). This result has motivated much research interest in the area of using neural networks as a nonlinear tool to analyze complex nonlinear systems. Other various possibilities include fully connected architectures like the Hopfield model (Fig. 1b) (Hopfield, 1982), self-organizing feature maps (Fig. 1c) (Kohonen, 1990), associative search networks, etc. By means of extension and/or combination of network architectures and learning rules, new models have been developed. The counterpropagation model (Hecht–Nielsen, 1988) is a combination of the self-organizing feature map mentioned above and the

Adaptive Resonance Theory models (ART; Carpenter & Grossberg, 1987). While these models vary in their details, all of them possess the key observed properties of the neurons in the biological brain: Neurons are slow, with the relevant computation time being on the order of milliseconds compared to the modern computer operations that occur in nanoseconds (or 1 million times faster). The brain, however, performs massive parallel processing, which is in contrast to the von Neumann machines, the conventional digital computers in which the instructions are executed sequentially, and this parallel processing provides the brain with its speed. The neurons in the brain have reciprocal or feedback connections and so a typical processing cycle includes a flow of stimuli in both directions. Information is stored in a distributed fashion with no central control. This has implications described below under graceful degradation. Learning occurs in this massively parallel system by the incremental adjustment of synaptic strengths between the neurons by repeated trials. Such a hardware architecture is found to possess the following properties:

Content Addressability. Information in memory can be accessed based on nearly any attribute of the representation one is trying to retrieve. In contrast, such implementations on standard computers suffer from combinatorial explosions when the amount of data stored increases.

Graceful Degradation. This characteristic of neural networks ensures that an incomplete or incorrect (noisy) input does not cause a catastrophic error in the output, unlike other digital systems. Thus neural networks are claimed to be more reliable in real time noisy environments. This property also results in a gradual loss of performance, graceful degradation, when individual neurons are damaged, without any catastrophic failure as in the case of serial processing.

Retrieval From a Partial Description. A neural network can retrieve a particular memory from a partial description of its properties. A consequence of these properties is that a neural network is more robust in noisy environments with incomplete information. Such a scenario could exist when scales are administered to a varied set of respondents who may not answer all questions accurately.

Default Assignment. Sometimes we come across an input/output pair that has not been presented to the network. In such occurrences, the network can give plausible guesses, that is, it can interpolate as well as extrapolate.

Spontaneous Generalization. Networks tend to retrieve what is common to a set of memories that will collectively match a retrieval cue that is too general to capture in any one memory. This is an alternative to explicitly storing a generalization. The use of a set of memories has two advantages over explicit storage. First, it does not require any special generalization formation mechanism. Second, it can provide us with generalizations on unanticipated lines, on demand.

Combining Statistical and Neural Network Methods

Accompanying a neural network analysis with a statistical analysis combines two powerful disciplines and is useful for four reasons. First, a statistical analysis helps to validate the neural network model. Recommendations that are robust across methods of analysis may endure longer than recommendations based on one methodology alone. Second, an inspection of unique conclusions, those that derive from one methodology but not the other, may give insights into possible inadequacies of the design, the sampling techniques, or the data. Results from either of the approaches not replicated by the other may be due to reasons such as the failure to follow assumptions and inappropriate modeling. Data that are wrong or extreme can cause problems; different techniques for both methodologies have varying sensitivity to unusual data values. Basic statistical techniques such as graphs, histograms, and box plots help screen invalid data before any methodology is attempted. Unique conclusions may also stem from differences between the mathematical and statistical models used. Third, including both network and statistical analyses adds to our understanding of how each performs. Finally, because some readers may be familiar with statistical methods but not neural network methods, by including statistical analyses one may reach some readers that one would have missed otherwise.

When considering neural networks and statistical analyses, it may help to think of a two by two table: the two columns are the methodologies, neural networks and statistics, and the rows are data types, real and simulated. This is a simplification; there are more than two dimensions, and each of the two columns has several subcolumns: Networks have many different architectures, and statistics can be partitioned a number of ways. Likewise the rows can be further subdivided.

Consider the statistics column. The statistical methodology you choose reflects the structure of the problem you investigate. In studies where the relative size of sensitivity slopes is of interest, we have used multiple analyses of variance and simultaneous confidence intervals. Although confidence intervals are often inspected to see if they contain zero, they can be used to test for some other value. The structure of the problem should motivate the analysis. If the problem is best described as a prediction model, then a linear or nonlinear model or set of models may be of interest. Scatterplots may suggest the particular form of the line(s) or curve(s) that would fit the model well. You might begin by approximating with a linear model, where the output is the dependent variable and the inputs are independent variables. A linear model can represent a variety of curves. However, because multicollinearities inflate the variances of predicted values and of parameter estimates, you may consider a principal components regression, using the principal components as the independent variables in the model. Statistics offers a rich set of resources for a variety of problems and statistical techniques are being continually developed. Time spent with a statistical consultant is surely worthwhile.

Consider the rows of the two by two table. Real data can be distorted by adding random or systematic error, and the resulting networks can be inspected to see how robust the network is to invalid data, how a distortion in selected variables affects the output, and how large a distortion can become before the network output becomes unreliable. Simulated data can be varied with representative values for means, variances, and covariance structure to see the effect on output. You can get estimates for simulations from your previous experience, from the literature, or by using estimates from a small sample before the entire data set has been collected. To keep the number of possible combinations manageable, the important variables are typically varied 2 or 3 times.

Modeling, Validation, and Sensitivity Analysis

The methodology followed for a typical problem involving the study of behavior using scales and interviews on a sample population is described in general terms first followed by the details of two case studies illustrating their usage. The overall problem in model development is to first define the set of inputs and outputs. By inputs we mean all the variables (scales) that affect the outcomes of interest (outputs). For example, in Case Study I dealing with adolescents, the inputs are personality (as measured by the Millon Adolescent Personality Inventory), parental bonding (Parental Bonding Questionnaire), social support (Social Support Questionnaire), gender, and DICA variables; and the output is Hopelessness (Kazdin Hopelessness Scale).

The first step is then to carefully select all the inputs that affect the outcome in the study. For neural network models, the inputs need not be completely uncorrelated. The target sample of subjects for the study then needs to be selected. Care should be exercised in this sample selection to ensure that all the characteristics of interest are represented adequately in the sample. For instance, if substance abuse is of interest to the study, the sample should have at least 10% subjects reporting substance abuse. Typically, the larger the percentage the better. This leads to the question of sample size. Again, to achieve adequate representation of all the groups, the sample sizes should be large enough as determined by the expertise of the investigators. The sample sizes depend on, for example, the quality of data, the number of inputs, and the network design. The scales (survey instruments) are then administered to all the subjects and their responses machine coded. Once the data are obtained, a training file consisting of such input–output pairs or patterns for all the subjects in the sample, is created. The file is then normalized by using the mean and standard deviations for each variable. This normalized training file is used to train the selected neural network model repeatedly for several epochs. The number of epochs required depends on the complexity of the problem. Because neural networks also suffer from overtraining, the usual methodology for training is to select a random sample of 80% of the training patterns for training the network and the remaining 20% for testing the network. The total error for the test sample is monitored as a function of the training epochs and typically the testing errors increase after an optimum number of training epochs. This optimal number of epochs is selected then as the cutoff for training the entire sample. The process of ensuring that the testing errors are kept small is termed network model validation.

After being trained in the manner described above, a neural network acts as an expert for predictions. If a new case history of a subject is presented to the network, it should be able to predict the outcome of interest for the subject, based on the training that it has received, much as an expert would. An expert would probably have problems drawing inferences from such a large number of variables; a neural network handles the complexity easily. More importantly, as explained below, the neural model can describe the relative importance of each input variable, which may be a difficult problem for an individual expert.

Sensitivity. A sensitivity analysis identifies the dominant factors that affect the outcomes of interest. In a novel sensitivity method using neural networks, developed by the authors, the network is presented with the case history (pattern) of each of the surveyed subjects and queried to determine how changing each of the inputs effects the output (outcomes of interest). This is a powerful way to change the value of one variable and to see the overall impact on the system while keeping the other variables fixed. The methodology thus quantifies the relative importance of each of the input variables by considering one variable at a time, keeping the others constant. Each variable is perturbed from the lowest value to the highest value of that input (which the net has been exposed to during training) and a rate of change of the output(s), that is, a measure of sensitivity, is computed for each variable. This rate of change is then averaged across all the case histories. A sensitivity study can be performed for both continuous and binary variables.

Statistical Analysis. Simultaneous 99% confidence intervals are then computed for the means of the slopes of the input variables using Bonferroni adjustments to obtain the appropriate t value for rejections. The overall level of significance is thus less than or equal to the preset alpha level (0.01). The intervals are inspected to see which did not contain any of the region of zero or in some cases $-\beta$ to $+\beta$ as determined by the researchers. Also, a Hotelling T^2 could be used to test the multivariate hypothesis that all input variable means are equal.

To illustrate the usage of these modeling and analysis techniques, two case studies are presented pertaining to two different areas in psychiatry. The first study (Reid, Nair, Kashani, & Rao, 1994) was a successful application of neural networks in adolescent psychiatry to determine the relative impact of personality factors, parental bonding, social support, gender, and some DICA variables on hopelessness. We show how the sensitivity analysis we developed permits clinical researchers to change the severity of each factor, and find the nonlinear effect on the outcome variable of interest. If clinicians are able to change a factor clinically, such studies give an estimation of the expected result. If clinicians are not able to change a factor clinically, they can expect what the change would be through such studies as this. The second case study (Reid, Nair, Mistry, & Beitman, 1995) pertains to the area of adult psychiatry where the effectiveness of stages of change and Adinazolan SR is studied for Panic Disorder in a randomized double-blind study.

Case Study I: Relationship of Personality, Parental Bonding, Social Support and DICA Variables to Adolescent Hopelessness

This case study (Kashani, Nair, Rao, & Reid, in press) which is briefly described here to illustrate neural network modeling, has inputs consisting of both binary and continuous variables, and a single continuous output. The data set consists of responses from 150 adolescents, selected from a systematic sample of over 1,700 high school students. Each adolescent was administered the Millon Adolescent Personality Inventory (Millon, Green, & Meagher, 1982), the Parental Bonding Questionnaire (Parker, Tupling, & Brown, 1979), the Social Support Questionnaire (Sarason, Levine, Basham, & Sarason, 1983), the Hopelessness Scale for Children (Kazdin, Rodgers, & Colbus, 1986), and was also interviewed by a trained clinician on DICA (Herjanic & Reich, 1982). We included the following Millon personality scales: Cooperative, Forceful, Sensitive, Social Tolerance, Family Rapport, Impulse Control, and Societal Conformity. The binary DICA diagnosis scales included were Oppositional disorder, Conduct disorder, and Anxiety. We also included a Psychosocial Stress scale from the DICA, a Boolean combination of the Dysthmic disorder (DD) and Major Depressive disorder (MDD) scales and a similar combination of Alcohol and Drug scales. We also included gender as an input.

Several studies using such scales have been performed by the researchers in the area of adolescent hopelessness (Kashani, Dandoy, & Reid, 1992). Kashani, Reid, and Rosenberg (1989) found that children who have high levels of hopelessness are at greater risk for suicide and depression and also for overall psychopathology. The neural network models presented here help to further some of the studies and provide quantitative representation of the various factors that influence hopelessness, as described below.

Modeling and Analysis

The network that modeled the complex relationships between the variables in the study had 19 inputs, 1 output (Hopelessness), and 3 neurons and 1 neuron respectively, in the two hidden layers. Seven observations were deleted due to missing data. The adolescents' responses to 20 variables thus represents 143 training patterns for the neural network.

The 19 inputs to the model were: Gender; the binary DICA variables Oppositional, Conduct Disorder, Alcohol and Drug, Anxiety, Depression (MDD & DD), and Psychosocial Stress; and the continuous scales of Cooperative, Forceful, Sensitive, Personal Esteem, Social Tolerance, Family Rapport, Impulse Control, Societal Conformity, Parental Care, Parental Overprotection, Satisfaction Rating, and Number of Supportive People. Only the DICA variables that had frequencies above 10% or were otherwise deemed important, were retained. The sole continuous output was the Hopelessness score.

The novel sensitivity approach (Kashani et al., in press) described in the previous section is effectively utilized to prioritize the 19 inputs based on their importance as far as hopelessness is concerned. The process uses the following methodology, after the neural network training process is complete: the network is queried about several hypothetical scenarios where, for instance, only the input Forceful (of the 19 inputs) is changed, all other 18 inputs remaining the same. The neural network model responds by predicting the effect on hopelessness due to the change in scores on the Forceful scale. This process is repeated for each of the 143 patterns (adolescent responses). The changes in hopelessness predicted by the neural network model are averaged to yield a slope, which represents the average change in hopelessness to be expected for a unit change in the forceful score. This process is then repeated for all the inputs, generating slopes for each of the 19 inputs. The slopes from such an analysis that were statistically significant and the inputs associated with them are noted. The significant inputs were determined using standard statistical methods as follows: The means of the slopes of the 19 input variables were used to compute simultaneous 99% confidence intervals using Bonferroni adjustments to obtain the appropriate t value for rejections. The overall level of significance is thus less than or equal to the preset α-level (0.01). The intervals were inspected to see which did not contain zero. We also ran a Hotelling T^2 to test the multivariate hypothesis that all 19 means were equal.

Results

The neural network model was trained first with the 143 adolescent responses (patterns) using the statistical method of dividing the dataset in an 80/20 split as described earlier, that is, 80% of the patterns were randomly selected for training the network, and the remaining 20%, which the network had not seen, were used to test how well the network had trained. This is a test to ensure that the neural network possesses the capability to generalize. The network predictions were found to be optimal in such a test after 150,000 epochs of training, since they agreed with the actual Hopelessness score to within ±25% for 79% of the adolesents (belonging to the test group) after training for the optimum number of epochs. The network model was then developed by training a network using the entire 100% of the dataset patterns for the optimum number (150,000 in this case) of epochs determined for training.

The trained network was then used to perform the sensitivity analysis. Table 1 summarizes the results of the sensitivity analysis for the dataset studied. Figure 2 shows the change in the hopelessness score (from which the slope is determined) as two of the significant variables, Parental Care and Social Tolerance are varied from their minimum to maximum values. Using statistical methods, as cited, the following six were found to be the significant inputs from among the 19 considered (with the corresponding slopes in brackets): Forceful (−23.1), Sensitive (22.0), Impulse Control (−17.4), Social Tolerance (11.9), Cooperative (−11.7), and Parental Care (−8.2). Thus, the personality trait Forceful has the highest slope (−23.1), that is, on average, the Hopelessness score will decrease by 23.1 (slope =

Table 1. Sensitivity Analysis for Case Study I: Significant input variables identified and their slopes

Input variable	Mean slope
Forceful	−23.1
Sensitive	22.0
Impulse Control*	−17.4
Social Tolerance*	+11.9
Cooperative	−11.7
Parental Care	−8.2

* Reversed scales, i.e., increasing values indicate increasing pathology.

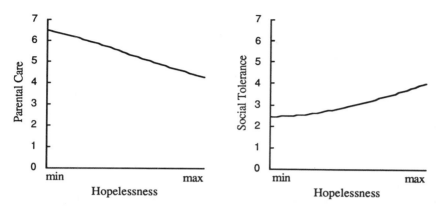

Figure 2. Variation of Hopelessness with respect to the input variables Parental Care and Social Tolerance.

−23.1) across the range of the Forceful score. The negative sign indicates that high scores on the Forceful scale (which indicate a tendency to be more aggressive and to dominate others) results in a decrease in hopelessness. All other slopes are interpreted accordingly. Thus, for the dataset studied, the neural network model revealed that a dominant and aggressive person was less likely to be hopeless. The second largest slope was associated with the personality trait Sensitive indicating that being more sensitive leads to increased hopelessness. For Impulse Control and Social Tolerance variables, higher scores are associated with greater pathology. As expected, Hopelessness increased as Social Tolerance increased (slope = 11.9). However, it decreased as Impulse Control increased (slope = −17.4) possibly because higher scores on Impulse Control, too, are associated with a tendency towards aggressiveness. As expected, Hopelessness also decreased as Parental Care increased (slope = −8.2). For the dataset considered, gender and the DICA variables were not found to be significant, that is, they were less important, compared to the personality and environmental variables.

Discussion

The sensitivity analysis methodology described in this chapter allowed for the identification of the input variables that had the greatest impact on Hopelessness. Such an analysis can be used to arrive at important conclusions in any similar study. Some of the conclusions we arrived at, using the slope values are described next for the case study.

Other factors remaining the same, clinicians can expect a decrease in Hopelessness by concentrating the treatment plan to consider those variables having the greatest impact on Hopelessness. Of the continuous personality, parental and social support variables, the personality trait of Forcefulness, as cited, had the greatest slope (in absolute value). This positive effect of dominant and aggressive behavior as shown in the Forceful personality trait, and Impulse Control, in countering hopelessness, is of clinical interest. Both these traits exhibit a tendency to dominate and be aggressive and the model showed that they were also associated with a lesser degree of hopelessness. Whether some personality traits can protect the individual against hopelessness or, on the contrary, whether chronic hopelessness impacts not only the behavior but also some personality factors, remains to be seen. In addition, whether a tendency to dominate or to be aggressive (not related to personality) is protective and its specific impact on hopelessness needs further exploration. Additionally, the inverse relation between hopelessness and assertion might imply that people who are able to assert themselves might be protected from hopelessness. Therefore assertion training can be considered as part of the treatment plan for the adolescent with hopelessness. These results can be considered as hypothesis generating for future studies.

Individuals with high Sensitive scores feel guilt, discontent, and pessimism, traits associated with hopelessness and low self-esteem. The positive slope between Sensitive and Hopelessness was the second highest in absolute value among the set of variables considered. Social Tolerance, the fourth largest slope in absolute value in the study, is associated with indifference to the feelings of others. A treatment plan that encourages interaction with others and concern about their feelings should also decrease hopelessness. As expected, the depressed adolescents reported more hopelessness than nondepressed subjects. This result supports previous findings in this regard. However, the relationship between substance abuse and hopelessness has not been investigated in the past and is of utmost significance because the study provides data that the adolescent with high scores on Hopelessness could be at risk for alcohol and drug abuse. The reader is referred to the paper by Kashani et al. (in press) for additional details pertaining to the psychiatric aspects of the problem addressed in this case study.

Case Study II: Effectiveness of Stages of Change and Adinazolam SR in Panic Disorder

Prochaska described four stages of change (SOC) that people move through on their way toward stable, healthy behavior: Precontemplation, Contemplation, Action, and Maintenance (Prochaska, DiClemente, & Norcross, 1992). People in the Precontemplation stage are not seriously thinking about changing. People in the Contemplation stage are thinking about changing. The Action stage involves a conscious ongoing effort to change behavior, and the Maintenance stage is the period following the Action stage in which people try to maintain their changed behavior.

Researchers developed the SOC questionnaire (McConnaughy, Prochaska, & Velicer, 1993; McConnaughy, DiClemente, Prochaska, & Velicer, 1989) for each of the four SOC scales. We hypothesized that SOC would also predict patients' change in a randomized controlled medication trial for panic disorder as measured by the Snaith Clinical Anxiety Scale (CAS) (Snaith, Baugh, Clayden, Husain, & Sipple, 1982), the Hamilton Anxiety Scale (HAM-A) (Hamilton, 1969), patient diary reports of panic attack frequency (PAF), the Clinical Global Impression scale (CGI) (Guy, 1976), and the Phobia Severity Scale (PSS) (Sheehan, 1986).

Because little has been written about the relationship of SOC with anxiety outcome measures, the two purposes of this study were to see whether adinazolam SR was effective relative to placebo on five panic disorder measures after 4 weeks of treatment; and to identify the most important variables to predict outcome at week 4 including the patient's readiness to change by modeling these relationships using neural networks, and to determine how changing the input variables affected five panic disorder outcomes.

Method

Patients who had at least one panic attack each week for 4 weeks prior to baseline were interviewed with the Structured Clinical Interview for the Diagnostic and Statistical Manual for Mental Disorders-III-Revised (DSM-III-R); 206 of these met the DSM-III-R criteria for panic disorder with agoraphobia. After the interview, there was a 2 week treatment washout, followed by a 1 week single-blind placebo phase. Of these 206 patients, 133 also completed the SOC questionnaire. They were then randomly assigned to either treatment or placebo groups. Because of incomplete data for 9 of the treatment patients and 11 of the placebo patients, the final sample after the random assignment had 58 patients in the drug treatment group and 55 in the placebo group.

Our goals were to determine whether adinazolam SR was more effective than placebo in reducing anxiety in any of the five anxiety measures after 4 weeks, and also to determine the relationship between adinazolam SR and the four stages of change variables. We trained two neural networks: one used drug patients and the other used placebo patients. The design of both networks was the same: gender, depression, agoraphobia, patients' responses to the 32 SOC questions, and five anxiety measures at baseline as inputs, and 5 anxiety measures at week 4 as outputs. The patients' responses to the inputs formed 58 and 55 training patterns for the two neural networks. We wrote the software in C language (Mistry & Nair, 1993). The errors dropped exponentially during training and were within plus or minus 1 percent for each of the patterns after 50,000 epochs of training.

Sensitivity Analysis. A sensitivity analysis reveals which factors most affect patients' anxiety level after 4 weeks. It is a measure of how much change in outputs may be expected for a given change in inputs. For each of the two networks (placebo and treatment groups) we changed each of the 4 SOC scales to see how that change would affect each of the 5 anxiety outcomes after 4 weeks. Each SOC scale (Precontemplation, Contemplation, Action, and Maintenance) was changed (perturbed) from its minimum to maximum value for every patient and an average rate of change of outcome scores was computed for each scale. This let us see how each of the outcomes changed as each input was changed. In addition, for each of the five anxiety outcome scores, an analysis of covariance (ANCOVA) was performed to test the effectiveness of the drug and placebo nets using initial scores as the covariate. Linear statistical models also evaluated the effect of individual SOC scales when combined in a model with drug/placebo to predict anxiety changes.

Results

Validation Study. The network predictions agreed with the actual five anxiety outcome measures to ±5% for about 90% of the training data set and to within ±15% for the remaining 10% of the training data set. This was considered good because the data set was randomly divided. A large number of observations are typically needed for improving the predictive characteristics of the network.

The sensitivity results were complex. In brief, the neural network models demonstrated the greater effectiveness of adinazolam SR over placebo after 4 weeks for certain measures; and they also showed that stages of change predicted change for several anxiety measures, particularly for the drug group.

Drug and Placebo Neural Networks. The means of change in neural network outcome scores for the drug group were relatively higher for CAS, HAM-A, and CGI scales compared to the placebo group. ANCOVAs indicated that the CAS and HAM-A scores were significantly lower at week 4 among the patients treated with adinazolam SR compared to the patients treated with placebo ($p < 0.002$, $p < 0.04$, respectively). For the PSS and PAF scores a similar trend was observed, but the difference in results between the drug and placebo groups was not significant.

Sensitivity Analysis. For the drug group, the neural network model showed that high Contemplation scores were associated with greater change in CAS scores compared to high Precontemplation scores (Fig. 3). The sensitivity functions (Fig. 3) from the neural network model clearly show the relative amount of change in outcome for each of the four SOC variables. Beitman et al. (in press), who combined drug and placebo groups in a regression model, did not detect the association between Contemplation and change of CAS outcome that the neural network model did. For the placebo group a similar trend was observed, but the amount of change in CAS score was less than that in the drug group.

Beitman et al. (in press) also reported that patients in the Precontemplation stage had little change in CAS, HAM-A, and panic attack frequency, and that patients in the Contemplation group were more likely to change in CGI scores from baseline to posttest a month later. The agreement of the neural network sensitivity analysis with Beitman's results validate the relatively new approach of sensitivity analysis and also show its effectiveness for this type of nonlinear modeling and analysis problem. In sum, the neural network model showed that stages of change predicted outcome in a medication trial.

Precontemplation scores predicted Clinical Anxiety decreases and Hamilton Anxiety decreases; Maintenance scores predicted Clinical Global Impression decrease, and Precontemplation, Contemplation, and Action scores all were related to decreases in Phobia Severity scores. Sensitivity analyses revealed that patients in the Precontemplation stage had little change in CAS, HAM-A, and panic attack variables, and that patients in the Contemplation stage were more likely to change in CGI scores from baseline to week 4. In other words predisposition to change has a powerful influence on outcome of short-term treatment of panic

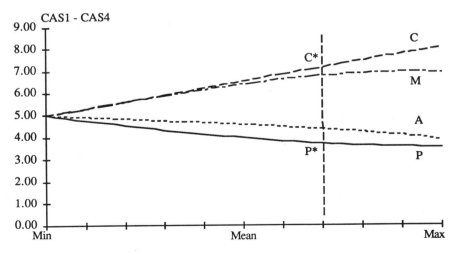

Figure 3. Sensitivity analysis for the CAS differences variable using the drug network.

disorder. This finding is consistent with previous studies (Prochaska et al., 1992). Clinicians should consider enhancing the effect of medication by assisting patients to move to a readiness to change state.

Panic disorder patients who were not yet predisposed to change were least likely to have a good outcome after 4 weeks of medication treatment. It may be possible to develop psychotherapeutic techniques that will help these "reluctant changers" progress along the stages of change continuum. If so, such techniques may become an adjunct to pharmacotherapy for selected patients.

Discussion and Future Research

The conventional statistical methods are effective with randomized control trials or in a correlational study, or to model relationships among a small number of variables. When the number of variables investigated (inputs and outputs) is large, nonlinear multivariate statistics is one appropriate tool for modeling the relationships. However, the method does not guarantee a valid model and becomes difficult to interpret for large numbers of variables. Neural networks and fuzzy logic possess the potential for quantifying complex mapping characteristics in a compact and elegant manner, as cited earlier. The two case studies presented here provide empirical data that the application of artificial neural networks is useful in psychiatry. This approach enhances the clinician's and the researcher's ability to study and handle multivariate problems, and enables us to see how a change in one input variable may potentially affect the outcome.

The neural modeling approach and the novel sensitivity approach outlined here for determining the relative importance of factors that relate to a certain phenomenon or property are promising and useful for clinical diagnoses and treatment and intervention plans in mental health.

Future Research

Clinicians often combine information from screening instruments with a clinical interview. The information gathered from clinical interviews is qualitative and usually very useful in diagnosis and determining treatment. Although there are several instruments that attempt to record important information from a clinical interview, more work needs to be done in identifying the kinds of interview information clinicians feel is useful and how they arrive at such expert decisions.

Hybrid Architectures. Artificial intelligence techniques that combine the power of neural networks to analyze numerical data and the ability of fuzzy logic to capture expert knowledge in the form of "if . . . then . . ." statements, are being investigated by several researchers currently. Because psychiatric studies involve both numerical data (using scales) and the participation of expert psychiatrists for reliable diagnosis, such architectures would be of considerable significance to the mental health community.

Fuzzy Logic. Fuzzy logic deals with imprecise qualities like *most, many, few, slightly*, etc., that are found in real-world situations (Zadeh, 1983; Klir & Folger, 1988). For example, a psychiatrist could say "if the patient acts very defiant and the patient strongly denies violent acts, then increase the patient's lie score by a little," where the membership functions of fuzzy sets *very defiant, strong denial*, and *a little* are determined from the expert's knowledge base. Fuzzy logic has several potential applications in psychiatry such as capturing such imprecise information, and the design of better scales (survey instruments), to cite two.

As mentioned, we are also investigating fuzzy logic coding and development of a knowledge base pertaining to adolescent mental health problems. Such a knowledge base will have considerable significance in diagnosis when coupled with data sets gathered using scales. The knowledge engineering process of eliciting expert knowledge about adolescents' mental health problems and transforming it into if–then fuzzy rules is the first step. Several questions pertaining to the development of such complex models in child psychiatry can be examined: How should variables that are not quantifiable numerically be considered? What are the inputs/outputs for such problems? How to code data in linguistic form, for example did the child really know the topic: Are children reliable reporters? (Herjanic, Herjanic, Brown, & Wheatt, 1975). Can the child answer questions such as: Do you have a short attention span? How do we incorporate similar assessment inputs, for example from parents, police, and school records? How would observational inputs from the expert interviewer be incorporated (these include body gestures, cooperativeness, etc.)? Such questions make the problem much more complex as compared to a regular learning problem. It appears that a neural network alone may not be able to incorporate these complex relationships, and architectures capable of accepting qualitative and quantitative data such as hybrid fuzzy–neural systems may be needed. Hybrid neurofuzzy architectures are still in the research stage in the expert system community, but we believe that such hybrid neurofuzzy architectures hold considerable significance to the psychiatric community in diagnosis, prediction, and interpretation of both normal and abnormal behaviors.

References

Beitman, B.D., Beck, N.C., Deuser, W.E., Carter, C.S., Davidson, J.R.T., & Maddock, R.J. Patient stage of change predicts outcome in a panic disorder medication trial. *Anxiety* (in press).

Carpenter, G., & Grossberg, S. (1987). A massively parallel architecture for a self-organizing neural pattern recognition machine. *Computer Vision, Graphics, and Image Processing, 37*, 54–115.

Cohen, J.D., & Servan–Schreiber, D. (1992). Introduction to neural network models in psychiatry. *Psychiatry Annals, 22*, 113–118.

Davidson, J.R.T., Beitman, B.D., Greist, J.H., Maddock, R.J., Lewis, C.P., Sheridan, A.Q., Carter, C.S., Ranga, K., Liebowitz, M.R., & Haack, D.G. (in press). Adinazolam SR treatment of panic disorder: A double-blind study. *Journal of Clinical Psychopharmacology*.

Guy, W. (1976). *ECDEU Assessment Manual for Psychopharmacology* (DHEW Publication number (ADM 76-338) US Alcohol, Drug Abuse, Mental Health Administration, Rockwell, Maryland, pp. 217–222.

Hamilton, M. (1969). Diagnosis and rating of anxiety. *British Journal of Psychiatry, 3*, 76–79.

Hecht–Nielsen, R. (1988). Application of counterpropagation networks. *Neural Networks, 1*, 131–139.

Herjanic, B., & Reich, W. (1982). Development of a structured psychiatric interview for children: Agreement between child and parent on individual symptoms. *Journal of Abnormal Child Psychology, 10*, 307–324.

Herjanic, B., Herjanic, M., Brown, F., & Wheatt, T. (1975). Are children reliable reporters? *Journal of Abnormal Child Psychology, 3*, 41–48.

Hoffman, R.E., & McGlashan, T.H. (1993). Parallel distributed processing and the emergence of schizophrenic symptoms. *Schizophrenia Bulletin, 19*, 119–140.

Hornik, K., Stinchcombe, M., & White, H. (1990). Universal approximation of an unknown function and its derivatives using multilayer feedforward networks. *Neural Networks, 3*, 551–560.

Hopfield, J.J. (1982). Neural networks and physical systems with emergent collective computational abilities. *Proceedings of the National Academy of Science, 79*, 2554–2558.

Kashani, J.H., Reid, JC., & Rosenberg, T.K. (1989). Levels of hopelessness in children and adolescents: A developmental perspective. *Journal of Consulting and Clinical Psychology, 57*, 496–499.

Kashani, J.H., Dandoy, A.C., & Reid, J.C. (1992). Hopelessness in children and adolescents: An overview. *Acta Paedopsychiatrica, 55*, 33–39.

Kashani, J.H., Nair, S.S., Rao, V.G., & Reid, J.C. (in press). Relationship of personality environmental, and DICA variables to adolescent hopelessness: A sensitivity approach using neural networks. Journal of the American Academy of Child and Adolescent Psychiatry.

Kazdin, A.E., Rodgers, A., & Colbus, D. (1986). The hopelessness scale for children: Psychometric characteristics and concurrent validity. *Journal of Consulting and Clinical Psychology, 54*, 241–245.

Kippenhan, J.S., Barker, W.W., Pascal S., Nage, J., & Duara, R. (1992). Evaluation of a neural network classifier for PET scans of normal and Alzheimer's disease subjects. *Journal of Nuclear Medicine, 33*, 1459–1467.

Kirk, R.E. (1982). *Experimental design* (2nd ed.). Belmont, CA: Wadsworth.

Klir, G.J., & Folger, T.A. (1988). *Fuzzy sets, uncertainty, and information.* Englewood Cliffs, NJ: Prentice Hall.

Kohonen, T. (1990). The self-organizing map. *Proceedings of the IEEE, 78*, 1464–1480.

McCord–Nelson, M., & Illingworth, W.T. (1991). *A practical guide to neural nets*. Reading, MA: Addison–Wesley.

McConnaughy, E.A., Prochaska, J.O., & Velicer, W.F. (1983). Stages of change in psychotherapy: Measurement and sample profiles. *Psychotherapy: Theory, Research, and Practice, 20*, 368–375.

McConnaughy, E.A., DiClemente, C.C., Prochaska, J.O., & Velicer, W.F. (1989). Stages of change in psychotherapy: A follow-up report. *Psychotherapy, 26*, 494–503.

Millon, T., Green, G.J., & Meagher, R.B. (1982). Millon Adolescent Personality Inventory Manual. Interpretive Scoring Systems, National Compute Systems Inc., Minneapolis, Minnesota.

Mistry, S.I., & Nair, S.S. (1993). Nonlinear HVAC computations using neural networks. *ASHRAE Transactions, 99/1*, 775–784.

Neter, J., Wasserman, W.W., & Kutner, M.H. (1989). *Applied linear regression models* (2nd ed.). Homewood, IL: Irwin.

Parker, G., Tupling, H., & Brown, L.B. (1979). A parental bonding instrument. *British Journal of Medical Psychology, 52*, 1–10.

Prochaska, J.O., DiClemente, C.C., & Norcross, J.C. (1992). In search of how people change. *American Psychologist, 47*, 1102–1114.

Reid, J.C., Nair, S.S., Kashani, J.H., & Rao, V.G. (1994). Detecting dysfunctional behavior in adolescents: The examination of relationships using neural networks. In J. Ozbolt (Ed.), *Proceedings of the Eighteenth Annual Symposium on Computer Applications in Medical Care*. Philadelphia, PA: Hanley & Belfus, 743–746.

Reid, J.C., Nair, S.S., Mistry, S.I., & Beitman, B.D. (in press). Effectiveness of stages of change and adinazolam SR in panic disorder: A neural network analysis. Journal of Anxiety Disorders.

Rumelhart, D., & McClelland, J. (1987). *Parallel distributed processing: Explorations in the microstructure of cognition*. Cambridge, MA: MIT Press.

Sarason, I.G., Levine, H.M., Basham, R.B., & Sarason, B.R. (1983). Assessing social support: The social support questionnaire. *Journal of Personality and Social Psychology, 44*, 127–139.

Servan–Schreiber, D., & Cohen, M.D. (1992). A neural network model of catecholamine modulation of behavior. *Psychiatric Annals, 22*, 125–130.

Sheehan, D.V. (1986). *The anxiety disease*. Bantam Books: New York.

Snaith, R.P., Baugh, S.J., Clayden, A.D., Husain, A., & Sipple, M.A. (1982). The clinical anxiety scale. *British Journal of Psychiatry, 141*, 518–523.

Spitzer, R.L., & Williams, J.B.W. (1987). *Structured clinical interview for DSM-III-R-Upjohn version (SCID-UP-R)*. New York: Biometrics Research Division, New York State Psychiatric Institute.

Waldrop, M.M. (1993). Cognitive neuroscience: A world with a future. *Science, 261*, 1805–1806.

Zadeh, L.A. (1983). The role of fuzzy logic in the management of uncertainty in expert systems. *Fuzzy Sets and Systems, 11*, 199–228.

Part IV
Computer Acceptance and Planning for the Future

24
Computer Use and Attitudes in Community Mental Health Clinics
Kenric W. Hammond and Jack J. O'Brien

Computer-based technology, with its ability to store, retrieve, and analyze information and deliver it to users on an unprecedented scale, has the potential to revolutionize the operation of businesses and social service organizations. Big mainframe computers already have accomplished this upheaval in the telephone, financial, and airline industries, among others. Increasingly affordable personal computers are penetrating new markets, including many small organizations. These new customers are fast learning about the obstacles to adopting computer-based technology as well. Resistence to change, false expectations of what technology can accomplish, fuzzy objectives, insufficient training, and incompatible software systems can make the changeover to computers a nightmare.

Community mental health clinics (CMHCs) are typical of small organizations that may benefit from introducing computer-based technology. Such benefits include tracking of client records, seeking and justifying reimbursement from third parties, quality of care assurance, the complex task of coordinating services with other providers, and the need to run more efficiently by automating routine manual tasks such as test administration and mailings. In this chapter we will explore the first steps that community mental care agencies in two states have taken in this direction.

There have been a number of surveys of potential and actual CMHC users of computer-based technology designed to elicit attitudes toward the use of computers as well as to measure computer usage and type of usage. Surveys can assist management and staff to better anticipate and plan for difficulties in implementing computer systems. Gorodezky and

This study was funded by a grant from the Washington Institute for Mental Illness Research and Training. We would like to thank the members of the advisory committee of this project for their time and effort.

Hedlund (1982) published a review of articles on computers in CMHCs that listed the computer applications and the few surveys of computer use and attitudes. To our knowledge, however, there has been only one attitude and use survey of CMHC computing in the past decade. Peters (1990) reported on a survey administered to 207 staff members of a community mental health service in the Vancouver, British Columbia area. This survey consisted of 15 items assessing attitudes about the use of computers at work, along with a variety of items concerning demographic information. Most respondents were generally positive, with 87% expressing favorable attitudes. There was considerable variation across professions, with physicians and psychologists holding more negative attitudes, and administrative and support staff expressing more positive thoughts.

Here we report on a series of surveys administered to 559 CMHC staff and clients in the states of Idaho and Washington. The survey items covered attitudes toward using computer systems as well as actual use in the clinics.

Methods

Survey Development

We developed six instruments, five of which were directed at various job classifications within the CMHC: direct service providers, support staff, clinic directors, finance managers, and computer experts (the person in charge of or most knowledgeable about the computer-based system), and one for CMHC clients. An advisory board consisting of 16 representatives of CMHCs in Washington and Idaho corresponding to the target survey groups assisted us with the design of the survey; in addition, we solicited the opinions of other interested stakeholders.

During the spring of 1991 we contacted the executive directors of each of the 92 Washington state CMHCs, asking them if they would distribute the surveys of their staff and clients. We received responses from 45 Washington state CMHCs, for a 49% response rate. In addition, each of the 7 Idaho state CMHC regions participated. A total of 559 responses were obtained from 260 direct service providers, 138 support staff, 55 clients, 37 clinic directors, 35 finance managers, and 34 computer experts.

For purposes of analysis, we divided the responding CMHCs in two ways. First, we separated the Washington state CMHCs from the Idaho state CMHCs. The two states have very different CMHC structures. Washington state contains a relatively large number of private agencies operating under a contract with the state. In Idaho, there are seven mental health regions, with all functions operated by the state and centralized in the seven regional offices. Second, we divided the Washington state CMHCs according to the size of their budget. Twelve CMHCs reported an annual budget of under $1,000,000; 18 reported a budget over $1,000,000. The remaining 15 CMHCs did not divulge budgetary information.

Results

Current and Projected Use of Computer Systems

A number of questions concerning current and future use of computer-based systems were directed at clinic directors and the computer experts as the CMHCs. All CMHCs reported some computer use; just over half (51%) said they contracted at least some services to outside vendors. About a fifth (19%) reported extensive use of in-house computers. Extensive use was reported more often by large CMHCs, but CMHC size was not associated with outside contracting.

The same question was also asked of CMHC directors and computer experts, but for a date 5 years in the future. The most striking finding was that extensive internal use is projected to rise from 19 to 74% of CMHCs; contracts with outside computer services vendors are expected to decline from 21 to 53%. Both large and small CMHCs intend to make extensive use of in-house computer systems.

Personal computers, either stand-alone or linked to a remote vendor were present in virtually all CMHCs. Both configurations were used in most settings, with little difference according to agency size. Both states have centralized reporting systems to which CMHCs feed data. Almost half (47%) of the large Washington state CMHCs possessed a system of networked personal computers, as opposed to none of the smaller CMHCs.

The CMHC directors and computer experts were asked what their system configuration would look like in 5 years. In-house networks (86%) and linkage of data with a Regional Support Network (86%) are expected to be the most popular. Larger CMHCs are leaning more than smaller CMHCs toward acquiring more complex systems (88 versus 75%).

Table 1 presents responses to a query about which management reports were computerized, and, if not, whether the capability was sought. Reports on payroll, client characteristics, staff activity, income statements, accounts receivable/payable, target population statistics, and fee collection monitoring were computerized in at least 60% of the CMHCs. From a third to a quarter of the CMHCs expressed a desire to computerize staff characteristics, quality assurance, data on pharmacy/medications, target population statistics, fund raising, volunteer services, equal employment opportunity data, credentials updating, and training. Fund raising, volunteer services, and data on pharmacy/medications were not seen as necessary to computerize by an additional third of the CMHCs.

Table 1. Prevalence of Management Reports Generated in CMHCs

Report	Currently Produced		Not Produced	
	Manually	Computer	Could Use	Do Not Need
Client characteristics	14	71	12	2
Staff activity	29	69	2	0
Income statement	20	68	7	5
Accounts receivable/payable	22	68	10	0
Fee collection monitoring	25	60	15	0
Payroll	10	71	12	7
Staff characteristics	28	31	26	15
Quality assurance	54	10	34	2
Pharmacy/medications	31	10	26	33
Target population statistics	10	60	31	0
Fund raising	21	8	36	36
Volunteer services	28	10	30	33
EEO data	34	22	31	13
Credentials updating	38	13	33	15
Training	54	8	28	10

Note: All responses are given in percent. EEO, equal employment opportunity.

CMHC directors and computer experts were asked to describe whether their facilities would be inclined to switch their current computer systems and what the potential barriers were to such a change. More than two-thirds (69%) said they would like to switch, but most facilities indicated that cost was a deterrent to changing their systems. Monetary cost, staff training, and investment in the current system were all seen as substantial barriers to a desired changeover.

Attitudes and Satisfaction

Clinic directors and computer experts were asked to estimate staff members' and clients' attitudes toward the use of computers in CMHCs. These leaders expressed that their financial, accounting, and clerical employees would generally be expected to have favorable attitudes, and that direct service providers would have more reservations. Therapists would have the most doubts, according to the directions. A majority of the respondents were uncertain of the attitudes held by clients.

We also asked CMHC clinic directors to rate their level of satisfaction with the flow of information in selected areas. On a 1 to 5 scale with 5 denoting a high level of satisfaction, the directors were least satisfied with the flow of information in the personnel and human services functions (a score of 2.5) and most satisfied in the billing and accounting functions (3.1). Directors of large Washington state CMHCs were less satisfied than those in small CMHCs; Idaho directors were more satisfied than Washington state directors.

Direct service providers were also asked about their attitudes toward computer-based systems. First, we inquired what specific benefits a computer-based system could bring to their work. As shown in Figure 1, more than half said that such a system would result in more efficient use of their time (68%), that client records would be available in the computer when paper records were missing (58%), and that they would have an enhanced ability to track clients and analyze patterns (57%). Only 35% thought that there would be fewer mistakes, and 41% thought they would have more time for clients. Better and more informed decisions would result, in the opinion of 44% of the respondents. Direct service providers in small Washington state CMHCs were less likely to see advantages than those in large CMHCs; Idaho caregivers were more enthusiastic than their Washington state counterparts.

Staff predictions of benefits of a computer-based system broke down according to prior experience with computers. Those who used a computer in their work foresaw the most benefits, but those who said they needed a great deal of computer training were not appreciably more negative than the total sample.

We also asked direct service providers how they felt about using their current computer system. Their responses indicated that, of the possible features asked, legibility and access to information were the most favorably reported on. Most respondents preferred the idea of a computer system to a paper-based system, but there was less agreement that computer systems could be better than paper records, or that they would decrease the cost of care.

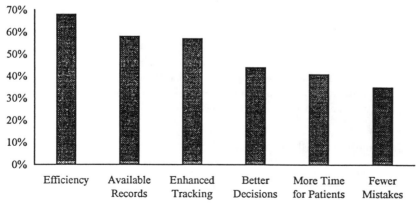

Figure 1. Direct Service Provider Expectations of Clinical Computing.

A further question had to do with how direct service providers felt a computer-based system "providing on-line storage and retrieval of patient records, including diagnoses, care plans, psychological tests and medications" could help them in various aspects of their work. Although most respondents expressed that such a system would be valuable, the consensus was that computers were of use mainly as a record- and chart-keeping system. There was more doubt about more complex areas, such as diagnosis, treatment planning, and team treatment coordination. Those who used a computer in their work favored the idea of a clinical package most; those who said they needed a great deal of computer training had a relatively negative opinion. Ownership of a computer did not greatly increase the chance of acceptance. Like other respondents, clinical staff were very unsure of client reactions to a computer-based system.

Support staff members, when asked how the felt about using a computer system, generally had more positive attitudes about their facility's computer system than did direct service providers asked the same question. As with the direct service providers, support staff responses did not appear to systematically vary according to facility type.

We asked similar questions of various staff groups, varying the items within the questions depending on the respondent's functions. Direct service providers, support staff, and finance and accounting managers were asked to quantify the importance they attached to various features in a computer-based system. Apart from specific functions desired, all respondent groups expressed a desire for systems that were simple and easy to use.

Satisfaction with various aspects of the current computer system was compared among direct service providers, support staff, finance and accounting managers, and computer experts. The results are shown in Figure 2, with a scale of 1 to 4, where 1 represents *very dissatisfied* and 4 *very satisfied*. The word processing function of system received the highest marks from all, as did the facility's Information System staff. The scheduling/appointment modules available to the respondents uniformly met with disfavor. Whether the computer system fit with their job duties produced a wide variation in responses according to job classification. Direct service providers were fairly dissatisfied, whereas the other groups were much more favorable. The responses to the computer training they had received were similarly distributed.

Confidentiality and Client Attitudes

We also inquired of the clinic directors about the steps CMHCs take with respect to the privacy of client information. Written privacy policies and signed employee privacy statements are in place in most CMHCs (95%), but specific safeguards such as passwords (57%), backups kept in secure

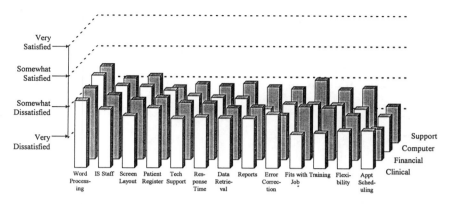

Figure 2. Satisfaction with Computer Services by Staff Category (Is, Information System).

locations (57%), and securing of terminals (43%), are less widely followed. Less than half of the facilities in our sample (43%) stated that they had implemented five or more of seven standard security steps presented in the survey question.

As shown in Table 2, a substantial number of clients expressed concern about the protection of their records if their CMHC had a computer-

Table 2. Client Attitudes Toward Use of a Computer-Based System in a CMHC

	n	Yes (%)
All respondents	55	
Important information about me would not be forgotten.	35	63.6
The staff would have easier access to my personal file.	33	60.0
I would not have to give the same information again.	31	56.4
It would allow me to register faster.	28	50.9
The privacy of my record would be less safe.	27	49.1
It would be easier for people with hearing impairments.	27	49.1
It would give the staff more time with me.	25	45.4
It would give me easier access to my record.	24	43.6
I could get billing information the same day.	21	38.2
I would not be sure where my records would end up.	20	36.4
Anyone could look at my file.	19	34.5
I prefer to use the computer for interviews and tests.	12	21.8
The system would be cold and impersonal.	12	21.8
I would like it if the system were in color.	11	20.0
I have had problems with lack of privacy of my records.	11	20.0
It would take more time and make work.	7	12.7
The staff would pay more attention to the computer than to me.	5	9.1

based system. About half thought that the privacy of their record would be less safe. Opinion was divided about the benefits of such a system. They felt records would be less likely to be lost and the clinic staff would have easier access to records, but more than half thought that computer use would not translate to more time with clients.

Discussion

We have reported on the results of six surveys administered to 559 CMHC members and clients in Washington and Idaho states concerning computer use and attitudes toward computer-based systems. The respondents were not randomly selected, but we went to some effort in instructing clinic directors to distribute surveys to staff without regard to computer use or knowledge.

The results were grouped into three sections. The first pertained to current and projected use of computers and computer-based systems. In this section, clinic directors and computer experts reported that, although computers were used in nearly all facilities, it was not extensive, and over half employed outside vendors for much of the necessary work. About 70% of CMHCs perform basic reporting, personnel, and accounting functions using computer-based systems. The clinic directors and computer experts foresaw a radical change in computer-based configuration within the next 5 years, resulting in extensive use of in-house personal computers, networked both to each other and to state mental health departments, and breaking sharply with outside data processing service vendors.

Most directors were ready to upgrade their systems immediately, and this was reflected in their dissatisfaction with the flow of information within the CMHC. A potential road block to further computerization was staff resistance. As reported in the second section of the results, however, most CMHC staff members voiced fairly positive attitudes toward the growing computerization of facility activities. More than half of the direct service providers who responded were of the opinion that computer-based systems would be more efficient, reliable, and of more help in tracking clients. Opinion was divided as to whether better care would be provided. Those who already worked with computers had a more favorable opinion of such systems than those who had little experience.

Our findings were similar to that of Peters (1990), at least in those respects where the surveys measured similar phenomena. Administrative and support staff members expressed more positive attitudes toward computers in both surveys. This may be due to the more established and better developed programs tailored to the functions performed by these employee groups. Software development for mental health evaluation and treatment programs is still in its infancy.

Those with prior computer experience held more favorable attitudes than those who needed training. This finding was also similar to that of Peters (1990). Notwithstanding, there was a great deal of dissatisfaction on the part of CMHC directors with the current computer-based systems. Many would gladly switch immediately if they could, with the primary direction of the changeover being to personal computers networked to each other and the state system, and away from contracts with outside vendors.

Many respondents expressed frustration over the lack of training to use computer systems. This issue may turn out to be crucial in winning over support of professional staff, in particular, and if so, addressing it could save a lot of effort and money when implementing a new system. The same goes for the performance of the system. If a system does not perform up to expectations, staff members will quickly become disenchanted. Preparation, both in terms of system planning and training, cannot be overemphasized. Adequate system performance and training both demand the support of the top administration (Gorodezky & Hedlund, 1982). The directors who responded to this survey appeared to appreciate the need for such support.

In the third section, although a written privacy policy was in place at nearly all CMHCs, practical steps to secure client records and other data were sporadically implemented. Clients themselves expressed concern that confidentiality might suffer or at least not improve with the implementation of a comprehensive computer-based system. Increased effort needs to be devoted to educating clients and CMHC staff about information security, involving them in the confidentiality process, and especially, tightening up privacy procedures.

Our findings indicate that CMHCs recognize that advances in computer technology have the potential to make their operations more efficient and to serve clients more effectively. Lack of resources and information, the slow pace of software development, and staff resistance seem to be the main stumbling blocks in implementing computer-based systems. CMHC directors appear to be moving away from contracting with outside vendors in favor of building modular in-house systems that will be constructed in steps as resources become available. The CMHCs seem to be moving toward systems that link clinicians together with a networked personal computer on every desk. This development demands that client records be portable.

CMHC directors are able to exercise more control over facility operations with in-house systems. Concomitant with this control is the responsibility to install safeguards to ensure client and staff confidentiality. Periodic study of security measures taken by CMHCs will help to monitor that appropriate precautions are being taken.

Finally, software development to help CMHCs serve clients appears to lag behind hardware advances. The market has been slow to recognize the potential in this area, or if it has, to adequately satisfy its customers. A coordinated effort on the part of CMHC information systems purchasers may be needed to communicate their requirements so that software development firms can better meet their needs.

References

Gorodezky, M.J., & Hedlund, J.L. (1982). The developing role of computers in community mental health centers: Past experience and future trends. *Journal of Operational Psychiatry*, *13*, 94–99.

Peters, R. (1990). Attitudes of community mental-health staff toward computers. *Canadian Journal of Community Mental Health*, *9*, 155–162.

25
Severely Mentally Ill Client Acceptance of Automated Assessments in Mental Health
Matthew G. Hile and Bruce W. Vieweg

Numerous automated systems have been developed for mental health settings. However, questions continue to arise about their acceptability, particularly with regard to direct client use. Failure to accurately answer these questions of acceptability can lead to great inefficiencies and poor decisions. For example, recently the first author was initially required, by state and Federal authorities, to forgo the development of an automated client-based data collection system because it might interfere with the client-assessor bonding. This occurred even though the alternative systems were more expensive, less reliable, and much less efficient. It was not until days before the implementation of the nonautomated system, after key officials had left the government, that the decision was rescinded and automated assessment permitted.

The notions that clients will resist computers and that computers will interfere with the therapeutic relationship are often cited by clinicians as reasons to avoid such use. However, these concerns have been widely disproved in the past. A variety of studies in the 1970s and 1980s found that many clients preferred automated assessments (Erdman, Greist, Klein, Jefferson, & Getto, 1981; Farrell, Camplair, & McCullough, 1987; Klingler, Johnson, & Williams, 1976; Schwartz, 1984; Wagman, 1980). The question continues to be asked, however, and more recent studies have explored these issues in more detail.

Ford and Vitelli (1992) reported on the Computerized Adjunct to Psychotherapy (CAP) program, a set of automated assessments and clinical interventions used at the Millbrook Correctional Center in Ontario, Canada. Inmates use commercial and in-house software to assess stress levels and chemical dependency, learn problem solving and stress management skills, and to develop more complete discharge plans. After completing the CAP, the authors assessed 72 inmates using the Millbrook Computer Attitudes Questionnaire, an 18-item Likert scale.

In general, inmates strongly approved of the CAP programs indicating that they found them interesting (82%), enjoyable (83%), and a good use of time (94%). They found that the automated programs increased self-understanding (78%) and increased their store of useful information (86%). When specifically comparing human and automated counseling, 49% of the inmates found it easier to be honest with a computer than with a human counselor. They equally preferred computer counseling (29%) to human counseling (32%) but learned more in sessions with the computer (35%) than with the human counselors (25%). These results indicate a strong positive attitude toward both automation in general and automation relative to human counselors.

Spinhoven, Labbe, and Rombouts (1993) evaluated the responses of 452 consecutive psychiatric outpatients asked to attend an additional session for a computerized psychological assessment. Of the 343 patients actually asked, 54% refused the additional session. Patients who refused were significantly older and less well educated than those who volunteered, but did not differ in terms of gender, level of psychopathology, or Diagnostic and Statistical Manual of Mental Disorders-III-Revised (DSM-III-R) diagnosis.

Few of the clients who volunteered to complete the automated assessments had negative attitudes (Spinhoven et al., 1993). Only 4% thought the task difficult, only 5% reported that it was "unpleasant", 21% would have preferred paper-and-pencil testing, 20% found that they were "tense" or "very tense" during the automated testing, while only 5% rated the computer experience "negatively". As was true of initial agreement to participate, neither diagnosis nor level of psychopathology were related to attitudes. Using a multiple regression model, the authors examined the level of acceptance of those individuals who agreed to complete the automated assessment. They found that four patient characteristics, age, sex, education, and computer experience, accounted for 30% of the variance in computer attitudes.

These authors conclude by stating that "(t)he 54% refusal rate suggests that a computerized assessment is not feasible for all psychiatric outpatients as part of a standard intake procedure" (Spinhoven et al., 1993, p. 444). However, more correctly, their results suggest that 54% of the psychiatric outpatients are unwilling to invest additional time and energy in the assessment process. Their results do not speak to the feasibility of general automated assessment for psychiatric outpatients. For these patients, the relevant psychiatric variables were identical across individuals who refused to participate, who evaluated the experience negatively, and who evaluated the experience positively. This suggests that clients' behavior and attitudes were likely due to nonclinically relevant differences. These results also suggest the importance of examining the effect of various demographic variables, including age, gender, and education, on attitudes in a system where all patients are required to undergo automated assessment as part of their therapeutic experience.

Petrie and Abell (1994) asked 150 consecutively admitted hospitalized parasuicide patients to volunteer for an automated assessment. Unlike the previous study, all but five (3%) of these individuals agreed to participate. Most of these patients preferred the automated (52.3%) to the clinician (17.4%) interviews, although many (30.3%) had no preference. No significant demographic differences were found between patients who preferred either automated or clinician interviews. Differences were found, however, on some clinically relevant dimensions. Patients who preferred the automated questionnaire had lower self-esteem, and higher levels of hopelessness and suicidal ideation. These clinical differences are signs of increased suicidal risk suggesting that automated assessments are more acceptable, and perhaps more effective, for clients in greater need.

Sawyer, Sarris, Quigley, Baghurst, and Kalucy (1990) evaluated the attitudes of parents seeking treatment from a child psychiatric service before and after they underwent automated or paper-and-pencil assessments. After the child and their parents were seen by a clinician, half of the 140 parents received an automated assessment and half an identical paper-and-pencil assessment. Parents who completed the automated assessment significantly increased their preference for both the automated assessment alone and a combination of clinician and automated assessment. Their preference for a paper-and-pencil-based assessment significantly decreased from pretest levels. The preferences of parents who received the written assessment did not change.

Parents in both groups also completed a semantic differential scale after their initial clinician interview and following their automated or paper-and-pencil assessment. The groups did not differ on the dimensions of logical–illogical, clear–confusing, interesting–boring, short–long, relaxing–threatening, fast–slow, and valuable–worthless. The clinical interview was rated more positively than both of the others on the dimensions of humanlike–mechanistic, friendly–cold, personal–impersonal, and pleasant–unpleasant. Additionally, the clinical interview was evaluated more positively than the automated assessment on the accurate–inaccurate dimension. However, even in the dimensions that showed the greatest differences, parent ratings of the automated assessment fell between neutral and moderate in terms of mechanistic, cold, and impersonal. On all other dimensions the average rating of the automated assessment was toward the more "positive" dimension (e.g., relaxing, valuable, etc.).

The results from Sawyer et al. (1990) suggest a number of important conclusions. First, the experience of automated assessment will positively influence the attitudes of those who use it. Requiring automated assessments may have beneficial effects in addition to the information gained. Second, even though automated assessments may be negatively compared with clinician assessments, consumer attitudes are generally positive toward these systems. Third, the three dimensions where automated assessment faired most poorly (viz., humanlike–mechanistic, friendly– cold, personal–impersonal) reflect the fact that the computer is not a person. These results should be neither unexpected nor necessarily nega- tive. Because Quintanar, Crowell, Pryor, and Adamopoulos (1982) found that respondents tend to be more honest and revealing with programs perceived as mechanistic, this perception by parents may indicate that such systems are more accurate than traditional clinical interviews.

These four reports continue the history of studies demonstrating posi- tive client responses toward automated assessments. However, each does so on a relatively limited scale. With the limited sample sizes, the authors focused on the responses to individual questions and not on the patterning of those results. In this chapter we address that lack by reporting on the satisfaction of 1,883 severely mentally ill clients who completed an automated assessment battery.

Description and Background of C/MIS

The Clinical/Management Information System (C/MIS) is a microcom- puter-based application that was developed to support the efforts of Great Rivers Mental Health Services, a Missouri Department of Mental Health facility located in St. Louis County, MO. It was collaboratively developed by the staff of Great Rivers Mental Health Services and the University of Missouri affiliated Missouri Institute of Mental Health (see Hile & Hedlund, 1989, for a detailed description of the development of C/MIS).

C/MIS stresses the assessment and monitoring of client progress and change over the course of treatment in either a purchase of service or direct service clinical model. C/MIS collects structured clinical information from three sources for use in both individual treatment planning and, in the aggregate, evaluation purposes. The three sources are clients, case managers, and treatment providers. Information is largely collected directly from clients via computer interviewing. The automated section of the clinical intake process takes from 45 minutes to 1.5 hours, depending on the individual being assessed.

The development of C/MIS was controlled by the clinicians and admin- istrators who would ultimately use its information in their decision making. While one could assume that the data needs of these two groups are disparate, the fact is that although their view of these data may be different, the data themselves are the same. Clinicians use individual client assessment information in treatment planning and to monitor individual client change. Administrators use those same data in the aggregate to evaluate overall programs, the entire facility, and specific program outcomes.

Three principles have guided C/MIS development.

1. Collect only those data whose need can be clearly justified by their support of the individual clinician's unique data requirements, the needs of administrators and quality assurance officers for aggregate clinical information, or that is required for clinical or administrative purposes.
2. Do not duplicate data entry.
3. Keep hardware requirements to a minimum.

Hardware and Software

C/MIS operates either on a single microcomputer, or in a multiuser environment on a local area network. The program is written in compiled Clipper, Version 5.2, and all data are stored in dBASE III+ data bases. The single user version requires at least an IBM XT-compatible microcomputer, 512K RAM, a floppy disk drive, and a hard disk. Both color and monochrome monitors are supported. A networked or attached printer is required to print reports.

Components

C/MIS collects information from its three sources at different times during the treatment process. It collects information from the client at admission, during the annual follow-up during treatment, and at the termination of treatment. It collects information from case managers at admission and at annual follow-up. It collects progress information from treatment providers quarterly.

Data collected from clients include an admission questionnaire, resources questionnaire, medical history questionnaire, social work assessment, St. Louis Symptom Checklist (Evenson, Holland, Mehta, & Yasin, 1980), Missouri Alcoholism Severity Scale (Evenson, Reese, & Holland, 1982), and the FACES Quality of Life Scale. Information collected from case managers include the Brief Psychiatric Rating Scale (BPRS; Overall & Gorham, 1962), the Global Assessment Scale (GAS; Endicott, Spitzer, Fleiss, & Cohen, 1976), and DSM diagnoses. Data collected from providers include quarterly progress notes that include medication and dosages, DSM diagnoses, a 5-point global improvement scale, and the BPRS. The Community Adjustment Profile Scale, completed by a relative of the client, is included as an optional assessment. C/MIS data is used to produce numerous standard reports.

Satisfaction Instrument

The Client Satisfaction with Automated System[1] (CSAS) scale is a 13-item questionnaire developed for the C/MIS project. It is the last automated instrument collected by C/MIS. Clients respond to its items using a 5-point Likert scale (viz., *Strongly agree, Agree, Don't know, Disagree*, and *Strongly disagree*). The items are:

1. I was able to use the computer without difficulty.
2. The instructions on how to answer the questions were clear.
3. I enjoyed using the computer to answer the questions.
4. I would rather answer these questions to a person than to the computer.
5. I would not like to answer any questions on the computer again.
6. I was able to be more truthful to the computer than I would have been with a person.
7. The computer interview was too long.
8. I was able to describe my problems and feelings quite well.
9. The computer did not ask me about things I think are important.
10. The computer questions were thorough and complete.
11. I do not think that answering all these questions was helpful.
12. I did not have a problem understanding the questions.
13. I was satisfied with the computer program and the questions it asked.

Questions were created to reflect many of the concerns raised by clinicians and the literature concerning automated assessments. They address the client's understanding of the system, its ability to adequately assess the important domains, and their general attitudes toward its use. There is also an option for each interviewee to type a brief (approximately 80 character) comment into the computer. More that 50% of clients type such brief comments.

Client Acceptance

The results presented below represent all of the client acceptance data from one center since data were first collected in 1990 (Fig. 1). It is clear, from the sample description provided in Table 1, that the population completing this questionnaire is quite impaired. Sixty-five percent have a history of prior inpatient treatment, 62% have had previous outpatient treatment, and the average GAS score of 51 places the group at the very bottom of the "Moderate functioning" category. DSM-III-R diagnosis was available for approximately 70% of the sample. Approximately 80% of these clients had diagnoses that are categorized as indicating a "serious

---

[1] This questionnaire or any of its items may be freely used for any noncommercial purpose.

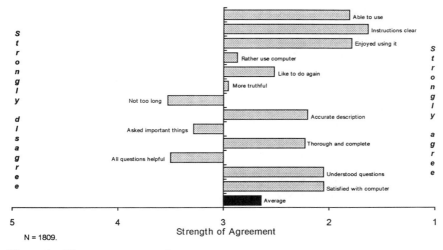

Figure 1. Client acceptance of automated assessment.

mental illness."[2] Nearly a third of these clients had a diagnosis of schizophrenia. The relatively high percentage of clients who report being "never married or divorced" (67%), and the very high number of clients reporting being "unemployed" (78%), also attest to the "chronic" and serious nature of the mental illness of these individuals.

The scale's normative information, and its relationship to various demographic variables, is presented in Table 2. For all analyses, the four negatively worded questions (numbers 5, 7, 9, and 11) were reverse scored. On all items, therefore, responses closer to 1 reflect more positive attitudes.

Differences between groups on the various questions is detailed below:

1. *Was able to use computer without difficulty.* Women rated their experience as more positive than did men, high school graduates were more positive than non high school grads, whites were more positive than African Americans, and younger individuals were more positive than older persons.

---

[2] Severe mental illness diagnostic categories, as described in Missouri's *Comprehensive Mental Health Plan for Adults*, are: Schizophrenic disorder (295.1, 295.2, 295.3, 295.6, 295.9); Delusional disorder (297.10); Schizoaffective disorder (295.7); Bipolar disorder (296.4, 296.5, 296.6, 296.7); Atypical psychosis (298.90); Major Depression, recurrent (296.3); Dementia or other organic condition complicated with delusional disorder, mood disorder, or severe personality disorder (290.20, 290.21, 290.12, 290.13, 290.42, 290.43, 294.10); Obsessive Compulsive Disorder (300.30); Post Traumatic Stress Disorder (309.89); Borderline Personality Disorder (301.83); Multiple Personality Disorder (300.14); Generalized Anxiety Disorder (300.02); and Severe Phobic Disorder (300.21, 300.22, 300.23).

Table 1. Sample Description

Variable	%
$n = 1,883$	55.3
Female	55.3
White	68.5
African American	29.0
Less than high school education	26.4
High school education	32.1
Some college	20.7
College graduate	5.6
Prior outpatient care	62.1
Prior inpatient care	65.4
Never married	43.0
Divorced	24.0
Unemployed	36.0
Age	Mean = 37.42, SD = 10.7
Average GAS score[a]	Mean = 51.88, SD = 11.48

[a] Global Assessment Scale, GAS, has a range of scores from 0 to 100. An average score of 52 would place a client just above the serious symptom range in the "moderate" symptoms or "moderate difficulty in social, occupational, or school functioning."

2. *Instructions were clear.* High school graduates, whites, and younger clients found the instructions clearer.
3. *Enjoyed using the computer.* Women enjoyed the computer process more than men.
4. *Would rather answer such questions to a person than a computer.* Women agreed more than men with this item and younger clients were more positive than older clients.
5. *Would like to answer questions on the computer again.* High school graduates and whites were more apt to agree with this item.
6. *Was able to be more truthful to the computer.* Men, high school graduates, and younger clients agreed more with this statement.
7. *Interview was not too long.* Women and whites agreed more with this item.
8. *Was able to describe problems and feelings quite well.* African Americans agreed with this statement more than did whites.
9. *Computer asked about important things.* No significant differences.
10. *Computer questions were thorough and complete.* Those with less than a high school diploma agreed more, as did African Americans.
11. *Answering these questions was helpful.* No significant differences.

Table 2. Relationship Between Scale Items and Four Demographic Variables

Item	All Clients	Age[a]	Sex		Education		Race	
			Male	Female	Less Than High School	More Than High School	White	African American
	(n = 1,883)	(n = 1,883)	(n = 828)	(n = 1,040)	(n = 351)	(n = 834)	(n = 1,287)	(n = 542)
Was able to use computer without difficulty	1.87 (0.94)	0.11†	1.95 (0.99)	1.80* (0.89)	2.01 (0.99)	1.73* (0.91)	1.80* (0.91)	2.03 (0.99)
Instructions were clear	1.68 (0.74)	0.08†	1.70 (0.74)	1.65 (0.74)	1.71 (0.72)	1.60* (0.76)	1.64* (0.71)	1.75 (0.79)
Enjoyed using the computer	1.85 (0.91)	0.04	1.93 (0.92)	1.79* (0.90)	1.87 (0.93)	1.74 (0.90)	1.82 (0.90)	1.87 (0.92)
Would rather answer to a computer than to a person	2.84 (1.2)	0.06†	2.92 (1.18)	2.77* (1.22)	2.92 (1.23)	2.85 (1.23)	2.82 (1.20)	2.85 (1.21)
Would like to answer questions on computer again	2.5 (1.20)	0.07†	2.58 (1.17)	2.46 (1.21)	2.66 (1.21)	2.46* (1.22)	2.46* (1.16)	2.61 (1.25)
Was able to be more truthful to a computer	2.9 (1.2)	0.15†	2.86* (1.18)	3.01 (1.23)	2.80 (1.22)	2.06* (1.24)	2.97 (1.18)	2.89 (1.29)
Interview was not too long	2.5 (1.0)	0.04	2.59 (1.05)	2.43* (1.01)	2.54 (1.07)	2.42 (1.01)	2.42* (0.96)	2.65 (1.15)
Was able to describe problems and feelings quite well	2.3 (0.98)	-0.02	2.25 (0.98)	2.26 (0.98)	2.10 (0.88)	2.25 (1.0)	2.34 (1.0)	2.03* (0.88)
Computer asked me about important things	2.7 (1.0)	0.05	2.69 (1.04)	2.72 (1.04)	2.73 (1.09)	2.71 (1.05)	2.72 (1.0)	2.66 (1.12)
Computer questions were thorough and complete	2.8 (0.92)	0.04	2.30 (0.93)	2.27 (0.91)	2.10* (0.81)	2.28 (0.97)	2.35 (0.93)	2.09* (0.88)
Answering these questions was helpful	2.5 (0.94)	0.00	2.29 (0.95)	2.49 (0.93)	2.56 (0.97)	2.46 (0.93)	2.49 (0.91)	2.62 (1.0)
I did not have a problem understanding these questions	2.1 (0.95)	0.07†	2.07 (0.95)	2.07 (0.96)	2.19 (1.02)	2.0* (0.96)	2.04 (0.95)	2.13 (0.99)
Was satisfied with the computer program and the questions it asked	2.1 (0.83)	0.00	2.14 (0.83)	2.10 (0.82)	1.99 (0.75)	2.07 (0.86)	2.14 (0.83)	2.04 (0.80)

[a] Age is the only continuous variable on this table, therefore the Pearson's r is used to measure its relationship to the scale items.

* Indicates response with a significantly higher agreement, $p < 0.01$ (t test independent samples, one tailed).

† Pearson r, two tailed, $p < 0.01$.

12. *Did not have a problem understanding these questions.* High school graduates and older clients had less difficulty in understanding questions.
13. *Was satisfied with the computer program and questions asked.* No significant differences.

Factor Analysis

SPSS for Windows (Version 6.1) was used to factor analyze the acceptance ratings for the 1,809 assessments. All factors having an eigenvalue greater than 1 were extracted and rotated using Varimax. The resulting solution is provided in Table 3 together with scale reliabilities (alphas). Table 4 provides the mean and standard deviations for the three relevant demographic groups for the instrument's four factors.

The factor analysis identified three multiitem factors and one single item factor. The items on each factor are indicated in bold on Table 3. Factor 1, *ease of use and enjoyment*, accounted for the greatest proportion of the variance (28.6%). Items important to this factor included the ability to use the computer, the clarity of instruction, the enjoyment of using the system, and the ability to understand the questions. Factor 2, *interview completeness*, described 13% of the variance. It dealt with the ability to describe one's problems and feelings well, the opinion that the computer asked important questions that were both thorough and complete, and the overall satisfaction with the computer program. The third multiitem factor, *negative attitudes*, accounted for 10.9% of the variance. It dealt with the individuals who would rather be interviewed by a person than a computer, their preference for using the computer again, the idea that the interview was too long, and beliefs that the questions were or were not helpful. The final factor, *truthful*, contains only a single item, able to be more truthful to the computer. This item accounts for 8.2% of variance.

In our four factor solution, the item, "Rather answer questions to a person than to a computer," was kept with the other items indicating negative attitudes toward C/MIS. This occurred despite the fact that it loaded somewhat more heavily on factor 4 (0.58) than on factor 3 (0.55). This was done for two reasons. First, this item logically fits with the other items indicating negative attitudes. By keeping it with these items, the factor has a clear meaning. Second, if the only item on factor 4, "Able to be more truthful to computer," is dropped from the scale, a three factor solution is returned and "Rather answer questions to a person than to a computer" loads with the other "negative attitude" items.

Factor scores were computed for each participant by averaging the items loading on the four factors. These factor scores were analyzed with regard to the demographic variables age, sex, race, and education (see

Table 3. CSAS Factor Loadings and Scale Reliabilities

Item	Factor 1 Ease of Use and Enjoyment	Factor 2 Interview Completeness	Factor 3 Negative Attitudes	Factor 4 Truthful
Able to use without difficulty	**0.80403**	-0.04125	0.16126	0.09485
Instructions were clear	**0.77941**	0.20600	0.09055	-0.05808
Enjoyed using the computer	**0.65393**	0.24086	0.27043	0.23460
Rather answer questions to person than to a computer	0.05038	-0.00565	**0.55208**	0.58942
Would not like to use computer again	0.20334	-0.16008	**0.68071**	0.08700
Able to be more truthful to computer	0.04403	0.24598	-0.17286	**0.80569**
Computer interview was too long	0.19180	0.03377	**0.69476**	0.00944
Able to describe problems and feelings quite well	0.15384	**0.76048**	0.03372	0.15876
Computer did not ask about important things	-0.14703	**0.52605**	0.45953	-0.22251
Questions were thorough and complete	0.19750	**0.80429**	0.05598	0.10072
Did not think answering questions was helpful	0.02547	0.25947	**0.67411**	-0.12111
Did not have a problem understanding questions	**0.66624**	0.21446	0.00131	-0.03767
Satisfied with the computer program and the questions	0.37922	**0.68258**	0.09884	0.12392
Percent of variance explained (sum = 61.3%)	28.6	13.5	10.9	8.2
Scale alpha (full 13-item scale α = 0.76)	0.76	0.70	0.62	—

Note: Bold numbers indicate items on each factor.

Table 4. Factor Scale Means and Standard Deviations for Three Demographic Groups

Factor	All Clients	Sex		Education		Race	
		Male	Female	Less Than High School	More Than High School	White	African American
	(n = 1,873)	(n = 828)	(n = 1,037)	(n = 498)	(n = 1,126)	(n = 1,286)	(n = 541)
1: Ease of use and enjoyment	1.87 (0.68)	1.91 (0.69)	1.83* (0.67)	1.99 (0.73)	1.79* (0.66)	1.83* (0.67)	1.94 (0.72)
2: Interview completeness	2.34 (0.69)	2.34 (0.67)	2.34 (0.67)	2.29 (0.64)	2.36 (0.72)	2.39 (0.71)	2.20* (0.61)
3: Negative attitudes	2.59 (0.75)	2.67 (0.73)	2.54* (0.78)	2.69 (0.76)	2.57* (0.77)	2.55* (0.71)	2.68 (0.83)
4: Truthful[a]	2.94 (1.2)	2.86* (1.18)	3.01 (1.23)	2.80 (1.22)	2.06* (1.24)	2.97 (1.18)	2.89 (1.29)

[a] The scores used for Factor 4, Truthful, are the scores for the single item "Was able to be more truthful to a computer."
* Indicates response with a significantly higher agreement, $p < 0.01$ (t test for independent samples, one tailed).

Table 5. Correlations Between CSAS Factors and Selected Demographic and Diagnostic Variables

Variable	Factor 1 Ease of Use and Enjoyment	Factor 2 Interview Completeness	Factor 3 Negative Attitudes	Factor 4 Truthful
Age	0.16*	0.04	0.09*	0.12*
GAS	−0.17*	−0.07*	−0.11*	0.07*
BPRS				
Total	0.05	0.08*	−0.02	−0.07*
Anxious depression	0.02	0.14*	−0.12*	−0.03
Thinking disturbance	0.13*	−0.02	0.15*	−0.08*
Withdrawal– Retardation	0.08*	0.01	0.06	−0.06
Hostile– Suspiciousness	0.08*	0.11*	0.01	−0.08

* Pearson r, two tailed, $p < 0.01$.

Tables 4, 5). Factor 1 was significantly different based on age, sex, educational level, and race. Factor 2 differed based on race and factor 3 differed again on age, sex, education, and race. Factor 4 differed in terms of age, sex, and education. While these various comparisons are statistically significant, the mean differences are quite small. Thus the practical or programmatic significance of these demographic factors is negligible.

Also examined was the relationship between the factors and two staff evaluations of psychiatric impairment, the GAS and the BPRS. Table 5 summarizes those analyses. For the GAS, more impaired clients had higher levels of enjoyment, thought the assessments more complete, felt that they were able to be less truthful, and held more negative attitudes. The BPRS results, however, were a mirror image of these with three of the four correlations being related in the *opposite* direction. On the BPRS, the more impaired clients thought the assessments less complete and felt that they were able to be more truthful. Although not significant, the correlation's sign was also reversed for ease of use.

Review of Client Typed Comments

A cursory review of the comments typed by clients at the end of the CACS are generally positive toward the C/MIS program and computers. Approximately 40% of clients typed at least a single word of comment following the structured assessment. Of these 800 comments, approximately 25% were generally positive, 17% generally negative, 4% made very specific suggestions of ways that the assessment could be improved, and approximately 13% made strange, peripheral, or other comments.

Positive comments included: "Enjoyed the computer, efficiency with privacy"; "I think the computer made me think about a lot of things in my life"; "Using the computer was fun"; "I thought it was nice to use the computer to put our own data in."

Negative comments included: "The computer is not the answer to people who are mentally ill"; "Format is too narrow"; "Talking with a social worker is better."

Specific suggestions included: "Incest survivor not in questions"; "I think it could have touched more on childhood problems"; "Need to add 'bicycling' as a method of commuting in the community."

Strange, peripheral, or other type of responses included: "God is good. Jesus can work it out. Have faith in yourself"; "Icar [sic] on highway and in inclement weather was my fear of driving"; "I wish everybody had two [sic] wear my face for a while."

Discussion

In public mental health, serious mentally ill clients can complete automated direct clinical assessments. Indeed, more than half of those clients prefer automated to human assessment. It can be clearly seen by these data that, in general, clients found the experience enjoyable, and that they would like to do it again. It was particularly reinforcing to the C/MIS development team that these clients found C/MIS to be solid, complete, and understandable. The instructions were clear and clients were able to use the system without difficulty. Unlike the Spinovan et al. (1993) study, our results found that automated assessment can be successfully used for all psychiatric outpatients as part of standard intake procedures.

As one would expect, there were clients, the majority of clients it seems, who did not think that *all* the questions were helpful or that the system asked *all* of the important things. On the other hand, many people felt that the instrument was too long. To understand the significance of these responses, they ought to be compared to more traditional assessments. Yet to our knowledge, no comparable data has been collected on paper-and-pencil assessments nor on human interviews. It is not unreasonable to assume that clients would judge more traditional assessments similarly. The Sawyer et al. (1991) study bears on this point. In it, the attitudes of parents who completed automated assessments were compared with the attitudes of those who completed traditional paper-and-pencil assessments. Parents who used the automated assessment increased their preference for them and decreased their preference for traditional assessments. Because parents who completed paper-and-pencil assessments did not change, this change probably did not result from dissonance reduction but from increased understanding. These results suggest that if they were directly compared, automated assessments will be seen more favorably than traditional written assessments.

We found a variety of significant differences in demographic variables of age, sex, race, and education. However, with this study's large sample size small, nonclinically significant differences might well be statistically significant. The average mean difference between the various groups was 0.23, less than one-quarter of a response unit. Only one difference, between those with and without a high school education to the questions "Was able to be more truthful to a computer," was greater than a third of a response unit. Thus, while these differences were statistically significant, they are small enough to be clinically irrelevant.

Differences were also found between acceptance and staff ratings of psychiatric impairment. These results are consistent with the Petrie and Abell (1994) study. Those authors found, as we did with the Anxious Depression scale of the BPRS, that more depressed clients preferred automated assessments. However, there is good reason to suspect the clinical significant of these results. First, the correlations between client acceptance and the GAS and BPRS total score were, in three of the four factors, reversed. Second, all of the correlations in total were quite small. Even the largest correlation, between the GAS and factor 1 (ease of use and enjoyment), accounts for only 3% of the factor's variance. Based on these reasons, the differences found for these variables are judged to be clinically irrelevant.

From these results, we believe that there is no appreciative difference in client acceptance of automated assessment based on age, sex, race, education level, or level of psychiatric impairment.

Although we are satisfied with the evaluation scale, anecdotally clients have reported difficulty with its negatively worded questions. Specifically, question 7 about the computer interview being too long proved difficult for these SMI clients to understand. As a result, future versions of this questionnaire will be modified to have all questions answered in the same direction. The new wording of the effected questions is:

5. I would like to answer questions on the computer again.
7. The computer interview was the right length for me.
9. The computer asked me about things I think are important.
11. I think that answering all these questions was helpful.

Summary

This is the first large-scale analysis of client automated assessment with seriously mentally ill clients being served in outpatient settings. Using automated assessment with these individuals has been an effective means of capturing important client information in a way that is quite acceptable to those individuals. It is clear from the results that this methodology can be used routinely with these individuals and that their acceptance of it is not effected by demographic variables or level of psychiatric impairment.

References

Erdman, H.P., Greist, J.H., Klein, M.H., Jefferson, J.W., & Getto, C. (1981). The computer psychiatrist: How far have we come? Where are we heading? How far dare we go? *Behavior, Research, Methods & Instrumentation, 13*, 393–398.

Endicott, J., Spitzer, R.L., Fleiss, J.L., & Cohen, J. (1976). The Global Assessment Scale: A procedure for measuring overall severity of psychiatric disturbance. *Archives of General Psychiatry, 33*, 766–771.

Evenson, R.E., Holland, R.A., Mehta, S., & Yasin, F. (1980). Factor analysis of the Symptom Checklist-90. *Psychological Reports, 46*, 695–699.

Evenson, R.E., Reese, P.J., & Holland, R.A. (1982). Measuring the severity of symptoms in outpatient alcoholics. *Journal of Studies on Alcohol, 43*, 839–842.

Farrell, A.D., Camplair, P.S., & McCullough, L. (1987). Identification of target complaints by computer interview: Evaluation of the computerized assessment system for psychotherapy evaluation and research. *Journal of Consulting and Clinical Psychology, 55*, 691–700.

Ford, B.D., & Vitelli, R. (1992). Inmate attitudes toward computerized clinical interventions. *Computers in Human Behavior, 8*, 223–230.

Hile, M.G., & Hedlund, J. (1989). Development of a management information system for a purchase of service setting. *Computers in Human Services, 5*, 71–82.

Klingler, D.E., Johnson, J.H., & Williams, T.A. (1976). Strategies in the evolution of an on-line computer-assisted unit for intake assessment of mental health patients. *Behavior, Research, Methods & Instrumentation, 8*, 95–100.

Overall, J.E., & Gorham, D.R. (1962). Brief Psychiatric Rating Scale. *Psychological Reports, 10*, 799–812.

Petrie, K., & Abell, W. (1994). Responses of parasuicides to a computerized interview. *Computers in Human Behavior, 10*, 415–418.

Quintanar, L.R., Crowell, C.R., Pryor, J.B., & Adamopoulos, J. (1982). Human–computer interaction: A preliminary social psychological analysis. *Behavior, Research, Methods & Instrumentation, 14*, 212–220.

Sawyer, M., Sarris, A., Quigley, R., Baghurst, P., & Kalucy, R. (1990). The attitude of parents to the use of computer-assisted interviewing in a child psychiatry service. *British Journal of Psychiatry, 157*, 675–678.

Schwartz, M.D. (1984). Reviews of assessment of psychiatric patients' problems by computer interviews. In M.D. Schwartz (Ed.), *Using computers in clinical practice*. New York: Haworth Press.

Spinhoven, P., Labbe, M.R., & Rombouts, R. (1993). Feasibility of computerized psychological testing with psychiatric outpatients. *Journal of Clinical Psychology, 49*, 440–447.

Wagman, M. (1980). PLATO DCS: An interactive computer system for personal counseling. *Journal of Counseling Psychology, 27*, 16–30.

26
Barriers to Telemedicine in Psychiatry
John Bennett, Milton P. Huang, and Norman E. Alessi

Telepsychiatry is the practice of psychiatry using a telecommunication link for the purpose of delivering clinical care. Telecommunications allow for access to care and consultation when a patient or other consultee are in a place other than the same location as the provider. Within the context of recent media attention given to telemedicine (TM), little attention has been shown to telepsychiatry. Instead, attention has been given to other medical applications, in particular cardiology, radiology, pathology, and emergency medicine. More broadly, issues concerning TM are being discussed as it becomes apparent that the implementation of TM is not progressing as rapidly or extensively as hoped (Sanders & Tedesco, 1993). These discussions do not attempt to deal with the specific and unique factors concerning the practice of psychiatry and the barriers that might exist in this field.

Telepsychiatry, the first TM application, would appear to be an area in which TM would have its broadest base of support. Access to psychiatry services are difficult, especially in rural areas, and especially in child psychiatry. There also appear to be fewer technological barriers, given our limited use of procedural instruments, increased reliance on standardized diagnostic criteria, and increasingly standardized psychiatric care. Yet telepsychiatry has not been reported on in any of the leading psychiatric journals for over a decade.

Certainly the difficulties that TM has encountered are contributing to the difficulties being encountered by telepsychiatry. Although TM has been promoted as a means of providing accessible, affordable, high quality medical care to people underserved by the present health care delivery system, and has received hundreds of millions of dollars in grants and other support to develop and deploy integrated regional TM systems, the actual utilization of TM has been much less than anticipated. According to a recent survey of the 10 most clinically active TM programs in North America, fewer than 2,000 patients were seen by physicians in interactive teleconsultations in 1993 (Allen, 1993). These numbers suggest that powerful barriers and impediments are interfering with the optimal utilization of TM systems. If telepsychiatry is to be more extensively utilized, it will be necessary to identify, understand, and successfully address the barriers and impediments that are affecting telemedicine, as well as those that pertain specifically to telepsychiatry.

In this chapter we define telepsychiatry and briefly summarize the history of the field. We examine areas where factors may serve as potential barriers to the development of TM, including economic, legal, cultural/organizational, the human interface, and the absence of standards. Particular attention will be paid to their implications as they pertain to telepsychiatry.

Definition of Telepsychiatry

Telepsychiatry (literally, psychiatry at a distance), and more generally TM, can be broadly defined as any technical arrangement or organization facilitating direct or indirect medical or psychiatric care taking place over a distance. For the purposes of this chapter, the definition will be narrowed to those arrangements or organizations involving the interactive use of television, telecommunications, and computer-based technologies to provide direct and indirect medical care: real-time audiovisual telecommunications that link psychiatrists and patients, medical specialists, primary care physicians, and other medical staff.

The primary technological components of interactive telepsychiatric videoconferencing systems typically include video cameras, microphones and noise canceling systems, monitors, analog–digital conversion equipment, compression–decompression utilities (codec), specially architectured and designed rooms, and a carrier medium. The carrier medium may involve one or a combination of three carrier solutions, including: analog video (cable or satellite); telephony utilizing either modem, Integrated Service Digital Networks (ISDN), T1, T3 lines, or satellite connections; and/or computer-based systems characterized by Ethernet, Fiber Distributed Data Interface (FDDI), or Asynchronous Transfer Mode (ATM). These solutions should have the ability to tie in conferencing or multipoint connections between participnts in addition to providing point to point connections. Unlike telepsychiatry, TM systems may also include digitized and telemetered diagnostic equipment, such as electronic stethoscopes, otoscopes, endoscopes, etc. Further, the ability to transmit and receive graphical and image-based data, such as EKGs, X-rays, EEGs, etc., operating in parallel systems or integrated into the video conferencing system, are often components of a telemedicine system (Sanders & Tedesco, 1993).

Although technology is central in providing distant communication and the transfer of information in telepsychiatry, telepsychiatry cannot be adequately analyzed or understood if definitions are limited to elements of the technological arrays. Telepsychiatry is in fact a "bundled" or "package" system defined by:

1. Medical, organizational, and economic configurations that develop with each implementation and determine the specific organization of care, service pathways, and economic arrangements;
2. manpower requirements necessary for appropriate clinical, technical, scheduling, and other arrangements;
3. clinical protocols and other methods for integrating TM patients into larger medical care networks; and,
4. the nature of behavior styles and interpersonal standards of conduct appropriate to the context of medical videoconferencing (Bashshur, 1978).

Therefore one would anticipate that in addition to technological issues, difficulties within any of these areas might also lead to the development of barriers to the implementation of TM.

In general, telepsychiatry is most frequently exemplified by two major functions: clinical care and distant education. In each of these functions, telecommunication technology brings people and resources together, bridges distance and time, and provides access to medical care, consultation, and information that might not otherwise be available in a timely manner, or only available at significant inconvenience or cost. Examples of clinical care within telepsychiatry include direct clinical care and consultation. In telepsychiatry, direct clinical care might include a diagnostic evaluation of a depressed adult at a rural Community Mental Health Agency by a psychiatrist in a university department of psychiatry. Telepsychiatric consultation could also be used in a commitment hearing, linking a state mental health facility, the referring psychiatrist, and probate judge via live video. Distant education can include a broad range of applications including the teaching of medical students from a main classroom setting to their off-campus rotation site, providing lecture materials for continuing medical education or providing information for patients concerning their own or a family member's illness.

History of Telepsychiatry

The histories of TM and telepsychiatry are inextricably intertwined. The first applications of TM were in fact in psychiatry. The first documented use of TM occurred in 1959 at the Nebraska Psychiatric Institute (Wittson & Benschoter, 1972). This effort resulted in grant support for a study to determine the value of telepsychiatry. These efforts demonstrated the effectiveness of the system in the evaluation of patients and in its use for either group or individual therapy (Wittson, Affleck, & Johnson, 1961). Technical and fiscal issues were noted as barriers. Subsequent reports appeared in the literature documenting the continued utilization of the

Nebraska system and the development and utilization of similar systems at the Harvard and Dartmouth Medical Schools and Mount Sinai School of Medicine (Benschoter, 1967; Menolascino & Osborne, 1970; Solow, Weiss, Bergen, & Sanborn, 1971; Dwyer, 1973; Straker, Mostyns, & Marshall, 1976). Television and telecommunications systems were utilized to study the feasibility of providing remote diagnosis and interactive medical care between a physician at one location and a patient at another, distant location. To our knowledge only one controlled study occurred during this time to support the use of telepsychiatry (Doniger, Tempier, Lalinec–Michaudg, & Meunier, 1986). The conclusion of this study was, "bi directional CCTV (closed circuit television) interviews can be an effective method of mental health care delivery." It was thought that CCTV could be used for all clinical and educational purposes.

Subsequently, other physicians were able to demonstrate that the quality of some telemedical data (e.g., X rays, visual methods of physical exam) were sufficient to make some diagnoses and provide some medical treatments safely and reliably using the existing technology (Bashshur & Lovett, 1977). Concerns were simultaneously raised about the absence of actual face-to-face encounters between physician and patient and the impossibility of such traditional practices as "laying-on-of-hands" in these telemedical encounters (Dwyer, 1973). Technological obstacles also interfered with more widespread experimentation and implementation of TM, including high cost of equipment, high rates of maintenance and repair, and difficulty tailoring the studio-based television and telecommunications equipment of the day to the specific needs of a medical context (Maxmen, 1978).

Little TM activity occurred from the mid-1970s until a resurgence in the early 1990s, except in the U.S. Space Program that bridged this period. NASA continued to provide medical care, conduct medical research, and demonstrate the ability to utilize digital medical telemetry to reliably monitor significant aspects of astronaut health and physiological function in the distant space environment (Bashshur, 1983).

The late 1980s and early 1990s brought a resurgence in interest, funding, application, and study of telemedicine. This renewal came as converging forces of the National Information Infrastructure (NII) and Health Care Reform (HCR) emerged as potent forces on the political landscape and high technology applications were offered as potential means to improve access to high quality medical care and reduce budget busting health care costs predicted for the future. The NII aimed at utilizing advanced telecommunications technology to rejuvenate the American economy and improve competitiveness in the international economic arena (Gore, 1991). HCR promoted the goals of increasing access to medical care, maintaining the quality of health care, and reducing health care costs, by opening health care markets to free market competition and utilizing advanced technology in the provision, management, and administration of health care systems. While the political landscape promoted renewed interest in TM as a means of achieving HCR goals, technological improvements reduced the costs of equipment while improving the reliability and stability of teleconferencing operations. In the period from the mid-1970s to the early 1990s, videoconferencing technology moved from analog-based video systems to computer-based, digitally compressed video formats, making it possible to map TM more effectively onto existing telecommunications infrastructures, primarily telephone lines.

Through the early 1990s telemedicine received increasing support in the form of grants, cost partnerships, and other funding, and TM networks proliferated. High profile TM links between hospitals and universities in the United States and Russia and other countries competed for attention in the press with stories about the information superhighway. By the end of the 1993/1994 fiscal year, TM was receiving more than $200 million (U.S.) yearly in funding for equipment and clinical operations in networks deployed in at least 26 states, with links to many foreign countries. TM applications included teleradiology and telepathology, as well as a full range of clinical specialties, including psychiatry.

Today there are a number of telepsychiatric sites within the United States. Table 1 lists programs identified as having active telepsychiatric programs (Allen & Allen, 1994). These programs offer a broad range of services including court evaluations, neuropsychiatric testing, and counseling to adults as well as children. The number of consultations range from 1 to well over 210 in the time interval of the survey. In addition to these programs many others are now entertaining the installation of telemedicine facilities within their institutions including Emory University, Ossawotamie State Hospital (KS), Southwest Virginia Mental Institute (GA), Indian Health Service (SD), Tennessee Psychiatric Clinic (TN), and Laureate Psychiatric Clinic (OK).

Barriers to TM and Telepsychiatry

Despite the recent growth of TM, there appear to be several barriers that must be overcome for the full implementation of TM within medicine. These will undoubtedly have implications for the implementation of telepsychiatry as well. The following will focus on these barriers as they apply to medicine, with special attention to their implications concerning psychiatry.

Economic Barriers

The major economic considerations that may pose as barriers to the implementation of TM are cost, reimbursement, and cost effectiveness.

Table 1. Programs With Active Telepsychiatric Programs

Institution (State)	No. Sites	No. Psychiatrists	Number of Consultations in 1994	Average Length of Consultation
Norfolk Regional Center (NE)	1	1	210	1 hr + 15–20 min F/U
University of South Carolina (SC)	2	1	144	90 min
Eastern Montana Telemed Project (MT)	5	1	58	30–60 min
Eastern Oregon Human Services Consortium (OR)	45	5	24	20–60 min
University of Kansas Medical Center (KS)	2	1	20	20–120 min
East Carolina University (NC)	2	2	10	60 min
Medical College of Georgia (GA)	2	8	5	60 min
Harvard University Research Group (MA)	1	5	2	30–60 min
South Dakota Services Center (SD)	15	7	1	60 min
University of Calgary (Canada)	1	4	10	40 min
Totals	76	35	484	530
Average	7.6	3.5	48.8	

Cost. There are many infrastructure costs involved in the establishment and maintenance of a telepsychiatric site. Although the cost of the telepsychiatric consultation office may be less, prices for components of the TM consultation room may run between $100,000 and $500,000 (U.S.), depending on the array of equipment necessary (Shoor, 1994). Further, carrier costs may run up to $1,500 per month for leased telephone lines, in addition to charges per session. Total costs, that include such items as staffing and personnel, transmission costs, maintenance and upkeep, periodic hardware and software upgrading costs, etc. add to the provider's price tag. The costs for either single TM applications or for integrated regional TM systems can be prohibitive, and stand in the way of full implementation. When one considers investment and total costs in the context of returns on investment, especially in the absence of clear reimbursement strategies, the net benefits of TM from a business perspective are not clear and act as a serious obstacle to implementation.

Reimbursement. Currently, reimbursement for TM lacks broad-based support. HCFA and some major insurers, for example, have agreed to reimburse some TM systems in limited ways, primarily for the purpose of study (BNA Medicare Report, 1993). HCFA makes it clear, however, that its limited support is not to be taken as general policy, and only certain arrangements for the delivery of services will be supported. HCFA will reimburse only for patients seen with a physician present at both ends of the teleconsultation. HCFA considers interactive TM an experimental technology that has "not been shown to be safe and effective" (BNA Medicare Report, 1993) and is reluctant, in the absence of clinical trials, to reimburse for services not involving the direct personal contact between physician and patient. HCFA's support for TM is crucial. TM's inability so far to receive reasonable levels of consistent reimbursement, from HCFA and other payers, acts as a serious brake to further implementation.

Cost Effectiveness. Given cost concerns, there is no substitute for cost-benefit and cost-effectiveness analyses of telemedicine compared to alternative delivery systems. The absence of such analysis impedes decision making about reimbursement. Bashshur (1994) writes,

> One of the most critical policy concerns with regard to the development of telemedicine is its effect on the cost of care. The extensive focus on cost issues in telemedicine is justifiable, given historically that high technology in health care has led to increase costs. Nonetheless, scientific research in this field has been hampered by the lack of consensus on a precise definition of telemedicine and its specific role in health care delivery, as well as the limited availability of fully operational optimal systems on which to collect and analyze valid and reliable data. With little sound research or policy analysis, policy decisions at this time must rely on anticipated potential benefits and logical speculation.

The absence of systematic analysis and study will continue to impede the development and diffusion of TM.

Legal Barriers

There are several legal areas that become of concern when dealing with TM. These include state licensure and credentialing, confidentiality, liability, and malpractice.

State Licensure and Credentialing. If you are providing psychiatry consultation services via TM from your office or clinic in one state to a patient in another state, in which state do the consultation services take place? In your state because you are the originator of services? Or in the patient's state, because the problems is located in the patient? Or both? How these questions are answered is crucial regarding issues of licensure.

The current state licensure system does not resolve questions such as these.

If the issue is defined in terms of the patient's state of residence, providing psychiatry consultation to a patient in a neighboring state where the consulting physician is not licensed could result in civil and criminal penalties. Mandating that psychiatrists be licensed in all the states in which their patients may reside would be impossibly cumbersome. Equally so, mandating that TM practice be restricted to those patients who live within the state boundaries of the local health care facility would place unreasonable limits on the application and reach for which the technology was designed. Credentialing is an issue that poses similar difficulties. How does a consulting specialist conduct a consultation with a patient in a rural hospital where he/she is not credentialed to practice?

Confidentiality. There is no easy and inexpensive way of determining the presence or absence of persons other than the therapist and patient in either videoconferencing room. Videoconferencing often requires the presence, at least at the beginning and end of sessions, of various technical personnel. There are several ways in which the networking capabilities of TM can lead to the exposure of private patient information (Norton, Lindborg, & Delaplain, 1993). Nonmedical technicians will often be involved in setting up or running video equipment and will see the patient during the interview. Other personnel such as medical students and consultants may be off-screen and able to observe the interview. Videotapes of the interview could be easily made. Finally, the actual transmission of the signal through a network is subject to possible interception. Of course, part of the advantage of TM is the ability to bring multiple individuals from a distance into the consultation. But, this requires precautions to protect the patient's confidentiality in each of these cases. Technological solutions such as encryption and password protection can protect against some of these problems (Wright, 1994), but this problem also results from social and legal expectations of medical treatment (Brannigan, 1992). Although clinicians using TM devices will certainly need to inform their patients about the possible breaches in confidentiality, many may decide to simply avoid using these systems.

Malpractice and Liability. There have been no malpractice suits to date involving TM, probably because it has been used so little. But as TM grows it will inevitably come to the attention of attorneys. TM using compressed video technology and diagnosis at a distance rather than hands on and in person, will automatically come under the charge of being incomplete and/or inadequate. This is where standards and conventions will be most important. Although providing the best defense against suit (there would probably be no other area of medicine so completely recorded), videotape records of TM sessions, archiving, storing, and retrieving analog records would be time consuming and expensive, antithetical to the application of technology to medicine.

Absence of Standards

The implementation of TM is illustrative of a technology growing more quickly than relevant regulation or the development of standards. As a new and constantly changing technology, no current standards exist for implementing TM. The two areas that will require development of standards are connectivity and practice.

Connectivity. The need for connectivity standards arises from variations in computer hardware, physical networks, and communications protocols. Different local systems use different computer hardware and software. In fact, as administrators upgrade old systems, many networks have now become a mixture of old hardware and newer hardware that have difficulty in exchanging information (Walker, 1989). These local area networks of computers (LANs) need to be connected to wider networks to be able to use telepsychiatry at a distance. The implementation of such connections is slowed by both the physical complexity of interconnection as well as political obstacles regarding ownership. Many types of networks exist, connected in different configurations and moving information at different speeds. Private contractors often have a financial incentive to limit broader types of interconnection, preferring to keep users working only in the networks they provide (Parsons, 1992). In addition to problems in making physical connections, there is also a problem in having the systems agree about details of the information sent. Transmission protocols exist that can help standardize this part of the connection, requiring computers to speak the same language. These protocols still require further development at several levels of complexity. At a lower level, TM systems need to have standards for compression and decompression algorithms. Many standards exist with names like H.320 or H.261, but their use varies from vendor to vendor (Chimiak & Raliski, 1994). These networks also need to standardize the communication of higher level information about categories of patients, diagnoses, billing, etc. Health Level Seven (HL7) is one such high-level standards, but remains under development (Hettinger & Brazile, 1994). The Department of Veterans Affairs is an example of one organization that is implementing multiple data exchange protocols in its telecommunications efforts (Dayhoff & Maloney, 1992). Their implementation has been highly dependent on their ability to mandate particular standards for a communications infrastructure.

Practice. In addition to the above concerns regarding the regulation of the communications system, there is an important question about the development of a process of regulation to establish and maintain standards for the TM consultation. Currently there are no standards or definitions about what is provided in a TM consultation and many questions arise. What is the responsibility of the TM consultant? Are the elements of a TM consultation less or different than that of the physician who is physically persent? What of the case of the physician who provides supervision at a distance? Who is responsible for difficulties in the examination if technical difficulties arise or information is lost from the data stream? How should the consultant provide verification of his or her credentials? If the teleconsultation occurs in different hospitals or different states, where does the consultant need to be licensed or accredited? Many such questions will only be answered as more people use TM systems so that social and legal norms can be established. Given the fears of litigation that many practitioners reasonably have, many will decide to avoid TM until these questions are more clearly resolved.

No standards for interactive TM care exist at this point in time. This will make physicians wary of practicing TM on a routine basis, although exceptions may occur where circumstances are of such a nature (emergencies, disasters, etc.) that risks associated with TM are outweighed by the need to provide immediate care.

Interface Barriers

The introduction of telepsychiatry raises a number of questions as to its impact within the doctor–patient relationship, both for the patient and the doctor. Therefore, we will explore the potential impact on both of these individuals by the introduction of this technology as well as difficulties that can arise within the physician–consultant relationship.

The few reports of telepsychiatric care present primarily anecdotal and generally rosy pictures of the acceptability of this medium of care. In a Nebraska study, for example, investigators found that after initial hesitation there was almost universal acceptance of telepsychiatry: "A single utilization of the system was all it took to convert the doubtful" (Benschoter, 1967). Another study found that the use of television "has not proved to be a significant barrier in establishing rapport with the patient or in perceiving emotional nuances" (Solow et al., 1971). Dwyer also reports high levels of acceptance among patients and psychiatrists, and in some cases patients preferred telepsychiatry interviews over face-to-face sessions (Dwyer, 1973). In a controlled study, on the other hand, compared to face-to-face controls, telepsychiatry interviews tended to be significantly less satisfactory for patients, consultees, and consultants, even though both telepsychiatry and control interviews were rated positively (Dongier et al., 1986). Questions of privacy and confidentiality (see, for example, Wittson & Benschoter, 1972) are raised as important issues affecting acceptability.

In general, evidence concerning the acceptability of telepsychiatry is impressionistic and anecdotal in nature. Systematic clinical trials are necessary to understand acceptability and the effect of the technological interface in telepsychiatry on the entire range of clinical activities. These studies should consider effects from the points of view of the patients, consultants, and consultees, and address issues like the ones outlined below.

Patient. To what degree is the clinical situation altered by the introduction of telecommunication equipment? Will there be alterations in the likelihood that patients will reveal the same about themselves in a virtual setting as they might in person? Will they feel comfortable in establishing an ongoing relationship within this context? As noted it is important for the patient and physician to feel that the relationship is warm and professional (Norton et al., 1993). What attention must be given to the telepsychiatry studio and the clinical situation to convey organization and attention to the patient's needs? What are the effects of patient's having or not having control over cameras, focusing, etc. affecting the remote viewing of the psychiatrist? Also, within the psychiatric context, there is the need to maintain privacy and confidentiality, therefore not allowing the presence of technicians, etc. to interfere, and to find ways to insure the security of settings and channels from intrusion. What residual concerns about confidentiality and privacy remain after care is taken to insure them from a technical perspective?

Psychiatrists. Psychiatrists will also have to be comfortable with the technology involved in telepsychiatry, and because support personnel are inappropriate in this setting, hands-on technical operating of the system will be necessary for successful clinical interviewing. This will include moving, cueing, and focusing cameras as part of the clinical interview as well as making modifications in the style and pace of conversation in order to match the technical interface. Physicians who are "technophobic" or uncomfortable with the utilization of technological interfaces will be reluctant to engage in telepsychiatry. There will be an initial discomfort with the style of interactions necessary to communicate effectively through compressed video formats. What kinds of training or enculturation experiences are useful in developing familiarity and skill in telepsychiatry?

Psychiatrists using teleconferencing equipment will practice a form of medicine involving virtual and technologically mediated relationships with individuals and groups who are being treated at a distance. The interaction with the patient in telepsychiatry will require additional and different skills than those involved in other applications of TM. Reluctance and inhibition in these nonstandard interpersonal situations will produce deformations in clinical and personal conduct that may interfere with the goals of the interviewing process. What are the aspects of professional psychiatric care that are different in telepsychiatry than in face-to-face interviews?

Organizational and Cultural Barriers

The introduction of any new technology into an established culture has the potential not only for creating efficiencies and smoother operations, but also for creating inefficiencies, unexpected effects, and transformations in the structure of organizations and systems. Bashshur notes that "telemedicine has the potential for restructuring the system of delivering patient care (Bashshur, 1994). Resistance to new technologies, including TM, may not only be due to costs that are perceived to be involved, or time needed to master and utilize technologies (Connelly, Rich, Curley, & Kelly, 1990), but may also represent an apprehension that the technologies being deployed will fundamentally alter the way medicine and psychiatry is practiced and organized.

Optimized TM systems will assume and be an element in the pressure toward greater integration of health care delivery systems. What will be the effects of integration be on free standing clinics and hospitals? How will new protocols needed to triage TM patients into existing health care organizations affect those organizations? As issues of licensing and privileging are resolved, how will this affect medical staffing and organizational structures? How will the capacity to provide health care at a distance affect health care markets? Will telecommunications and the newly competitive health care marketplace favor rich providers and drive poorer providers out of business, or into the arms of large medical conglomerates for protection? Will the promise of utilizing TM as a means to maintain patients in their home communities and local hospitals (see, for example, Sanders & Tedesco, 1993) be realized, or will some providers use TM to increase market share, control resources, and assure patient flow?

None of these questions can be answered ahead of time, of course, but the early blush of cooperation and integration may be followed by competitive actions based on harsh economic realities. Organizations and institutions may need to protect themselves from electronic entry into their markets. States may see licensing reciprocity as a method of market penetration by providers across the border, and so on. Broad organizational issues such as these would certainly create barriers for the implementation of TM in general and telepsychiatry in particular.

Conclusion and Recommendations

The potential barriers to the acceptance and implementation of telepsychiatry are numerous and cover a broad range. If telepsychiatry is to succeed, it will need to do so in the larger context of TM. Fundamental to determining costs and future reimbursement is the need for systematic study of cost benefits and cost effectiveness, acceptability, and safety and effectiveness of telepsychiatry versus alternative delivery systems. The concerns of physicians and payers about the quality of medical care provided via telepsychiatry needs to be addressed through controlled clinical trials and standards setting, from both technological and clinical perspectives. Finally, marketplace and organizational concerns need to be addressed in order to maintain a process of deployment in a cooperative and integrative manner. With these efforts, telepsychiatry holds the potential of providing improved access to psychiatric care in cost-effective ways.

Acknowledgment. The authors are grateful to Dr. Rashid Bashshur for his knowledge, leadership, and consultation in the area of TM.

References

Allen, A. (1993). Editor's note. *Telemedicine Newsletter, 1*, 2–4.

Allen, D., & Allen, A. (1994). Telemental health services today. *Telemedicine Today, 2*, 1–24.

Bashshur, R. (1978). Public acceptance of telemedicine in a rural community. *Biosciences Communications, 4*, 17–38.

Bashshur, R. (1983). Telemedicine and health policy. In O.H. Gandy, P. Espinosa, & J.A. Ordover (Eds.), *Proceedings From the Tenth Annual Telecommunications Policy Research Conference* (pp. 347–360). Norwood, NJ: Ablex Publishing Corp.

Bashshur, R. (1994). Telemedicine effects: Cost, quality and access [Abstract of position paper]. Second National Aeronautics and Space Administration/ Uniformed Service University of the Health Sciences, International Conference on Telemedicine. September 8–10, 1994.

Bashshur, R., & Lovett, J. (1977). Assessment of telemedicine: Results of the initial experience. *Aviation Space Environment Medicine, 48*, 65–70.

Benschoter, R.A. (1967). Multi-purpose television. *Annals of the New York Academy of Sciences, 142*, 471–478.

Brannigan, V.M. (1992). Protecting the privacy of patient information in clinical networks: Regulatory effectiveness analysis. *Annals of the New York Academy of Sciences, 670*, 190–201.

Bureau of National Affairs. (1993). *BNA's Medicare Report, 4*, 972–975.

Chimiak, W., & Raliski, E. (1994). Telemedicine: The babeling tower. *Healthcare Informatics, April*, 39–46.

Connelly, D.P., Rich, E.C., Curley, S.P., & Kelly, J.T. (1990). Knowledge resource preferences of family physicians. *The Journal of Family Practice, 30*, 353–359.

Dayhoff, R., & Maloney, D. (1992). Exchange of veterans affairs medical data using national and local networks. *Annals of the New York Academy of Sciences, 670*, 50–66.

Dongier, M., Tempier, R., Lalinec–Michaud, M., & Meunier, D. (1986). Telepsychiatry: Psychiatric consultation through two-way television. A controlled study. *Canada Journal of Psychiatry, 31*, 32–34.

Dwyer, T.F. (1973). Telepsychiatry: Psychiatric consultation by interactive television. *American Journal of Psychiatry, 130*, 865–869.

Gore, A. (1991). Infrastructure for the global village. *Scientific American*, 150–153.

Hettinger, B.J., & Brazile, R.P. (1994). Health level seven: Standard for health care electronic data transmission. *Computers in Nursing, 12*, 13–16.

Maxmen, J.S. (1978). Telecommunications in psychiatry. *American Journal of Psychotherapy, 32*, 450–455.

Menolascino, F.J., & Osborne, R.G. (1970). Psychiatric television consultation for the mentally retarded. *American Journal of Psychiatry, 127*, 1684–1687.

Norton, S., Lindborg, C., & Delaplain, C. (1993). Consent and privacy in telemedicine. *Hawaii Medical Journal, 52*, 340–341.

Parsons, D. (1992). Progress and problems of interhospital consulting by computer networking. *Annals of the New York Academy of Sciences, 670*, 1–11.

Sanders, J.H., & Tedesco, F.J. (1993). Telemedicine: Bringing medical care to isolated communities. *Journal of the Medical Association of Georigia, 82*, 237–241.

Shoor, R. (1994). Long distance medicine. *Business & Health, 12*, 39–46.

Solow, C., Weiss, R., Bergen, B., & Sanborn, C. (1971). 24-Hour psychiatric consultation via TV. *American Journal of Psychiatry, 127*, 1684–1687.

Straker, N., Mostyn, P., & Marshall, C. (1976). The use of two-way TV in bringing mental health services to the inner city. *American Journal of Psychiatry, 133*, 1202–1205.

Walker, J.M. (1989). Integrating information systems with HL7. *Hospitals, July 5*, FB60–62.

Wittson, C.L., Affleck, D.C., & Johnson, V. (1961). Two-way television in group therapy. *Mental Hospitals, 2*, 22–23.

Wittson, C.L., & Benschoter, R. (1972). Two-way television: Helping the medical center reach out. *Amercian Journal of Psychiatry, 129*, 624–627.

Wright, B. (1994). Health care and privacy law in electronic commerce. *Healthcare Financial Management, 48*, 66–70.

A Selected Bibliography

Bruce W. Vieweg, James L. Hedlund, and Matthew G. Hile

General Reviews

Ager, A., & Bendall, S. (Eds.). (1991). *Microcomputers and clinical psychology: Issues, applications and future developments.* Chichester, UK: Wiley.

Bloor, R. (1988). *Computers in psychiatry.* London, UK: Education in Practice.

Crawford, J.L., Morgan, D.W., & Gianturco, D.T. (Eds.). (1974). *Progress in mental health information systems: Computer applications.* Cambridge, MA: Ballinger.

Erdman, H.P., Greist, J.H., Klein, M.H., Jefferson, J.W., & Getto, C. (1981). The computer psychiatrist: How far have we come? Where are we heading? How far dare we go? *Behavior Research Methods & Instrumentation, 13,* 393–398.

Glueck, B.C., & Stroebel, C.F. (1980). Computers and clinical psychiatry. In H.I. Kaplan, A.M. Freedman, & B.J. Sadock (Eds.), *Comprehensive textbook of psychiatry* (Vol. 1, 3rd ed., pp. 413–428). Baltimore, MD: Williams & Wilkins.

Greist, J.H., Carroll, J.A., Erdman, H.P., Klein, M.H., & Wurster, C.R. (1987). *Research in mental health computer applications: Directions for the future* (Mental Health Systems Reports, Series DN No. 8, DHHS Pub. No. [ADM] 87-1468). Washington, DC: Superintendent of Documents, U.S. Government Printing Office.

Greist, J.H., & Klein, M.H. (1981). Computers in psychiatry. In S. Arieti & H.K.H. Brodie (Eds.), *American handbook of psychiatry* (pp. 750–777). New York: Basic Books.

Hedlund, J.L., Vieweg, B.W., & Cho, D.W. (1985). Mental health computing in the 1980s, Part 1: General mental health information systems and clinical documentation. *Computers in Human Services, 1,* 3–33.

Hedlund, J.L., Vieweg, B.W., & Cho, D.W. (1985). Mental health computing in the 1980s, Part 2: Clinical applications. *Computers in Human Services, 1,* 1–31.

Hedlund, J.L., Vieweg, B.W., Wood, J.B., Cho, D.W., Evenson, R.C., Hickman, C.V., & Holland, R.H. (1981). *Computers in mental health: A review and annotated bibliography* (NIMH Series FN No. 7, DHHS Pub. No. [ADM] 81-

1090). Washington, DC: Superintendent of Documents, U.S. Government Printing Office.

Johnson, J.H. (Ed.). (1981). Computer technology and methodology in clinical psychology, psychiatry, and behavior medicine [Special issue]. *Behavior Research Methods & Instrumentation, 13*, 389–636.

Lieff, J.D. (1987). *Computer applications in psychiatry.* Washington, DC: American Psychiatric Press.

Rome, H.P. (1985). Computers and psychiatry: An historical perspective. *Psychiatric Annals, 15*, 519–523.

Schwartz, M.D. (Ed.). (1984). *Using computers in clinical practice: Psychotherapy and mental health applications.* New York: Haworth Press.

Sidowski, J.B., Johnson, J.H., & Williams, T.A. (Eds.). (1980). *Technology in mental health care delivery systems.* Norwood, NJ: Ablex.

General Mental Health Information Systems

Bertollo, D.N., Bank, R., Laska, E.M., Siegel, C., & Gulbinat, W. (1994). The NKI/WHO mental health information system. In G. Andrews, H. Dilling, T.B. Ustun, & M. Briscoe (Eds.), *Computers in mental health: 1994* (pp. 59–62). Geneva, Switzerland: World Health Organization.

Bronson, D.E., Pelz, D.C., & Trzcinski, E. (1988). *Computerizing your agencies' information system* (Sage Human Services Guide #54). Newbury Park, CA: Sage.

Cardinali, R., & Farrelly, C. (1991). Human resource management—Applying methodologies of information systems to the Department of Mental Health—a case study of the Connecticut Department of Mental Health. *New Technology in the Human Services, 5*, 6–11.

Carrilio, T.E., Kasser, J., & Moretto, A.H. (1985). Management information systems: Who is in charge? *Social Casework, 66*, 417–423.

Chapman, R.L. (1976). *The design for management information systems for mental health organizations: A primer* (NIMH Series FN No. 5). Washington, DC: Superintendent of Documents, U.S. Government Printing Office.

Cuvo, D., Hall, F., & Milder, G.R. (1988). Computerizing central intake. A means toward accountability. *Social Casework, 69*, 214–223.

Gardner, J.M., Souza, A., Scabbia, A., & Breuer, A. (1986). Microcare— Promises and pitfalls in implementing microcomputer programs in human service agencies. *Computers in Human Behavior, 2*, 147–156.

Glastonbury, B., LaMendola, W., & Toole, S. (1988). *Information technology and the human services.* Chichester, UK: Wiley.

Glueck, B.C. (1974). Computers at the Institute of Living. In J.L. Crawford, D.W. Morgan, & D.T. Gianturco (Eds.), *Progress in mental health information systems: Computer applications* (pp. 303–316). Cambridge, MA: Ballinger.

Grasso, A.J., & Epstein, I. (1989). The Boyesville experience: Integrating practice decision-making, program evaluation and management information. *Computers in Human Services, 4*, 85–94.

Hammond, K.W., & Gottfredson, D.K. (1984). The VA mental health information system package: Version 1. *Computer Use in Social Services Network, 4*, 6–7.

Hedlund, J.L., Sletten, I.W., Evenson, R.C., Altman, H., & Cho, D.W. (1977). Automated psychiatric information systems: A critical review of Missouri's Standard System of Psychiatry (SSOP). *Journal of Operational Psychiatry*, *8*, 5–26.

Hedlund, J.L., & Vieweg, B.W. (1982). Some utilization and maintenance issues with mental health information systems. In B.I. Blum (Ed.), *Proceedings of the Sixth Annual Symposium on Computer Applications in Medical Care* (pp. 130–134). New York: Institute of Electrical & Electronics Engineers.

Hinkle, J.E. (1988). Microcomputers in the adolescent treatment facility: Specifications and utilizations. *Children & Youth Services Review*, *10*, 253–261.

Johnson, J.H., & Williams, T.A. (1975). The use of on-line computer technology in a mental health admitting system. *American Psychologist*, *30*, 388–390.

Johnson, J.H., & Williams, T.A. (1980). Using on-line technology to improve service response and decision making effectiveness in a mental health admitting system. In J.B. Sidowski, J.H. Johnson, & T.A. Williams (Eds.), *Technology in mental health care delivery systems* (pp. 237–249). Norwood, NJ: Ablex.

Kennedy, R.S., Salamon, I., & McKegney, F.P. (1991). A new clinical information system for emergency psychiatry. In P.D. Clayton (Ed.), *Proceedings of the Fifteenth Annual Symposium on Computer Applications in Medical Care* (pp. 872–874). New York: McGraw–Hill.

Laska, E.M., & Bank, R. (Eds.). (1975). *Safeguarding psychiatric privacy: Computer systems and their uses*. New York: Wiley.

Leginski, W.A., Croze, C., Driggers, J., Dumpman, S., Geertsen, D., Kamis–Gould, E., Namerow, M.J., Patton, R.E., Wilson, N.Z., & Wurster, C.R. (1989). *Data standards for mental health decision support systems: A report to the task force to revise the data content and system guidelines of the mental health statistics improvement program* (NIMH Series FN No. 10, DHHS Pub. No. [ADM] 89-1589). Washington, DC: U.S. Government Printing Office.

Mead, D.G., Cain, M.W., & Steele, K. (1985). A computer data based management system for a family therapy clinic. In C.R. Figley (Ed.), *Computers and family therapy* (pp. 49–88). New York: Haworth Press.

Mezzich, J.E., Dow, J.T., Ganguli, R., Munetz, M.R., & Zettler–Segal, M. (1986). Computerized initial and discharge evaluations. In J.E. Mezzich (Ed.), *Clinical care and information systems in psychiatry* (pp. 14–58). Washington, DC: American Psychiatric Press.

Monnickendam, M.R., & Morris, A. (1989). Developing an integrated computerized case management system for Israeli defense forces: An evolutionary approach. *Computers in Human Services*, *5*, 133–149.

Nurius, P.S., & Hudson, W.W. (1993). *Human services practice, evaluation, and computers*. Pacific Grove, CA: Brooks/Cole Publishing Co.

Paton, J.A., & D'Huyvetter, P.K. (1980). *Automated management information systems for mental health agencies: A planning and acquisition guide* (NIMH Series FN No. 1, DHHS Pub. No. 80-797). Washington, DC: Superintendent of Documents, U.S. Government Printing Office.

Salamon, I., & Kennedy, R. (1992). Computer linkage of psychiatric emergency rooms. *Hospital & Community Psychiatry*, *43*, 397–399.

Schoech, D.J., Cavalier, A.R., & Hoover, B. (1993). Using technology to change the human services delivery system. *Administration in Social Work*, *17*, 31–52.

Seiffer, S. (1990). A microcomputer-based management information system for continuing treatment psychiatric rehabilitation programs. In D. Baskin (Ed.), *Computers in psychiatry and psychology* (pp. 143–156). New York: Brunner/Mazel.

Slavin, S. (Ed.). (1981). Applying computers in social service and mental health agencies: A guide to selecting equipment, procedures and strategies [Special issue]. *Administration in Social Work, 5*, 1–181.

Williams, T.A., Johnson, J.H., & Bliss, E.L. (1975). A computer-assisted psychiatric assessment unit. *American Journal of Psychiatry, 132*, 1074–1076.

Wodarski, J.S. (1988). Development of management information systems for human services: A practical guide. *Computers in Human Services, 3*, 37–49.

Mental Health Centers

Baskin, D., & Seiffer, S. (1990). A nationwide survey of computer utilization in community mental health centers. In D. Baskin (Ed.), *Computer applications in psychiatry and psychology* (pp. 159–170). New York: Brunner/Mazel.

Giannetti, R.A., Johnson, J.H., & Williams, T.A. (1978). Computer technology in community mental health centers: Current status and future prospects. In F.H. Orthner (Ed.), *Proceedings of the Second Annual Symposium on Computer Applications in Medical Care* (pp. 117–121). New York: Institute of Electrical & Electronics Engineers.

Hansen, K.E., Johnson, J.H., & Williams, T.A. (1975). Development of an on-line management information system for community mental health centers. *Behavior Research Methods & Instrumentation, 9*, 139–143.

Hershey, J.C., & Moore, J.R. (1975). The use of an information system for community health services planning and management. *Medical Care, 13*, 114–125.

Knesper, D.J., Quarton, G.C., Gorodezky, M.J., & Murray, C.W. (1978). A survey of the users of a working state mental health information system: Implications for the development of improved systems. In F.H. Orthner (Ed.), *Proceedings of the Second Annual Symposium on Computer Applications in Medical Care* (pp. 160–165). New York: Institute of Electrical & Electronics Engineers.

Kupfer, D.J., Levine, M.S., & Nelson, J.A. (1976). *Mental health information systems: Design and implementation*. New York: Marcel Dekker.

MacFadden, R.J. (1986). The microcomputer millennium: Transforming the small social agency. *Social Casework, 67*, 160–165.

Maypole, D.E. (1978). Developing a management information system in a rural community mental health center. *Administration in Mental Health, 6*, 69–80.

Nelson, B.H., & Pecarchik, J.R. (1974). A computerized program audit for community mental health centers. *Community Mental Health Journal, 10*, 102–110.

Newkham, J., & Bawcom, L. (1981). Computerizing an integrated clinical and financial record system in a CMHC: A pilot project. *Administration in Social Work, 5*, 97–112.

Paton, J.A., & Mayberry, D. (1978). Management information systems: Bringing the M and the IS together. In F.H. Orthner (Ed.), *Proceedings of the Second*

Annual Symposium on Computer Applications in Medical Care (pp. 190–197). New York: Institute of Electrical & Electronics Engineers.

Sherman, P.S. (1981). A computerized CMHC clinical and management information system: Saga of a "mini" success. *Behavior Research Methods & Instrumentation, 13*, 445–453.

Spector, P.E., & Voissem, N.H. (1984). An information system for mental health agencies: Some guidelines for non-programmers. *Administration in Mental Health, 12*, 15–25.

St. Clair, C., Siegel, J., Caruso, R., & Spivack, G. (1976). Computerizing a mental health center information system. *Administration in Mental Health, 4*, 10–18.

Substance Abuse Programs

Acker, C., Acker, W., & Shaw, G.K. (1984). Assessment of cognitive function in alcoholics by computer: A controlled study. *Alcohol & Alcoholism, 19*, 223–233.

Barber, J.G. (1991). Microcomputers and prevention of drug abuse. *M.D. Computing, 8*, 150–155.

Barber, J.G. (1993). An application of microcomputer technology to the drug education of prisoners. *Journal of Alcohol & Drug Education, 38*, 14–22.

Bernadt, M.W., Daniels, O.J., Blizard, R.A., & Murray, R.M. (1989). Can a computer reliably elicit an alcohol history? *British Journal of Addiction, 84*, 405–411.

Bloch, J.E. (1993). Computer management in a substance abuse resource center. *Computers in Human Services, 9*, 163–175.

Bosworth, K., & Yoast, R. (1991). DIADS: Computer-based system for development of school drug prevention programs. *Journal of Drug Education, 21*, 231–245.

Chang, M.M., Gino, A., Yahiku, P.Y., King, C.A., MacMurray, J.P., Ferry, L.H., Smith, L., Young, R., & Bozzetti, L. (1988). The alcohol treatment unit computerized medical record (ATU CMR): A clinician-entered inpatient record. In R.A. Greenes (Ed.), *Proceedings of the Twelfth Annual Symposium on Computer Applications in Medical Care* (pp. 717–721). Washington, DC: Institute of Electrical & Electronics Engineers.

Davis, L.J., Hoffmann, N.G., Morse, R.M., & Luehr, J.G. (1992). Substance Use Disorder Diagnostic Schedule (SUDDS): The equivalence and validity of a computer-administered and interview-administered format. *Alcoholism, 16*, 250–254.

Davis, L.J., & Morse, R.M. (1991). Self-administered alcoholism screening test: A comparison of conventional versus computer-administered formats. *Alcoholism: Clinical & Experimental Research, 15*, 155–157.

Duffy, J.C., & Waterton, J.J. (1984). Under reporting of alcohol consumption in sample surveys: The effect of computer interviewing in field work. *British Journal of Addiction, 79*, 303–308.

Elias, M.J., Dalton, J.H., Cobb, C.W., Lavoie, L., & Zlotlow, S.F. (1979). The use of computerized management information systems in evaluation. *Administration in Mental Health, 7*, 148–161.

Ford, W.E., & Luckey, J.W. (1983). Planning alcoholism services: A technique for projecting specific service needs. *International Journal of the Addictions, 18*, 319–331.

Gordon, S.M., Kennedy, B.P., & McPenke, J.D. (1988). Neuropsychologically impaired alcoholics: Assessment, treatment considerations, and rehabilitation. *Journal of Substance Abuse Treatment, 5*, 99–104.

Hays, R.D., Hill, L., Gillogly, J.J., Lewis, M.W., & Bell, R.M. (in press). Response times for the CAGE, Short-MAST, AUDIT, and JELLINEK Alcohol Scales. *Behavior Research Methods, Instruments, & Computers.*

Lucus, R.W., Mullin, P.J., Luna, C.B., & McInroy, DC (1977). Psychiatrists and a computer as interrogators of patients with alcohol related illnesses: A comparison. *British Journal of Psychiatry, 131*, 160–167.

Kadden, R., & Wetstone, S. (1982). Teaching coping skills to alcoholics using computer based education. In B.I. Blum (Ed.), *Proceedings of the Sixth Annual Symposium on Computer Applications in Medical Care* (p. 635). New York: Institute of Electrical & Electronics Engineers.

Meier, S.T., & Sampson, J.P. (1989). Use of computer-assisted instruction in the prevention of alcohol abuse. *Journal of Drug Education, 19*, 245–256.

Meier, S.T., & Wick, M.T. (1991). Computer-based unobtrusive measurement: Potential supplements to reactive self-reports. *Professional Psychology: Research & Practice, 22*, 410–412.

Moncher, M.S., Parms, C.A., Orlandi, M.A., Schinke, S.P., Miller, S.O., Palleja, J., & Schinke, M.B. (1989). Microcomputer based approaches for preventing drug and alcohol abuse among adolescents from ethnic-racial minority backgrounds. *Computers in Human Behavior, 5*, 77–93.

Orlandi, M.A., Dozier, C.E., & Marta, M.A. (1991). Computer-assisted strategies for substance abuse prevention: Opportunities and barriers. *Journal of Consulting & Clinical Psychology, 58*, 425–431.

Parades, A. (1977). Management of alcoholism programs through a computerized information system. *Alcoholism, 1*, 305–309.

Rathbun, J. (1993). Development of a computerized alcohol screening instrument for the university community. *Journal of American College Health, 42*, 33–36.

Sells, S.B., & Simpson, D.D. (1979). Implications for evaluation of dependency treatment based on data provided by a management information system. *Addictive Diseases, 9*, 80–94.

Thomas, B.S. (1991). Computer-assisted decision making: A strategy for primary prevention of substance abuse. *Journal of Pediatric Health Care, 5*, 257–263.

Wood, W., & Youatt, R. (1979). A computer feedback system for clinical research. *Computer Programs in Biomedicine, 9*, 80–94.

Zalkind, D., Zelon, H., Moore, M., & Kaluzny, A. (1979). Planning for management information systems in drug treatment organizations. *International Journal of the Addictions, 14*, 183–196.

Mental Retardation & Developmental Disabilities

Browning, P., White, W.A.T., Nave, G., & Barkin, P.Z. (1986). Interactive video in the classroom: A field study. *Education & Training of the Mentally Retarded, 21*, 85–92.

Carey, D.M., & Sale, P. (1994). Practical considerations in the use of technology to facilitate the inclusion of students with severe disabilities. *Technology and Disability*, *3*, 77–86.

Chen, S.H.A., & Bernard–Opitz, V. (1993). Comparison of personal and computer-assisted instruction for children with autism. *Mental Retardation*, *31*, 368–376.

Crawford, J.L., Conklin, G.S., McMahon, D.J., Vitale, S.J., Robinson, J.A., Geller, J., & DiStefano, O.R. (1978). An automated behavioral rehabilitation system for long term patients. In F.H. Orthner (Ed.), *Proceedings of the Second Annual Symposium on Computer Applications in Medical Care* (pp. 198–205). New York: Institute of Electrical & Electronics Engineers.

Desrochers, M.N., & Hile, M.G. (1993). SIDDS: Simulations in developmental disabilities. *Behavior Research Methods, Instruments, & Computers*, *25*, 308–313.

Dura, J.R., Mulick, J.A., Hammer, D., & Myers, E.G. (1990). Establishing independent microcomputer use in people with multiple handicaps, profound mental retardation, and a history of learning failure. *Computers in Human Behavior*, *6*, 177–183.

Gardner, J.E., & Bates, P. (1991). Attitudes and attributions on use of microcomputers in schools by students who are mentally handicapped. *Education & Training in Mental Retardation*, *26*, 98–107.

Gardner, J.M., & Breuer, A. (1985). Micropsych: Applications in a residential facility for developmentally disabled persons. *Professional Psychology*, *16*, 889–897.

Gardner, J.M., & Breuer, A. (1985). Reliability and validity of a microcomputer assessment system for developmentally disabled persons. *Education & Training of the Mentally Retarded*, *20*, 209–213.

Gurthrie, D., Heighton, R., Keeran, C.V., & Payne, D. (1976). Data bases and the privacy rights of the mentally retarded: Report to the AAMD task force on data base confidentiality. *Mental Retardation*, *14*, 3–7.

Hannaford, A.E., & Taber, F.M. (1982). Microcomputer software for the handicapped: Development and evaluation. *Exceptional Children*, *49*, 137–142.

Hile, M.G., Campbell, D.M., Ghobary B.B., & Desrochers, M.N. (1993). Development of knowledge bases and the reliability of decision support for behavioral treatment consultation for persons with mental retardation: The Mental-Retardation Expert. *Behavior Research Methods, Instruments & Computers*, *25*, 195–198.

Huiatt, R.D. (1980). The Adaptive Behavior Scale as a generalized application system and its inter-relation with other MSIS modules. In J.A. Johnsen (Ed.), *Proceedings of the Fifth Annual MSIS National User's Group Conference* (pp. 49–55). Orangeburg, NY: Rockland Research Institute.

Kratochwill, T.R., Doll, E.J., & Dickson, W.P. (1991). Use of computer technology in behavioral assessments. In T.B. Gutkin & S.L. Wise (Eds.), *The computer and the decision-making process* (pp. 125–154). Hillsdale, NJ: Erlbaum.

Lancioni, G.E., Smeets, P.M., & Oliva, D. (1988). A computer aided program to supervise occupational engagement of severely mentally retarded persons. *Behavioral Residential Treatment*, *3*, 1–18.

Margalit, M., & Weisel, A. (1990). Computer-assisted social skills learning for adolescents with mild retardation and social difficulties. *Educational Psychology*, *10*, 343–354.

Parette, H.P. (1991). The importance of technology in the education and training of persons with mental retardation. *Education & Training in Mental Retardation*, *26*, 165–178.

Parette, H.P., & VanBiervliet, A. (1992). Tentative findings of a study of the technology needs and use patterns of persons with mental retardation. *Journal of Intellectual Disability Research*, *26*, 7–27.

Plienis, A.J., & Romanczyk, R.G. (1985). Analyses of performance, behavior, and predictors for severely disturbed children: A comparison of adult vs. computer instruction. *Analysis and Intervention in Developmental Disabilities*, *5*, 345–356.

Ragghianti, S., & Miller, R. (1982). The microcomputer and special education management. *Exceptional Children*, *49*, 131–135.

Realon, R.E., Favell, J.E., & McGimsey, J.F. (1992). Computer prompts to improve social interactions and data collection. *Mental Retardation*, *30*, 23–28.

Repp, A.C., Singh, N.N., Karsh, K.G., & Deitz, D.E. (1991). Ecobehavioural analysis of stereotypic and adaptive behaviours: Activities as setting events. *Journal of Mental Deficiency Research*, *35*, 413–429.

Schoech, D., Cavalier, A.R., Hoover, B., Kondraske, G., & Brown, C. (1993). Integrating technology into service delivery for persons with developmental disabilites: An interim report. In W. LaMendola, B. Glastonbury, & S. Toole (Eds.), *A casebook of computer applications in the social and human services* (pp. 299–313). New York: Haworth Press.

Talbot, F., Pepin, M., & Loranger, M. (1992). Computerized cognitive training with learning disabled students: A pilot study. *Psychological Reports*, *71*(Pt. 2), 1347–1356.

Diagnosis and Classification

Ames, D. (1992). Psychiatric diagnosis made by the AGECAT system in residents of local authority homes for the elderly: Outcome and diagnostic stability after four years. *International Journal of Geriatric Psychiatry*, *7*, 83–87.

Benfari, R.C., Leighton, A.H., Beiser, J., & Coen, K. (1972). CASE: Computer assigned symptom evaluation: An instrument for psychiatric epidemiological application. *Journal of Nervous & Mental Disease*, *154*, 115–124.

Carroll, B. (1987). Artificial intelligence: Expert systems for clinical diagnosis: Are they worth the effort? *Behavioral Science*, *32*, 274–292.

Chen, H.Y., Luo, H.C., & Phillips, M.R. (1992). Computerized psychiatric diagnoses based on Euclidean distances: A Chinese example. *Acta Psychiatrica Scandinavica*, *85*, 11–14.

Comings, D.E. (1984). A computerized diagnostic interview schedule (DIS) for psychiatric disorders. In M.D. Schwartz (Ed.), *Using computers in clinical practice: Psychotherapy and mental health applications* (pp. 195–203). New York: Haworth Press.

Copeland, J.R.M., Dewey, M.E., Henderson, A.S., Kay, D.W.K., Neal, C.D., Harrison, M.A.M., McWilliam, C., Forshaw, D., & Shiwach, R. (1988). The Geriatric Mental State (GMS) used in the community: Replication studies of the computerized diagnosis AGECAT. *Psychological Medicine*, *18*, 219–223.

Erdman, H.P., Greist, J.H., Klein, M.H., & Jefferson, J.W. (1987). A review of computer diagnosis in psychiatry with special emphasis on DSM-III. *Computers in Human Services*, *2*, 1–11.

Erdman, H.P., Klein, M.H., Greist, J.H., Bass, S.M., Bires, J.K., & Machtinger, P.E. (1987). A comparison of the diagnostic interview schedule and clinical diagnosis. *American Journal of Psychiatry*, *144*, 1477–1480.

Farmer, A.E., Jenkins, P.L., Katz, R., & Ryder, L. (1991). Comparison of CATEGO-derived ICD-8 and DSM-III classifications using the Composite International Diagnostic Interview in severely ill subjects. *British Journal of Psychiatry*, *158*, 177–182.

First, M.B., Oplar, L.A., Hamilton, R.M., Linfield, L.S., Silver, J.M., Toshav, N.L., Kahn, D., Williams, J.B. W., & Spitzer, R.L. (1993). Evaluation in an inpatient setting of DTREE, a computer-assisted diagnostic assessment procedure. *Comprehensive Psychiatry*, *34*, 171–175.

Fleiss, J.L., Spitzer, R.L., Cohen, J., & Endicott, J. (1972). Three computer diagnosis methods compared. *Archives of General Psychiatry*, *27*, 643–649.

Glutting, J.J. (1986). The McDermott Multidimensional Assessment of Children: Applications to the classification of childhood exceptionality. *Journal of Learning Disabilities*, *19*, 331–335.

Greist, J.H., Klein, M.H., & Erdman, H.P. (1976). Routine on-line psychiatric diagnosis by computer. *American Journal of Psychiatry*, *133*, 1405–1408.

Greist, J.H., Mathisen, K.S., Klein, M.H., Benjamin, L.S., Erdman, H.P., & Evans, F.J. (1984). Psychiatric diagnosis: What role for the computer? *Hospital & Community Psychiatry*, *35*, 1089, 1090, 1093.

Hale, R.L., & Glassman, S.S. (1986). Using computers to construct, evaluate, and apply actuarial systems of classification: A methodology and example. *Computers in Human Behavior*, *2*, 195–213.

Hedlund, J.L., & Vieweg, B.W. (1987). Computer generated diagnosis. In C.G. Last & M. Hersen (Eds.), *Issues in diagnostic research* (pp. 241–269). New York: Plenum.

Hirschfeld, R., Spitzer, R.L., & Miller, R.G. (1974). Computer diagnosis in psychiatry: A Bayes approach. *Journal of Nervous & Mental Disease*, *158*, 399–407.

Johnson, J.H., Klingler, D.E., Giannetti, R.A., & Williams, T.A. (1977). The reliability of diagnoses by technician, computer and algorithm. *Journal of Clinical Psychology*, *36*, 447–451.

Mathisen, K.S., Evans, F.J., & Myers, K. (1987). Evaluation of a computerized version of the diagnostic interview schedule. *Hospital & Community Psychiatry*, *38*, 1311–1315.

McDermott, P.A., & Hale, R.L. (1982). Validation of a systems-actuarial computer process for multidimensional classification of child psychopathology. *Journal of Clinical Psychology*, *38*, 477–486.

Melrose, J.P., Stroebel, C.F., & Glueck, B.C. (1970). Diagnosis of psychopathology using stepwise multiple discriminant analysis. *Comprehensive Psychiatry*, *11*, 43–50.

Moreno, H.R., & Plant, R.T. (1993). A prototype decision support system for differential diagnosis of psychotic mood and organic mental disorders. *Medical Decision Making*, *13*, 43–48.

Mulsant, B.H. (1990). A neural network as an approach to clinical diagnosis. *M.D. Computing*, *7*, 25–36.

Murphy, J.M., Neff, R.K., Sobol, A.M., Rice, J.X., & Olivier, DC (1985). Computer diagnosis of depression and anxiety: The Stirling County study. *Psychological Medicine*, *15*, 99–112.

Nurius, P.S., & Hudson, W.W. (1989). Computers and social diagnosis: The client's perspective. *Computers in Human Services*, *5*, 21–35.

Overall, J.E., & Higgins, C.W. (1977). An application of actuarial methods in psychiatric diagnosis. *Journal of Clinical Psychology*, *33*, 973–980.

Overall, J.E., & Hollister, L.E. (1964). Computer procedures for psychiatric classification. *Journal of the American Medical Association*, *187*, 583–588.

Schmid, W., Bronish, T., & Von Zerssen, D. (1982). A comparative study of PSE/CATEGO and DiaSiKa: Two psychiatric diagnostic systems. *British Journal of Psychiatry*, *141*, 292–295.

Sletten, I.W., Ulett, G.A., Altman, H., & Sundland, D. (1970). The Missouri Standard System of Psychiatry (SSOP): Computer generated diagnoses. *Archives of General Psychiatry*, *23*, 73–79.

Spitzer, R.L., & Endicott, J. (1968). DIAGNO: A computer program for psychiatric diagnosis utilizing the differential diagnostic procedure. *Archives of General Psychiatry*, *18*, 746–756.

Spitzer, R.L., & Endicott, J. (1969). DIAGNO II: Further developments in a computer program for psychiatric diagnosis. *American Journal of Psychiatry*, *125*(Suppl.), 12–21.

Spitzer, R.L., & Endicott, J. (1974). Computer diagnosis in automated record-keeping systems: A study of clinical acceptability. In J.L. Crawford, D.W. Morgan, & D.T. Gianturco (Eds.), *Progress in mental health information systems: Computer applications* (pp. 73–105). Cambridge, MA: Ballinger.

Spitzer, R.L., Endicott, J., Cohen, J., & Fleiss, J.L. (1974). Constraints on the validity of computer diagnosis. *Archives of General Psychiatry*, *31*, 197–203.

Stein, S.J. (1987). Computer-assisted diagnosis for children and adolescents. In J.N. Butcher (Ed.), *Computerized psychological assessment: A practitioners guide* (pp. 145–158). New York: Basic Books.

Strauss, J.S., Bartko, J.J., & Carpenter, W.T. (1973). The use of clustering techniques for the classification of psychiatric patients. *British Journal of Psychiatry*, *122*, 531–540.

Strauss, J.S., Gabriel, K.R., Kokes, R.F., Ritzler, B.A., Van Ord, A., & Tarana, E. (1979). Do psychiatric patients fit their diagnoses? Patterns of symptomatology as described with the biplot. *Journal of Nervous & Mental Disease*, *167*, 105–113.

Stroebel, C.F., & Glueck, B.C. (1972). The diagnostic process in psychiatry: Computer approaches. *Psychiatric Annals*, *2*, 58–77.

Turrina, C., Siciliani, O., Dewey, M.E., Fazzari, G.C., & Copeland, J.R.M. (1992). Psychiatric disorders among elderly patients attending a geriatric medical day hospital: Prevalence according to clinical diagnosis (DSM-III-R) and AGECAT. *International Journal of Geriatric Psychiatry*, *7*, 499–504.

van den Brink, W., Koeter, M.W., Ormel, J., Dijkstra, W., Giel, R., Gloof, C.J., & Wohlfarth, T.D. (1989). Psychiatric diagnosis in an outpatient population: A comparative study of PSE-CATEGO and DSM-III. *Archives of General Psychiatry*, *46*, 369–372.

Wing, J.K. (1985, May). *New developments after twenty-five years of the PSE.* Paper presented in the Symposium on New Diagnostic Interviews, American Psychiatric Association Annual Meeting, Dallas, TX.

Wing, J.K., Cooper, J.E., & Sartorius, N. (1974). *Measurement and classification of psychiatric symptoms: An instruction manual for the PSE and CATEGO systems.* London: Cambridge University Press.

Wittchen, H. (1993). Computer scoring of CIDI diagnoses. *International Journal of Methods in Psychiatric Research, 3,* 101–107.

Wyndowe, J. (1987). The microcomputerized Diagnostic Interview Schedule: Clinical use in an outpatient setting. *Canadian Journal of Psychiatry, 32,* 93–99.

Yokley, J.M., & Reuter, J.M. (1989). The computer-assisted child diagnostic system: A research and development tool. *Computers in Human Behavior, 5,* 277–295.

Zetin, M., Warren, S., Lanssens, E., & Tominaga, D. (1987). Computerized psychiatric diagnostic interview. In W.W. Stead (Ed.), *Proceedings of the Eleventh Annual Symposium on Computer Applications in Medical Care* (pp. 292–298). Los Angeles: Institute of Electrical & Electronics Engineers.

Mental Status

Hinkle, J.S. (1992). The mental status examination via computer: An evaluation of the Mental Status Checklist computer report. *Measurement & Evaluation in Counseling & Development, 24,* 188–189.

Hyler, S.E., & Bujold, A.E. (1994). Computers and psychiatric education: The "Taxi Driver" mental status examination. *Psychiatric Annals, 24,* 13–19.

Jones, J.R., & McWilliam, C. (1989). The Geriatric Mental State Schedule administered with the aid of a microcomputer: A pilot study. *International Journal of Geriatric Psychiatry, 4,* 215–219.

Slaughter, J.R., Hesse, B.W., & Turner, C.W. (1988). Computerized mental status testing in the elderly. In R.A. Greenes (Ed.), *Proceedings of the Twelfth Annual Symposium on Computer Applications in Medical Care* (pp. 58–62). Washington, DC: Institute of Electrical & Electronics Engineers.

Sletten, I.W., Ernhart, C.B., & Ulett, G.A. (1970). The Missouri automated mental status examination: Development, use and reliability. *Comprehensive Psychiatry, 11,* 315–327.

Spitzer, R.L., & Endicott, J. (1971). An integrated group of forms for automated case records: A progress report. *Archives of General Psychiatry, 24,* 540–547.

Weitzel, W.D., Morgan, D.W., Guyden, T.E., & Robinson, J.A. (1973). Toward a more efficient mental status examination: Free-form or operationally defined. *Archives of General Psychiatry, 28,* 215–218.

Zheng, Y., Yang, W., Phillips, M.R., Dai, C., & Zheng, H. (1988). Reliability and validity of a Chinese computerized diagnostic instrument. *Acta Psychiatrica Scandinavica, 77,* 81–88.

Automated Nursing Notes

Evenson, R.C., & Cho, D.W. (1987). The Missouri Inpatient Behavior Scale. *Journal of Clinical Psychology, 43,* 100–110.

Evenson, R.C., & Cho, D.W. (1987). Norms for the Missouri Inpatient Behavior Scale: Sex, race and age differences in psychiatric symptoms. *Psychological Reports*, *60*, 803–807.

Glueck, B.C., Gullotta, G.P., & Ericson, R.P. (1980). Automation of behavior assessments: The computer produced nursing note. In J.B. Sidowski, J.H. Johnson, & T.A. Williams (Eds.), *Technology in mental health care delivery systems* (pp. 183–197). Norwood, NJ: Ablex.

Morgan, D.W., Crawford, J.L., & Frenkel, S.I. (1973). An automated patient behavior checklist. *Journal of Applied Psychology*, *58*, 393–396.

Stein, R.F. (1969). An exploratory study in the development and use of automated nursing reports. *Nursing Research*, *18*, 14–21.

Willer, B., & Stasiak, E. (1973). Automated nursing notes in a psychiatric institution. *Journal of Psychiatric Nursing*, *11*, 27–29.

Psychological Testing

Acker, W. (1981). A microcomputer administered neuropsychological assessment system for use with chronic alcoholics. *Substance & Alcohol Actions/Misuse*, *1*, 545–550.

Acker, W. (1983). A computerized approach to psychological screening: The Bexley–Maudsley Automated Screening and The Bexley–Maudsley Category Sorting Test. *International Journal of Man–Machine Studies*, *18*, 361–369.

Adams, K.M., & Heaton, R.K. (1987). Computerized neuropsychological assessment: Issues and applications. In J.N. Butcher (Ed.), *Computerized psychological assessment: A practitioners guide* (pp. 355–365). New York: Basic Books.

Aiken, L.R. (1991). Sixteen computerized perceptual performance tests for psychological assessment courses. *Educational & Psychological Measurement*, *51*, 649–653.

American Psychological Association. (1987). Appendix B: American Psychological Association guidelines for computer-based tests and interpretations. In J.N. Butcher (Ed.), *Computerized psychological assessment: A practitioners guide* (pp. 413–431). New York: Basic Books.

Anthony, W.Z., Heaton, R.K., & Lehman, R.A. (1980). An attempt to cross validate two actuarial systems for neuropsychological test interpretation. *Journal of Consulting & Clinical Psychology*, *48*, 317–326.

Bartram, D., Beaumont, J.G., Cornford, T., Dann, P.L., & Wilson, S.L. (1987). Recommendations for the design of software for computer based assessment. *Bulletin of the British Psychological Society*, *40*, 86–87.

Beaumont, J.G. (1982). System requirements for interactive testing. *International Journal of Man–Machine Studies*, *17*, 311–320.

Beaumont, J.G. (1985). The effect of microcomputer presentation and response medium on digit span performance. *International Journal of Man–Machine Studies*, *22*, 11–18.

Beaumont, J.G. (1985). Speed of response using keyboard and screen-based microcomputer response media. *International Journal of Man–Machine Studies*, *23*, 61–70.

Beaumont, J.G., & French, C.C. (1987). A clinical field study of eight automated psychometric procedures: The Leicester/DHHS project. *International Journal of Man–Machine Studies*, 26, 661–682.

Ben–Porath, Y.S., & Butcher, J.N. (1986). Computers in personality assessment: A brief past, an ebullient present, and an expanding future. *Computers in Human Behavior*, 2, 167–182.

Bersoff, D.N., & Hofer, P.J. (1991). Legal issues in computerized psychological testing. In T.B. Gutkin & S.L. Wise (Eds.), *The computer and the decision-making process* (pp. 225–243). Hillsdale, NJ: Earlbaum.

Burke, M.J., & Normand, J. (1987). Computerized psychological testing: Overview and critique. *Professional Psychology: Research and Practice*, 18, 42–51.

Butcher, J.N. (1987). *Computerized psychological assessment: A practitioners guide*. New York: Basic Books.

Butcher, J.N. (1987). The use of computers in psychological assessment: An overview of practices and issues. In J.N. Butcher (Ed.), *Computerized psychological assessment: A practitioners guide* (pp. 3–25). New York: Basic Books.

Butcher, J.N. (1987). Computerized clinical and personality assessment using the MMPI. In J.N. Butcher (Ed.), *Computerized psychological assessment: A practitioners guide* (pp. 161–167). New York: Basic Books.

Butcher, J.N. (1994). Psychological assessment by computer: Potential gains and problems to avoid. *Psychiatric Annals*, 24, 20–24.

Butcher, J.N., Keller, L.S., & Bacon, S.F. (1985). Current developments and future directions in computerized personality assessment. *Journal of Consulting & Clinical Psychology*, 53, 803–815.

Cavanaugh, J.L., Rogers, R., & Wasyliw, O.E. (1982). A computerized assessment program for forensic science evaluations: A preliminary report. *Journal of Forensic Sciences*, 27, 113–118.

Conoley, C.W., Plake, B.S., & Kemmerer, B.E. (1991). Issues in computer-based test interpretative systems. *Computers in Human Behavior*, 7, 97–101.

Crook, T.H., & Larrabee, G.J. (1988). Interrelationships among everyday memory tests: Stability of factor structure with age. *Neuropsychology*, 2, 1–12.

Crook, T.H., Youngjohn, J.R., & Larrabee, G.J. (1992). Multiple equivalent test forms in a computerized, everyday memory battery. *Archives of Clinical Neuropsychology*, 7, 221–232.

Davis, C., & Cowles, M. (1989). Automated psychological testing: Methods of administration, need for approval, and measures of anxiety. *Educational & Psychological Measurement*, 49, 311–320.

Elithorn, A., Mornington, S., & Stavrou, A. (1982). Automated psychological testing: Some principles and practice. *International Journal of Man–Machine Studies*, 17, 247–263.

Elwood, D.L., & Clark, C.L. (1978). Computer administration of the Peabody Picture Vocabulary Test (PPVT). *Behavior Research Methods & Instrumentation*, 10, 43–46.

Elwood, D.L., & Griffin, H.R. (1972). Individual intelligence testing without the examiner: Reliability of an automated method. *Journal of Consulting & Clinical Psychology*, 38, 9–14.

Exner, J.E. (1987). Computer assistance in Rorschach interpretation. In J.N. Butcher (Ed.), *Computerized psychological assessment: A practitioners guide* (pp. 218–235). New York: Basic Books.

Eyde, L.D., & Kowal, D.M. (1987). Computerised test interpretation services: Ethical and professional concerns regarding U.S. producers and users. *Applied Psychology: An International Review, 36,* 401–417.

Eyde, L.D., Kowal, D.M., & Fishburne, F.J. (1991). The validity of computer-based interpretations of the MMPI. In T.B. Gutkin & S.L. Wise (Eds.), *The computer and the decision-making process* (pp. 75–123). Hillsdale, NJ: Erlbaum.

Farrell, A.D. (1989). Impact of standards for computer-based tests on practice: Consequences of the information gap. *Computers in Human Behavior, 5,* 1–12.

Fowler, R.D. (1980). The automated MMPI. In J.B. Sidowski, J.H. Johnson, & T.A. Williams (Eds.), *Technology in mental health care delivery systems* (pp. 69–84). Norwood, NJ: Ablex.

Fowler, R.D. (1985). Landmarks in computer-assisted psychological assessment. *Journal of Consulting & Clinical Psychology, 53,* 748–759.

Fowler, R.D. (1987). Developing a computer-based test interpretation system. In J.N. Butcher (Ed.), *Computerized psychological assessment: A practitioners guide* (pp. 50–63). New York: Basic Books.

Fowler, R.D., & Butcher, J.N. (1986). Critique of Matarazzo's views on computerized testing: All sigma and no meaning. *American Psychologist, 41,* 94–96.

Goldberg, J.B. (1966). Computer analysis of sentence completions. *Journal of Personality Assessment, 30,* 37–45.

Golden, C.J. (1987). Computers in neuropsychology. In J.N. Butcher (Ed.), *Computerized psychological assessment: A practitioners guide* (pp. 344–354). New York: Basic Books.

Goldstein, G., Tarter, R.E., Shelly, C., & Hegedus, A. (1983). The Pittsburgh Initial Neuropsychological Testing System (PINTS): A neuropsychological screening battery for psychiatric patients. *Journal of Behavioral Assessment, 5,* 227–238.

Green, C.J. (1982). The diagnostic accuracy and utility of MMPI and MCMI computer interpretive reports. *Journal of Personality Assessment, 46,* 359–365.

Gutkin, T.B., & Wise, S.L. (Eds). *The computer and the decision making process.* Hillsdale, NJ: Erlbaum.

Gynther, M.D., Altman, H., & Sletten, I.W. (1973). Replicated correlates of MMPI two-point code types: The Missouri actuarial system [Monograph]. *Journal of Clinical Psychology, 29,* 263–289.

Hammond, K.W., & Gottfredson, D.K. (1984). The VA mental health information package: Version 1. *Computer Use in Social Services Network, 4,* 6–7.

Hansen, J.I.C. (1987). Computer-assisted interpretation of the Strong Interest Inventory. In J.N. Butcher (Ed.), *Computerized psychological assessment: A practitioners guide* (pp. 292–325). New York: Basic Books.

Harrell, T.H., & Lombardo, T.A. (1984). Validation of an automated 16PF administrative procedure. *Journal of Personality Assessment, 48,* 638–642.

Harris, W.G., Niedner, D., Feldman, C., Fink, A., & Johnson, J.H. (1981). An on-line interpretive Rorschach approach: Using Exner's comprehensive system. *Behavior Research Methods & Instrumentation, 13,* 588–591.

Hart, R.R., & Goldstein, M.A. (1985). Computer-assisted psychological assessment. *Computers in Human Services, 1,* 69–75.

Heaton, R.K., & Adams, K.M. (1987). Potential versus current reality of automation in neuropsychology: Reply to Kleinmuntz. *Journal of Consulting & Clinical Psychology, 55,* 268–269.

Heaton, R.K., Grant, I., Anthony, W.Z., & Lehman, R.A. (1981). A comparison of clinical and automated interpretation of the Halstead–Reitan Battery. *Journal of Clinical Neuropsychology*, *3*, 121–141.

Hedlund, J.L., & Vieweg, B.W. (1988). Automation in psychological testing. Psychiatric Annals, 18(4), 217–227.

Hofer, P.J. (1985). Developing standards for computerized psychological testing. *Computers in Human Behavior*, *1*, 301–315.

Hofer, P.J., & Green, B.F. (1985). The challenge of competence and creativity in computerized psychological testing. *Journal of Consulting & Clinical Psychology*, *53*, 826–838.

Holden, R.R., Fekken, G.C., & Cotton, D.H.G. (1990). Clinical reliabilities and validities of the microcomputerized Basic Personality Inventory. *Journal of Clinical Psychology*, *46*, 845–849.

Honaker, L.M. (1988). The equivalency of computerized and conventional MMPI administration: A critical review. *Clinical Psychology Review*, *8*, 561–577.

Hopwood, J.H., Wei, K.H., & Yellin, A.M. (1981). A computerized method for generating the Rorschach's structural summary from the sequence of scores. *Journal of Personality Assessment*, *45*, 116–117.

Hunt, E., & Pellegrino, J. (1985). Using interactive computing to expand intelligence testing: A critique and prospectus. *Intelligence*, *9*, 207–236.

Jackson, D.N. (1985). Computer-based personality testing. *Computers in Human Behavior*, *1*, 255–264.

Jacob, S., & Brantley, J.C. (1989). Ethics and computer-assisted assessment: Three case studies. *Psychology in the Schools*, *26*, 163–167.

Johnson, J.H., Giannetti, R.A., & Williams, T.A. (1979). Psychological Systems Questionnaire: An objective personality test designed for on-line computer presentation, scoring, and interpretation. *Behavior Research Methods & Instrumentation*, *11*, 257–260.

Johnson, J.H., & Williams, T.A. (1975). The use of on-line computer technology in a mental health admitting system. *American Psychologist*, *30*, 388–390.

Jones, D., & Stavrou, A. (1988). Computer automated psychological assessment of cognitive abilities. *New Technology in the Human Services*, *4*, 26–29.

Kahn, M.W., Fox, H., & Rhode, R. (1988). Detecting faking on the Rorschach: Computer versus expert clinical judgment. *Journal of Personality Assessment*, *52*, 516–523.

Karson, S., & O'Dell, J.W. (1987). Computer-based interpretation of the 16PF: The Karson clinical report in contemporary practice. In J.N. Butcher (Ed.), *Computerized psychological assessment: A practitioners guide* (pp. 198–217). New York: Basic Books.

Klee, S.H., & Garfinkel, B.D. (1983). The computerized continuous performance task: A new measure of inattention. *Journal of Abnormal Child Psychology*, *11*, 487–496.

Kramer, J.J. (1986). Epilogue: Why no standards for computer-based testing and test interpretation? *Computers in Human Behavior*, *1*, 317–320.

Kratochwill, T.R., Doll, E.J., & Dickson, W.P. (1985). Microcomputers in behavioral assessment: Recent advances and remaining issues. *Computers in Human Behavior*, *1*, 277–291.

Krug, S.E. (1993). *PSYCHWARE SOURCEBOOK: A reference guide to computer based products for assessment in psychology, education and business (4th ed.)*. Champaign, IL: Metritech.

LaBeck, L.J., Johnson, J.H., & Harris, W.G. (1983). Validity of a computerized on-line MMPI interpretive system. *Journal of Clinical Psychology, 39*, 412–416.

Lachar, D. (1974). *The MMPI: Clinical assessment and automated interpretation.* Los Angeles: Western Psychological Services.

Lachar, D. (1987). Automated assessment of child and adolescent personality. The Personality Inventory for Children (PIC). In J.N. Butcher (Ed.), *Computerized psychological assessment: A practitioners guide* (pp. 261–291). New York: Basic Books.

Lanyon, R.I. (1987). The validity of computer-based personality assessment products: Recommendations for the future. *Computers in Human Behavior, 3*, 225–238.

Lanyon, R.I., & Goodstein, L.D. (1982). Automated personality assessment. In R.I. Lanyon & L.D. Goodstein (Eds.), *Personality assessment* (pp. 219–237). New York: Wiley.

Larrabee, G.J., & Crook, T.H. (1988). A computerized everyday memory battery for assessing treatment effects. *Psychopharmacology Bulletin, 24*, 695–697.

Levy, A.J., & Barowsky, E.I. (1986). Comparison of computer-administered Harris–Goodenough Draw-a-Man Test with standard paper-and-pencil administration. *Perceptual & Motor Skills, 63*, 395–398.

Lockshin, S.B., & Harrison, K. (1993). Computer-assisted assessment of psychological problems. In A. Ager & S. Bendall (Eds.), *Microcomputers and clinical psychology: Issues, applications and future developments* (pp. 47–63). Chichester, UK: Wiley.

Lushene, R.E. (1981). Development of a psychological assessment system. In H.J. Heffernan (Ed.), *Proceedings of the Fifth Annual Symposium on Computer Applications in Medical Care* (pp. 422–425). New York: Institute of Electrical & Electronics Engineers.

Lynch, W. (1988). Computers in neuropsychological assessment. *Journal of Head Trauma Rehabilitation, 3*, 92–94.

Martin, T.A., & Wilcox, K.L. (1989). HyperCard administration of a block-design task. *Behavior Research Methods, Instruments, & Computers, 21*, 312–315.

Matarazzo, J.D. (1983). Computerized psychological testing [Editorial]. *Science, 221*, 323.

Matarazzo, J.D. (1985). Clinical psychological test interpretations by computer: Hardware outpaces software. *Computers in Human Behavior, 1*, 235–253.

Matarazzo, J.D. (1986). Computerized clinical psychological test interpretations. *American Psychologist, 41*, 14–24.

Matarazzo, J.D. (1986). Response to Fowler and Butcher on Matarazzo. *American Psychologist, 41*, 96.

Matarazzo, J.D. (1992). Psychological testing and assessment in the 21st century. *American Psychologist, 47*, 1007–1018.

McCullough, C.S. (1991). Evaluating the validity of multidimensional computer-based test interpretation programs. *Journal of School Psychology, 29*, 279–292.

Meier, S.T., & Wick, M.T. (1991). Computer-based unobtrusive measurement: Potential supplements to reactive self-reports. *Professional Psychology: Research & Practice, 22*, 410–412.

Merrell, K.W. (1985). Computer use in psychometric assessment: Evaluating benefits and potential problems. *Computers in Human Services, 1*, 59–67.

Moreland, K.L. (1985). Validation of computer-based test interpretations: Problems and prospects. *Journal of Consulting & Clinical Psychology*, *53*, 816–825.

Moreland, K.L. (1987). Computerized psychological assessment: What's available. In J.N. Butcher (Ed.), *Computerized psychological assessment: A practitioners guide* (pp. 26–49). New York: Basic Books.

Moreland, K.L., & Onstad, J.A. (1987). Validity of Millon's computerized interpretation system for the MCMI: A controlled study. *Journal of Consulting & Clinical Psychology*, *55*, 113–114.

Piotrowski, Z.A. (1980). CPR: The psychological X-Ray in mental disorders. In J.B. Sidowski, J.H. Johnson, & T.A. Williams (Eds.), *Technology in mental health care delivery systems* (pp. 85–108). Norwood, NJ: Ablex.

Roid, G.H. (1985). Computer-based test interpretation: The potential of quantitative methods of test interpretation. *Computers in Human Behavior*, *1*, 207–219.

Roper, B.L., Ben–Porath, Y.S., & Butcher, J. N. (1991). Comparability of computerized adaptive and conventional testing with the MMPI-2. *Journal of Personality Assessment*, *57*, 278–290.

Sampson, J.P. (1983). Computer-assisted testing and assessment: Current status and implications for the future. *Measurement & Evaluation in Guidance*, *15*, 293–299.

Samuels, R.M., & Herman, K. (1982). Microcomputers in clinical practice. In P.A. Keller & L.G. Ritt (Eds.), *Innovations in clinical practice: A source book* (Vol. 1). Sarasota, FL: Professional Resource Exchange, Inc.

Sanders, R.L. (1985). Computer-administered individualized psychological testing: A feasibility study. *International Journal of Man–Machine Studies*, *23*, 197–213.

Schoenfeldt, L.F. (1989). Guidelines for computer-based tests and interpretations. *Computers in Human Behavior*, *5*, 13–21.

Skinner, H.A., & Pakula, A. (1986). Challenge of computers in psychological assessment. *Professional Psychology: Research & Practice*, *17*, 44–50.

Swenson, W.M. (1985). The development of automated personality assessment in medical practice. *Psychiatric Annals*, *15*, 549–553.

Thompson, J.A., & Wilson, S.L. (1982). Automated psychological testing. *International Journal of Man–Machine Studies*, *17*, 279–289.

Vale, C.D. (1981). Design and implementation of a microcomputer based adaptive testing system. *Behavior Research Methods & Instrumentation*, *13*, 399–406.

Vale, C.D., & Keller, L.S. (1987). Developing expert computer systems to interpret psychological tests. In J.N. Butcher (Ed.), *Computerized psychological assessment: A practitioners guide* (pp. 64–83). New York: Basic Books.

Veldman, D.J., Menaker, S.L., & Peck, R.F. (1969). Computer scoring of sentence completion data. *Behavioral Science*, *14*, 501–507.

Watson, C.G., Thomas, D., & Anderson, P.E.D. (1992). Do computer-administered Minnesota Multiphasic Personality Inventories underestimate booklet-based scores? *Journal of Clinical Psychology*, *48*, 744–748.

Watts, K., Baddeley, A., & Williams, M. (1982). Automated tailored testing using Raven's Matrices and the Mill Hill Vocabulary Tests: A comparison with manual administration. *International Journal of Man–Machine Studies*, *17*, 331–334.

Weiss, D.J., & Vale, C.D. (1987). Computerized adaptive testing for measuring abilities and other psychological variables. In J.N. Butcher (Ed.), *Computerized psychological assessment: A practitioners guide* (pp. 325–343). New York: Basic Books.

White, D.M., Clements, C.B., & Fowler, R.D. (1985). A comparison of computer administration with standard administration of the MMPI. *Computers in Human Behavior, 1,* 153–162.

Wilson, S.L., Thompson, J.A., & Wylie, G. (1982). Automated psychological testing for the severely physically handicapped. *International Journal of Man–Machine Studies, 17,* 291–296.

Wylie, G.A., Wilson, S.L., & Wedgwood, J. (1984). The use of microcomputers in psychological assessment of physically disabled adults. *Journal of Medical Engineering & Technology, 8,* 224–229.

Yokley, J.M., Coleman, D.J., & Yates, B.T. (1990). Cost effectiveness of three child mental health assessment methods: Computer assisted assessment is effective and inexpensive. *Journal of Mental Health Administration, 17,* 99–107.

Zachary, R.A., & Pope, K.S. (1984). Legal and ethical issues in the clinical use of computerized testing. In M.D. Schwartz (Ed.), *Using computers in clinical practice: Psychotherapy and mental health applications* (pp. 151–164). New York: Haworth Press.

Interviewing

Allen, B., & Skinner, H.A. (1987). Lifestyle assessment using microcomputers. In J.N. Butcher (Ed.), *Computerized psychological assessment: A practitioners guide* (pp. 108–123). New York: Basic Books.

Ancill, R.J., Rogers, D., & Carr, A.C. (1985). Comparison of computerised self-rating scales for depression with conventional observer ratings. *Acta Psychiatrica Scandinavica, 71,* 315–317.

Angle, H.V., Ellinwood, E.H., & Carroll, J. (1978). Computer interview problem assessment of psychiatric patients. In F.H. Orthner (Ed.), *Proceedings of the Second Annual Symposium on Computer Applications in Medical Care* (pp. 137–148). New York: Institute of Electrical & Electronics Engineers.

Blouin, A.G., Perez, E.L., & Blouin, J.H. (1988). Computerized administration of the Diagnostic Interview Schedule. *Psychiatry Research, 23,* 335–344.

Bucholz, K.K., Robins, L.N., Shayka, J.J., Przybeck, T.R., Helzer, J.E., Goldring, E., Klein, M.H., Greist, J.H., Erdman, H.P., & Skare, S.S. (1991). Performance of two forms of a computer psychiatric screening interview: Version I of the DISSI. *Journal of Psychiatric Research, 25,* 117–129.

Canoune, H.L., & Leyhe, E.W. (1985). Human versus computer interviewing and psychotic subjects. *Journal of Personality Assessment, 49,* 103–106.

Carr, A.C., Ancill, R.J., Ghosh, A., & Margo, A. (1981). Direct assessment of depression by microcomputer. *Acta Psychiatrica Scandinavica, 64,* 415–422.

Carr, A.C., & Ghosh, A. (1983). Response of phobic patients to direct computer assessment. *British Journal of Psychiatry, 142,* 60–65.

Carr, A.C., & Ghosh, A. (1983). Accuracy of behavioural assessment by computer. *British Journal of Psychiatry, 142,* 66–70.

Erdman, H.P., Klein, M.H., & Greist, J.H. (1985). Direct patient computer interviewing. *Journal of Consulting & Clinical Psychology, 53,* 760–773.

Farrell, A.D., Camplair, P.S., & McCullough, L. (1987). Identification of target complaints by computer interview: Evaluation of the Computerized Assessment System for Psychotherapy Evaluation and Research. *Journal of Consulting & Clinical Psychology*, 55, 691–700.

Ferriter, M. (1993). Computer-aided interviewing in social work. *Computers in Human Services*, 9, 59–66.

Fowler, D.R., Finkelstein, A., Penk, W., Bell, W., & Itzig, B. (1987). An automated problem-rating interview: The DPRI. In J.N. Butcher (Ed.), *Computerized psychological assessment: A practitioners guide* (pp. 87–107). New York: Basic Books.

Giannetti, R.A. (1987). The GOLPH psychosocial history: Response-contingent data acquisition and reporting. In J.N. Butcher (Ed.), *Computerized psychological assessment: A practitioners guide* (pp. 124–144). New York: Basic Books.

Gonzalez, G.M. (1993). Computerized speech recognition in psychological assessment: A Macintosh prototype for screening depressive symptoms. *Behavior Research Methods, Instruments, & Computers*, 25, 301–303.

Greist, J.H., & Klein, M.H. (1980). Computer programs for patients, clinicians, and researchers. In J.B. Sidowski, J.H. Johnson, & T.A. Williams (Eds.), *Technology in mental health care delivery systems* (pp. 161–181). Norwood, NJ: Ablex.

Greist, J.H., Klein, M.H., & Van Cura, L.J. (1973). A computer interview for psychiatric patient target symptoms. *Archives of General Psychiatry*, 29, 247–253.

Johnson, J.H., & Williams, T.A. (1980). Using on-line computer technology to improve service response and decision-making effectiveness in a mental health admitting system. In J.B. Sidowski, J.H. Johnson, & T.A. Williams (Eds.), *Technology in mental health care delivery systems* (pp. 237–249). Norwood, NJ: Ablex.

Jones, J.R., & McWilliam, C. (1989). The Geriatric Mental State Schedule administered with the aid of a microcomputer: A pilot study. *International Journal of Geriatric Psychiatry*, 4, 215–219.

Levitan, R.D., Blouin, A.G., Nevarro, J.R., & Hill, J. (1991). Validity of the computerized DIS for diagnosing psychiatric inpatients. *Canadian Journal of Psychiatry*, 36, 728–731.

Lewis, G., Pelosi, A.J., Glover, E., Wilkinson, G., Stansfeld, S.A., Williams, P., & Shepherd, M. (1988). The development of a computerized assessment for minor psychiatric disorder. *Psychological Medicine*, 18, 737–745.

Mathisen, K.S., Evans, F.J., Meyers, K., & Kogan, L. (1985). Human factors influencing patient–computer interaction. *Computers in Human Behavior*, 1, 163–170.

McCullough, L., Farrell, A.D., & Longabaugh, R. (1986). The development of a microcomputer-based mental health information system. *American Psychologist*, 41, 207–214.

Nurius, P.S., & Hudson, W.W. (1988). Computer-based practice: Future dream or current technology. *Social Work*, 33, 357–362.

Parks, B.T., Mead, D.E., & Johnson, B.L. (1985). Validation of a computer administered marital adjustment test. *Journal of Marital & Family Therapy*, 11, 207–210.

Rogers, R.L., & Meyer, J.S. (1988). Computerized history and self-assessment questionnaire for diagnostic screening among patients with dementia. *Journal of the American Geriatrics Society*, *36*, 13–21.

Sawyer, M.G., Sarris, A., & Baghurst, P. (1991). The use of a computer-assisted interview to administer the Child Behavior Checklist in a child psychiatry service. *Journal of the American Academy of Child & Adolescent Psychiatry*, *30*, 674–681.

Sawyer, M.G., Sarris, A., & Baghurst, P. (1992). The effect of computer-assisted interviewing on the clinical assessment of children. *Australian & New Zealand Journal of Psychiatry*, *26*, 223–231.

Skinner, H.A., & Allen, B.A. (1980). Does the computer make a difference? Computerized versus face-to-face versus self-report assessment of alcohol, drug, and tobacco use. *Journal of Consulting & Clinical Psychology*, *51*, 267–275.

Slack, W.V. (1971). Computer-based interviewing system dealing with nonverbal behavior as well as keyboard responses. *Science*, *171*, 84–87.

Slack, W.V., Hicks, G.P., Reed, C.E., & Van Cura, L.J. (1966). A computer-based medical-history system. *New England Journal of Medicine*, *274*, 194–198.

Wilkinson, G., & Markus, A.C. (1989). PROQSY: A computerised technique for psychiatric case identification in general practice. *British Journal of Psychiatry*, *154*, 378–382.

Wyndowe, J. (1987). The microcomputerized Diagnostic Interview Schedule: Clinical use in an outpatient setting. *Canadian Journal of Psychiatry*, *32*, 93–99.

Psychotherapy

Anonymous. (1986). Computerized psychiatric interviewing: An adjunct to therapy whose pluses may outweigh its minuses. *Psychiatric News*, *21*, 29.

Binik, Y.M., Servan–Schreiber, D., Freiwald, S., & Hall, K.K. (1988). Intelligent computer-based assessment and psychotherapy: An expert system for sexual dysfunction. *Journal of Nervous & Mental Disease*, *176*, 387–400.

Binik, Y.M., Westbury, C.F., & Servan–Schreiber, D. (1989). Interaction with a "Sex-expert" system enhances attitudes toward computerized sex therapy. *Behavior Research & Therapy*, *27*, 303–306.

Bloom, B.L. (1992). Computer-assisted psychological intervention: A review and commentary. *Clinical Psychology Review*, *12*, 169–197.

Colby, K.M. (1980). Computer psychotherapists. In J.B. Sidowski, J.H. Johnson, & T.A. Williams (Eds.), *Technology in mental health care delivery systems* (pp. 109–117). Norwood, NJ: Ablex.

Colby, K.M. (1986). Ethics of computer assisted psychotherapy. *Psychiatric Annals*, *16*, 414–415.

Colby, K.M., Gould, R.L., & Aronson, G. (1989). Some pros and cons of computer-assisted psychotherapy. *Journal of Nervous & Mental Disease*, *177*, 105–108.

Colby, K.M., Watt, J.B., & Gilbert, J.P. (1966). A computer method of psychotherapy: Preliminary communication. *Journal of Nervous & Mental Disease*, *142*, 148–152.

Farrell, A.D., Camplair, P.S., & McCullough, L. (1987). Identification of target complaints by computer interview: Evaluation of the Computerized Assessment

System for Psychotherapy Evaluation and Research. *Journal of Consulting & Clinical Psychology*, *55*, 691–700.

Gould, R.L. (1992). Adult development and brief computer-assisted therapy in mental health and managed care. In J.L. Feldman & Fitzpatrick (Eds.), *Managed mental health care: Administrative and clinical issues* (pp. 347–358). Washington, DC: American Psychiatric Press.

Hilf, F.D., Colby, K.M., Smith, D.C., Wittner, W.K., & Hall, W.A. (1971). Machine mediated interviewing. *Journal of Nervous & Mental Disease*, *152*, 278–288.

Lawrence, G.H. (1986). Using computers for the treatment of psychological problems. *Computers in Human Behavior*, *2*, 43–62.

Murphy, J.W., & Pardeck, J.T. (1988). Technology and language use: Implications for computer mediated therapy. *Journal of Humanistic Psychology*, *28*, 120–134.

Plutchik, R., & Karasu, T.B. (1991). Computers in psychotherapy: An overview. *Computers in Human Behavior*, *7*, 33–44.

Servan-Schreiber, D., & Binik, Y.M. (1989). Extending the intelligent tutoring system paradigm: Sex therapy as intelligent tutoring. *Computers in Human Behavior*, *5*, 241–259.

Slack, W.V., & Slack, C.W. (1977). Talking to a computer about emotional problems: A comparative study. *Psychotherapy: Theory, Research, & Practice*, *14*, 156–164.

Starkweather, J.A., Kamp, M., & Monto, A. (1967). Psychiatric interview simulation by computer. *Methods of Information in Medicine*, *6*, 15–23.

Zarr, M.L. (1984). Computer-mediated psychotherapy: Toward patient-selection guidelines. *American Journal of Psychotherapy*, *38*, 47–62.

Zarr, M.L. (1994). Computer-aided psychotherapy: Machine helping therapist. *Psychiatric Annals*, *24*, 42–46.

Behavior Therapy

Allen, D.H. (1984). The use of computer fantasy games in child therapy. In M.D. Schwartz (Ed.), *Using computers in clinical practice: Psychotherapy and mental health applications* (pp. 329–334). New York: Haworth Press.

Aradi, N.S. (1985). The application of computer technology to behavioral marital therapy. In C.R. Figley (Ed.), *Computers and family therapy* (pp. 167–177). New York: Haworth Press.

Burda, P.C., Starkey, T.W., & Dominguez, F. (1991). Computer administered treatment of psychiatric inpatients. *Computers in Human Behavior*, *7*, 1–5.

Burling, T.A., Marotta, J., Gonzalez, R., Moltzen, J.O., Eng, A.M., Schmidt, G.A., Welch, R.L., Ziff, D.C., & Reilly, P.M. (1989). Computerized smoking cessation program for the worksite: Treatment outcome and feasibility. *Journal of Consulting & Clinical Psychology*, *57*, 619–622.

Burnett, K.F., Magel, P.E., & Harrington, S. (1989). Computer-assisted behavioral health counseling. *Journal of Counseling Psychology*, *36*, 63–67.

Burnett, K.F., Taylor, C.B., & Agras, W.S. (1992). Ambulatory computer-assisted behavior therapy for obesity: An empirical model for examining behavioral correlates of treatment outcome. *Computers in Human Behavior*, *8*, 239–248.

Carr, A.C., Ghosh, A., & Marks, I.M. (1988). Computer-supervised exposure treatment for phobias. *Canadian Journal of Psychiatry*, *33*, 112–117.

Chandler, G.M., Burck, H., Sampson, J.P., & Wray, R. (1988). The effectiveness of a generic computer program for systematic desensitization. *Computers in Human Behavior*, *4*, 339–346.

Clarke, B., & Schoech, D.J. (1984). A computer-assisted therapeutic game for adolescents: Initial development and comments. In M.D. Schwartz (Ed.), *Using computers in clinical practice: Psychotherapy and mental health applications* (pp. 335–353). New York: Haworth Press.

Dolan, P.M., & Shapiro, D. (1981). Interactive computer assistance for biofeedback and psychophysiological research: Pragmatics of development. *Behavior Research Methods & Instrumentation*, *13*, 311–322.

Finley, W.W., Etherton, M.D., Dickman, D., Farimian, D., & Simpson, R.W. (1981). A simple EMG-reward system for biofeedback training in children. *Biofeedback & Self-Regulation*, *6*, 169–180.

Fisher, S. (1986). Use of computers following brain injury. In F.A. McGuire (Ed.), *Computer technology and the aged* (pp. 81–93). New York: Haworth Press.

Ghosh, A., & Greist, J.H. (1988). Computer treatment in psychiatry. *Psychiatric Annals*, *18*, 246–250.

Holbrook, T. (1988). Computer technology and behavior therapy: A modern marriage. *Computers in Human Services*, *3*, 89–109.

Kenardy, J., & Adams, C. (1993). Computers in cognitive-behaviour therapy. *Australian Psychologist*, *28*, 189–194.

Kolotkin, R.L., Billingham, K.A., & Feldman, H.S. (1981). Computers in biofeedback research and therapy. *Behavior Research Methods & Instrumentation*, *13*, 532–542.

Kurleychek, R.T., & Glang, A.E. (1984). The use of microcomputers in the cognitive rehabilitation of brain-injured persons. In M.D. Schwartz (Ed.), *Using computers in clinical practice: Psychotherapy and mental health applications* (pp. 245–256). New York: Haworth Press.

Lambert, M.E. (1987). Mr. Howard: A behavior therapy simulation. *Behavior Therapist*, *10*, 139–140.

Lang, P.J. (1980). Behavioral treatment and bio-behavioral assessment: Computer applications. In J.B. Sidowski, J.H. Johnson, & T.A. Williams (Eds.), *Technology in mental health care delivery systems* (pp. 119–137). Norwood, NJ: Ablex.

Matthews, T.J., DeSanti, S.M., Callahan, D., Koblenz–Sulcov, C.J., & Werden, J.I. (1987). The microcomputer as an agent of intervention with psychiatric patients: Preliminary studies. *Computers in Human Behavior*, *3*, 37–47.

Matthews, T.J., Werden, J.I., & Koblenz–Sulcov, C.J. (1991). A client-run computer system for psychiatric ward management. *Advances in Behavior Research & Therapy*, *13*, 1–11.

McGuire, B.E. (1990). Computer-assisted cognitive rehabilitation. *Irish Journal of Psychology*, *11*, 299–308.

Noell, J., Biglan, A., Hood, D., & Britz, B. (1994). An interactive videodisc-based smoking cessation program: Prototype development and pilot test. *Computers in Human Behavior*, *10*, 347–358.

Resnick, H. (1988). "Busted": A computerized therapeutic game: Description, development and preliminary evaluation. In B. Glastonbury, W. LaMendola, & S. Toole (Eds.), *Information technology and the human services* (pp. 103–113). Chichester, UK: Wiley.

Schneider, S.J. (1986). Trial of an on-line behavioral smoking cessation program. *Computers in Human Behavior*, *2*, 277–286.

Schneider, S.J., Walter, R., & O'Donnell, R. (1990). Computerized communication as a medium for behavioral smoking cessation treatment: Controlled evaluation. *Computers in Human Behavior*, *6*, 141–151.

Selmi, P.M., Klein, M.H., Greist, J.H., Sorrell, S.P., & Erdman, H.P. (1990). Computer-administered cognitive-behavioral therapy for depression. *American Journal of Psychiatry*, *147*, 51–56.

Skilbeck, C. (1984). Computer assistance in the management of memory and cognitive impairment. In B. Wilson & N. Moffat (Eds.), *Clinical management of memory problems*. Kent, UK: Crown Helm Ltd.

Taylor, C.B., Agras, W.S., Losch, M., Plante, T.G., & Burnett, K. (1991). Improving the effectiveness of computer-assisted weight loss. *Behavior Therapy*, *22*, 229–236.

Tombari, M.L., Fitzpatrick, S.J., & Childress, W. (1985). Using computers as contingency managers in self-monitoring interventions: A case study. *Computers in Human Services*, *1*, 75–82.

Velicer, W.F., Prochaska, J.O., Bellis, J.M., DiClemente, C.C., Rossi, J.S., Fava, J.L., & Steiger, J.H. (1993). An expert system intervention for smoking cessation. *Addictive Behaviors*, *18*, 269–290.

Zicker, J.E., Tompkins, W.J., Rubow, R.T., & Abbs, J.H. (1980). A portable microprocessor-based biofeedback training device. *IEEE Transactions on Biomedical Engineering*, *27*, 509–515.

Psychiatric Records, Including Problem Oriented Medical Record and Treatment Planning

Ball, M.J., & Collen, M.F. (Eds.). (1992). *Aspects of the computer-based patient record*. New York: Springer–Verlag.

Bowes, N.L., Kenney, J.J., & Pearson, C.L. (1993). The impact of automation on attitudes and productivity in a human social services agency: An emerging issue for employee assistance program managers. In M. Leiderman, C. Guzetta, L. Strumigner, & M.R. Monnickendam (Eds.), *Technology in people services: Research, theory, and applications* (pp. 75–95). Binghamton, NY: Haworth Press.

Casper, E.S. (1989). A follow-up study of a management system to maximize medical records standards compliance. *Journal of Mental Health Administration*, *16*, 128–131.

Chang, M.M. (1987). Clinician-entered computerized triage records. *Hospital & Community Psychiatry*, *38*, 652–655.

Craig, T.J., Volaski, V., DiStefano, O., Alexander, M.J., Kadyszewski, P., Crawford, J.L., & Richardson, M.A. (1982). Automating the treatment planning process: How? Why? For whom? In B.I. Blum (Ed.), *Proceedings of the Sixth Annual Symposium on Computer Applications in Medical Care* (pp. 425–428). New York: Institute of Electrical & Electronics Engineers.

Droege, T., & Kahn, E.M. (1985). dbNotes-psych: A psychiatric note management system using dBase III. In M.J. Ackerman (Ed.), *Proceedings of the Ninth Annual Symposium on Computer Applications in Medical Care* (pp. 367–371). Washington, DC: Institute of Electrical & Electronics Engineers.

Ericson, R.P. (1984). An integrated medical information system. In J.E. Mezzich (Ed.), *Clinical care and information systems in psychiatry* (pp. 1–11). Washington, DC: American Psychiatric Press.

Fowler, D.R., Finkelstein, A., Penk, W., Bell, W., & Itzig, B. (1987). An automated problem-rating interview: The DPRI. In J.N. Butcher (Ed.), *Computerized psychological assessment: A practitioners guide* (pp. 87–107). New York: Basic Books.

Gifford, S., & Maberry, D. (1979). An integrated system for computerized patient records. *Hospital & Community Psychiatry, 30*, 532–535.

Hammond, K.W., King, C.A., Date, V.V., Prather, R.J., & Loo, L. (1988). GRAMPS: An automated ambulatory geriatric record. In R.A. Greenes (Ed.), *Proceedings of the Twelfth Annual Symposium on Computer Applications in Medical Care* (pp. 708–712). Washington, DC: Institute of Electrical & Electronics Engineers.

Hammond, K.W., & Munnecke, T.H. (1984). A computerized psychiatric treatment planning system. *Hospital & Community Psychiatry, 35*, 160–163.

Hay, W.M., Hay, L.R., Angle, H.V., & Ellinwood, E.H. (1977). Computerized behavioral assessment and the problem oriented record. *International Journal of Mental Health, 6*, 49–63.

Honigfeld, G., Pulier, M., Laska, E.M., Kaufl, R., & Ziek, P. (1974). An approach to problem oriented psychiatric records. In J.L. Crawford, D.W. Morgan, & D.T. Gianturco (Eds.), *Progress in mental health information systems: Computer applications* (pp. 107–120). Cambridge, MA: Ballinger.

Laska, E.M. (1981). Development in computerization of the psychiatric record. In C. Siegel & S.K. Fischer (Eds.), *Psychiatric records in mental health care* (pp. 271–296). New York: Brunner/Mazel.

Longabaugh, R. (1988). Does the POS/POMR have a future: A look at the Pros and Cons of the Problem Oriented Record. *POST, 7*, 1–3.

Madaric, M., Maletic, A., Zimonja–Kriskovic, J., Palmovic, R., & Illic–Supek, D. (1986). Psychiatric day hospital medical record processing. In R. Salamon, B. Blum, & M. Jorgensen (Eds.), *Proceedings of Medinfo 86* (pp. 818–821). Amsterdam: North Holland.

Modai, I., Walevski, A., Mark, M., Rabinowitz, J., & Munitz, H. (1991). Successful replacement of traditional psychiatric records with a multi-user computer system. *Medical Care, 29*, 1057–1060.

Modai, I., & Rabinowitz, J. (1993). Why and how to establish a computerized system for psychiatric case records. *Hospital & Community Psychiatry, 44*, 1093–1095.

Ormiston, S., Barrett, N., Binder, R., & Molyneux, V. (1989). A partially computerized treatment plan. Hospital & Community Psychiatry, *40*, 531–533.

Pulier, M.L., Honigfeld, G., & Laska, E.M. (1975). Problem orientation in psychiatry. In E.M. Laska & R. Bank (Eds.), *Safeguarding psychiatric privacy: Computer systems and their uses* (pp. 315–319). New York: Wiley.

Rabinowitz, J., Modai, I., Valevski, A., Zemishlany, Z., & Mark, M. (1993). Benefits of a structured format for paper and computerized psychiatric case records. *Hospital & Community Psychiatry*, *44*, 1095–1097.

Richardson, M.A., Craig, T.J., Simpson, F., Pass, R., McMahon, D., Kadyszewski, P., & Summers, I. (1982). Experimental automated treatment planning— Multiple data sources and multiple uses. In R.C. Insull & J.A. Sumner (Eds.), *Proceedings of the Seventh Annual MSIS National Users Group Conference* (pp. 151–158). Orangeburg, NY: Rockland Research Institute.

Roberts, B. (1980). A computerized diagnostic evaluation of a psychiatric problem. *American Journal of Psychiatry*, *137*, 12–15.

Ryback, R., Stout, R.L., & Hedlund, J.L. (1981). Computerization and the POR. In R.S. Ryback, R. Longabaugh, & D.R. Fowler (Eds.), *The problem oriented record in psychiatry and mental health care* (2nd ed., pp. 127–143). New York: Grune & Stratton.

Siegel, C., & Fischer, S.K. (Eds.) (1981). *Psychiatric records in mental health care*. New York: Brunner/Mazel.

Snyder, D.K., Lachar, D., & Wills, R. M. (1988). Computer-based interpretation of the Marital Satisfaction Inventory: Use in treatment planning. *Journal of Marital & Family Therapy*, *14*, 397–409.

Weaver, R.A., Christensen, P.W., Sells, J., Gottfredson, D.K., Noorda, J., Schenkenberg, T., & Wennhold, A. (1994). Computerized treatment planning. *Hospital & Community Psychiatry*, *45*, 825–827.

Weiss, K.M., & Chapman, H.A. (1993). A computer-assisted inpatient psychiatric assessment and treatment planning system. *Hospital & Community Psychiatry*, *44*, 1097–1100.

Client Tracking Including Treatment Monitoring and Case Management

Alexander, M.J., Siegel, C., Dlugacz, Y., & Fischer, S. (1983). Post implementation changes in physicians' attitudes toward an automated drug review system. In R.E. Dayhoff (Ed.), *Proceedings of the Seventh Annual Symposium on Computer Applications in Medical Care* (pp. 660–663). Silver Spring, MD: Institute of Electrical & Electronics Engineers.

Craig, T.J., & Conklin, G. (1981). Clinical considerations in the introduction of a computerized drug ordering and exception system. In H.G. Heffernan (Ed.), *Proceedings of the Fifth Annual Symposium on Computer Applications in Medical Care* (pp. 620–623). New York: Institute of Electrical & Electronics Engineers.

Craig, T.J., & Mehta, R.M. (1984). Clinician–computer interaction: Automated review of psychotropic drugs. *American Journal of Psychiatry*, *141*, 267–270.

Craig, T.J., Richardson, M.A., Pass, R., Simpson, F., & Summers, I. (1983). A simulation study of automated treatment planning in a mental hospital. In R.E. Dayhoff (Ed.), *Proceedings of the Seventh Annual Symposium on Computer Applications in Medical Care* (pp. 90–93). Silver Springs, MD: Institute of Electrical & Electronics Engineers.

Dlugacz, Y.D., Siegel, C., & Fischer, S. (1982). Clinicians' reactions to the drug ordering and drug exception reporting system. In R.C. Insull & J.A. Sumner

(Eds.), *Proceedings of the Seventh Annual MSIS National Users Group Conference* (pp. 179–186). Orangeburg, NY: Rockland Research Institute.

Greist, J.H., Klein, M.H., Gutman, A.S., & Van Cura, L.J. (1977). Computer measures of patient progress in psychotherapy. *Psychiatry Digest, 38*, 23–30.

Kline, L.J., & Cappello, C.A. (Eds.). (1987). *Issues in Patient Tracking: Proceedings of the Tenth MSIS National User's Group Conference.* Orangeburg, NY: Nathan S. Kline Institute for Psychiatric Research.

Laska, E.M., Craig, T.J., Siegel, C., & Wonderling, J. (1981). Long-term monitoring of psychopharmacological treatment in hospitalized patients. In G. Tognoni, C. Bellantuono, & M. Lader (Eds.), *Epidemiological impact of psychotropic drugs* (pp. 101–117). New York: Elsevier/North-Holland Biomedical Press.

Laska, E.M., Siegel, C., & Simpson, G.M. (1980). Automated review system for orders of psychotropic drugs. *Archives of General Psychiatry, 37*, 824–827.

Metzner, J.L. (1992). A survey of university–prison collaboration and computerized tracking systems in prison. *Hospital & Community Psychiatry, 43*, 713–716.

Mittel, N.S., Gardner, G.H., & Rose, B.W. (1981). Computerized monitoring of psychotropic drug orders: Some trends and revelations. *Hospital & Community Psychiatry, 32*, 277–278.

Overall, J.E., Faillace, L.A., Rhodes, H.M., Johnson, S.R., Volkow, N., Stone, M.A., & Cecil, S. (1987). Computer-based monitoring of clinical care in a public psychiatric hospital unit. *Hospital & Community Psychiatry, 38*, 381–386.

Schnitker, K., & Boeker, K. (1978). Assuring accountability in residential self-help skills programs. *Mental Retardation, 16*, 300–307.

Sherman, P.S. (1989). A micro-based decision support system for managing aggressive case management programs for treatment resistant clients. In W. LaMendola, B. Glastonbury, & S. Toole (Eds.), *A casebook of computer applications in the social and human services* (pp. 181–190). Binghamton, NY: Haworth Press.

Siegel, C., & Alexander, M.J. (1984). Acceptance and impact of the computer in clinical decisions. *Hospital & Community Psychiatry, 35*, 773–775.

Siegel, C., Laska, E.M., & Fischer, S. (1981). The Multi-State Information System drug exception system: A quality assurance tool. In H.G. Heffernan (Ed.), *Proceedings of the Fifth Annual Symposium on Computer Applications in Medical Care* (pp. 615–619). New York: Institute of Electrical & Electronics Engineers.

Sorrell, S.P., Greist, J.H., Klein, M.H., Johnson, J.H., & Harris, W.G. (1982). Enhancement of adherence to tricyclic antidepressants by computerized supervision. *Behavior Research Methods & Instrumentation, 14*, 176–180.

Stroebel, C.F., & Glueck, B.C. (1970). Computer derived global judgments in psychiatry. *American Journal of Psychiatry, 126*, 1057–1066.

Tupin, J.P., Overall, J.E., McKinley, C.K., Dreisbach, L.K., & Patrick, J.H. (1967). Computer monitoring and analysis of a psychiatric treatment program. *Mental Health, 51*, 414–418.

Vafeas, J.G. (1991). Personal computer based clinical systems: A goal oriented case management model. *Computers in Human Services, 8*, 21–36.

Expert Systems and Consultation Including Prediction, Decision Support Systems, and Artificial Intelligence

Barta, P., & Barta, W. (1988). DISPO advisor: Expert system for psychiatric disposition. In R.A. Greenes (Ed.), *Proceedings of the Twelfth Annual Symposium on Computer Applications in Medical Care* (pp. 22–25). Washington, DC: Institute of Electrical & Electronics Engineers.

Beaumont, J.G. (1991). Expert systems and the clinical psychologist. In A. Ager & S. Bendall (Eds.), *Microcomputers and clinical psychology: Issues, applications and future developments* (pp. 175–193). Chichester, UK: Wiley.

Bronzino, J.D., Morelli, R.A., & Goethe, J.W. (1988). OVERSEER: An expert system monitor for the psychiatric hospital. In R.A. Greenes (Ed.), *Proceedings of the Twelfth Annual Symposium on Computer Applications in Medical Care* (pp. 8–12). Washington, DC: Institute of Electrical & Electronics Engineers.

Carroll, J.A., Greist, J.H., Jefferson, J.W., Baudhuin, M.G., Hartley, B.L., Erdman, H.P., & Ackerman, D.L. (1986). Lithium Information Center: One model of a computer-based psychiatric information service. *Archives of General Psychiatry*, *43*, 483–485.

Colby, K.M. (1979). Computer simulation and artificial intelligence in psychiatry. In E.A. Serafetinides (Ed.), *Methods of biobehavioral research*. New York: Grune & Stratton.

Davis, G.E., Lowell, W.E., & Davis, G.L. (1993). A neural network that predicts psychiatric length of stay. *M.D. Computing*, *10*, 87–92.

Erdman, H.P. (1987). A computer consultation program for primary care physicians: Impact of decision-making model and explanation capability. *Medical Care*, *25*(Suppl.), 138–147.

Erdman, H.P., Greist, J.H., Gustafson, D.H., Taves, J.E., & Klein, M.H. (1987). Suicide risk prediction by computer interview: A prospective study. *Journal of Clinical Psychiatry*, *48*, 464–467.

Feldman, M.J., & Barnett, G.O. (1991). An approach to evaluating the accuracy of DXplain. *Computer Methods & Programs in Biomedicine*, *35*, 261–266.

Fluke, J.D., & O'Beirne, G.N. (1989). Artificial intelligence: An aide in child protective service caseload control systems. *Computers Human Services*, *4*, 101–109.

Frick, T.W. (1992). Computerized adaptive mastery tests as expert systems. *Journal of Educational Computing Research*, *8*, 187–213.

Garfield, D.A.S., Rapp, C., & Evans, M. (1992). Natural language processing in psychiatry: Artificial intelligence technology and psychopathology. *Journal of Nervous & Mental Disease*, *180*, 227–237.

Gelernter, D., & Gelernter, J. (1984). Expert systems and diagnostic monitors in psychiatry. In G.S. Cohen (Ed.), *Proceedings of the Eighth Annual Symposium on Computer Applications in Medical Care* (pp. 45–48). Silver Springs, MD: Institute of Electrical & Electronics Engineers.

Gingerich, W.J. (1990). Expert systems: New tools for professional decision making. *Computers in Human Services*, *6*, 219–230.

Gingerich, W.J. (1990). Developing expert systems. *Computers in Human Services*, *6*, 251–263.

Gingerich, W.J. (1990). Expert systems and their potential uses in social work. *Families in Society: The Journal of Contemporary Human Services*, *71*, 220–228.

Gingerich, W.J., & de Shazer, S. (1991). The BRIEFER project: Using expert systems as theory construction tools. *Family Process*, *30*, 241–250.

Glueck, B.C., & Stroebel, C.F. (1969). The computer and the clinical decision making process. II. *American Journal of Psychiatry*, *125*, 2–7.

Goldstein, R.B., Black, D.W., Nasrallah, A., & Winokur, G. (1991). The prediction of suicide: Sensitivity, specificity and predictive value of a multivariate model applied to suicide among 1906 patients with affective disorder. *Archives of General Psychiatry*, *48*, 418–422.

Greist, J.H., Gustafson, D.H., Stauss, F.F., Rowse, G.L., Laughren, T., & Chiles, J.A. (1974). Suicide risk prediction: A new approach. *Suicide & Life Threatening Behavior*, *4*, 212–223.

Greist, J.H., Jefferson, J.W., Ackerman, D.L., Baudhuin, M.G., Erdman, H.P., & Carroll, J.A. (1985). Lithium Information Center: The Lithium Library revisited. *Journal of Clinical Psychiatry*, *46*, 327–331.

Greist, J.H., Jefferson, J.W., Combs, A.M., Schou, M., & Thomas, A. (1977). The Lithium Librarian: An international index. *Archives of General Psychiatry*, *34*, 456–459.

Guastello, S.J., & Rieke, M.L. (1994). Computer-based test interpretations as expert systems—Validity and viewpoints from artificial intelligence theory. *Computers in Human Behavior*, *10*, 435–455.

Gustafson, D.H., Greist, J.H., Stauss, F.F., Erdman, H.P., & Laughren, T.P. (1977). A probabilistic system for identifying suicide attempters. *Computers & Biomedical Research*, *10*, 83–89.

Gustafson, D.H., Sainfort, F., Johnson, S.W., & Sateia, M. (1993). Measuring quality of care in psychiatric emergencies: Construction and evaluation of a Bayesian index. *Health Services Research*, *28*, 131–158.

Hale, M.S., & De L'aure, W. (1983). Microcomputer use of a consultation-liaison service. *Psychosomatics*, *24*, 1003–1007, 1011, 1015.

Hartman, D.E. (1986). Artificial intelligence or artificial psychologist? Conceptual issues in clinical microcomputer use. *Professional Psychology: Research & Practice*, *17*, 528–534.

Hedlund, J.L., Evenson, R.C., Sletten, I.W., & Cho, D.W. (1980). The computer and clinical prediction. In J.B. Sidowski, J.H. Johnson, & T.A. Williams (Eds.), *Technology in mental health care delivery systems* (pp. 201–235). Norwood, NJ: Ablex.

Hedlund, J.L., Vieweg, B.W., & Cho, D.W. (1987). Computer consultation for emotional crises: An expert system for "non experts." *Computers in Human Behavior*, *3*, 109–127.

Hofmeister, A.M., Althouse, R.B., Likins, M., Morgan, D.P., Ferrara, J.M., Jenson, W.R., & Rollins, E. (1994). SMH.PAL—An expert system for identifying treatment procedures for students with severe disabilities. *Exceptional Children*, *61*, 174–181.

Illovsky, M.E. (1994). Counseling, artificial intelligence and expert systems. *Simulation & Gaming*, *25*, 88–98.

Johri, S.K., & Guha, S.K. (1991). Set-covering diagnostic expert system for psychiatric disorders: The third world context. *Computer Methods and Programs in Biomedicine*, *34*, 1–7.

Mutschler, E. (1990). Computer assisted decision making. *Computers in Human Services, 6*, 231–250.

Overall, J.E., & Henry, B.W. (1972). Decisions about drug therapy: III. Selection of treatment for psychiatric inpatients. *Archives of General Psychiatry, 28*, 81–89.

Overall, J.E., Henry, B.W., Markett, J.R., & Emken, R.L. (1972). Decisions about drug therapy: I. Prescriptions for adult psychiatric outpatients. *Archives of General Psychiatry, 26*, 140–145.

Powsner, S.M., & Miller, P.L. (1993). Automated online transition from the medical record to the psychiatric literature. In J.H. Van Bemmel & A.T. McCray (Eds.), *Yearbook of medical informatics 1993: Sharing knowledge and information* (pp. 234–239). New York: Schattauer.

Schoech, D., Jennings, H., Schkade, L.L., & Hooper–Russell, C. (1985). Expert systems: Artificial intelligence for professional decisions. *Computers in Human Services, 1*, 81–115.

Schuerman, J.R. (1987). Expert consulting systems in social welfare. *Social Work Research & Abstracts, 23*, 14–18.

Schwab, A.J., Jr., Bruce, M.E., & McRoy, R.G. (1986). Using computer technology in child placement decisions. *Social Casework, 67*, 359–368.

Servan–Schreiber, D. (1986). Artificial intelligence and psychiatry. *Journal of Nervous & Mental Disease, 174*, 191–202.

Sharf, R.S. (1985). Artificial intelligence: Implications for the future of counseling. *Journal of Counseling & Development, 64*, 34–37.

Sicoly, F. (1989). Computer-aided decisions in human services: Expert systems and multivariate models. *Computers in Human Behavior, 5*, 47–60.

Stein, D.J., Patterson, R., & Hollander, E. (1994). Expert systems for psychiatric pharmacotherapy. *Psychiatric Annals, 24*, 37–41.

Steyaert, J. (1994). Soft computing for soft technologies: Artificial neural networks and fuzzy set theory for human services. *Computers in Human Services, 10*, 55–67.

Stroebel, C.F., & Glueck, B.C. (1970). Computer derived global judgments in psychiatry. *American Journal of Psychiatry, 126*, 1057–1066.

Velicer, W.F., Prochaska, J.O., Bellis, J.M., DiClemente, C.C., Rossi, J.S., Fava, J.L., & Steiger, J.H. (1993). An expert system intervention for smoking cessation. *Addictive Behaviors, 18*, 269–290.

Vogel, L.H. (1985). Decision support systems in the human services: Discovering limits to a promising technology. *Computers in Human Services, 1*, 67–80.

Watkins, W.M., & McDermott, P.A. (1993). Psychodiagnostic computing: From interpretive programs to expert systems. In T.B. Gutkin & S.L. Wise (Eds.), *The computer and the decision-making process* (pp. 11–42). Hillsdale, NJ: Erlbaum.

Winfield, M.J., Simpson, R., & Bayliss, R. (1989). Child-care placements: A knowledge systems approach. In W. LaMendola, B. Glastonbury, & S. Toole (Eds.), *A casebook of computer applications in the social and human services.* Binghamton, NY: Haworth Press.

Zahedi, F. (1994). An introduction to neural networks and a comparison with artificial intelligence and expert systems. *Interfaces, 21*, 25–38.

Modeling of Psychopathology

Colby, K.M. (1975). *Artificial paranoia*. New York: Pergamon Press.

Colby, K.M. (1976). Clinical implications of a simulation model of paranoid processes. *Archives of General Psychiatry, 33*, 854–857.

Colby, K.M., & Gilbert, J.P. (1964). Programming a computer model of neurosis. *Journal of Mathematical Psychology, 1*, 405–417.

Faught, W.S., Colby, K.M., & Parkison, R.C. (1977). Inferences, affects, and intentions in a model of paranoia. *Cognitive Psychology, 9*, 153–187.

Moser, U., Zeppelin, I.V., & Schneider, W. (1970). Computer simulation of a model of neurotic defense processes. *Behavioral Science, 15*, 194–202.

Reilly, K.D., Freese, M.R., & Rowe, P.B. (1984). Computer simulation modeling of abnormal behavior: A program approach. *Behavioral Science, 29*, 186–211.

Santo, Y., & Finkel, A. (1982). "Chris": A computer simulation of schizophrenia. In B.I. Blum (Ed.), *Proceedings of the Sixth Annual Symposium on Computer Applications in Medical Care* (pp. 737–741). New York: Institute of Electrical & Electronics Engineers.

Stein, D.J. (1994). Computational models of the mind and psychiatry. *Psychiatric Annals, 24*, 47–52.

Tompkins, S.S., & Messick, S. (1963). *Computer simulation of personality: Frontier of psychological theory*. New York: Wiley.

Program Evaluation, Quality Assurance, and Outcome Evaluation

Attkisson, C.C., McIntyre, M.H., Hargreaves, W.A., Harris, M.R., & Ochberg, F.M. (1974). A working model for mental health program evaluation. *American Journal of Orthopsychiatry, 44*, 741–753.

Block, W.E. (1975). Applying utilization review procedures in a community mental health center. *Hospital & Community Psychiatry, 26*, 358–360.

Bloom, B.L. (1972). Human accountability in a community mental health center: Report of an automated system. *Community Mental Health Journal, 8*, 251–260.

Cameron, J.C. (1976). Using a computer profile to assess quality of care in a psychiatric hospital. *Hospital & Community Psychiatry, 27*, 623.

Courtney, M.E., & Collins, R.C. (1994). New challenges and opportunities in child welfare outcomes and information technologies. *Child Welfare, 73*, 359–378.

Currie, P.C. (1994). Re-engineering the behavioral healthcare industry with information technology. *Behavioral Healthcare Tomorrow, 3*, 71–73.

Doenlen, H.A., & Craig, T.J. (1982). Use of computerized psychiatric diagnosis for case review. In R.C. Insull & J.A. Sumner (Eds.), *Proceedings of the Seventh Annual MSIS National Users Group Conference* (pp. 141–150). Orangeburg, NY: Rockland Research Institute.

Evenson, R.C. (1974). Program evaluation using an automated data base. *Hospital & Community Psychiatry, 25*, 80–83.

Evenson, R.C., Sletten, I.W., Hedlund, J.L., & Faintich, D.M. (1974). CAPS: An automated evaluation system. *American Journal of Psychiatry, 131*, 531–534.

Fiester, A.R., & Fort, D.J. (1978). A method of evaluating the impact of services at a comprehensive community mental health center. *American Journal of Community Psychology*, *6*, 291–302.

Fishman, D.B. (1980). A computerized, cost-effectiveness methodology for community mental health centers. In J.B. Sidowski, J.H. Johnson, & T.A. Williams (Eds.), *Technology in mental health care delivery systems* (pp. 43–63). Norwood, NJ: Ablex.

Gray, G.V., & Glazer, W.M. (1994). Psychiatric decision making in the 90s: The coming age of decision support. *Behavioral Healthcare Tomorrow*, *3*, 47–54.

Gustafson, D.H., Fainfort, F., Johnson, S.W., & Sateia, M. (1993). Measuring quality of care in psychiatric emergencies: Construction of a Bayesian index. *Health Services Research*, *28*, 131–158.

Helmick, E., Miller, S.I., Nutting, P., Shorr, G., & Berg, L. (1976). A monitoring and evaluation plan for alcoholism programs. *British Journal of Addiction*, *71*, 39–43.

Huber, G.A., Wolfe, H., & Hardwick, C.P. (1974). Evaluating computerized screening as an aid to utilization review. *Inquiry*, *11*, 188–195.

Kane, R.L., Bartlett, J., & Potthoff, S. (1994). Integrating an outcomes information system into managed care for substance abuse. *Behavioral Healthcare Tomorrow*, *3*, 57–61.

Kaplan, J.M., & Smith, W.G. (1974). An evaluation program for a regional mental health center. In J.L. Crawford, D.W. Morgan, & D.T. Gianturco (Eds.), *Progress in mental health information systems: Computer applications* (pp. 161–174). Cambridge, MA: Ballinger.

Miller, R.R., Black, G.C., Ertel, P.Y., & Ogram, G.F. (1974). Psychiatric peer review: The Ohio system. *American Journal of Psychiatry*, *131*, 1367–1370.

Murtaugh, C., Siegel, C., Fischer, S., Alexander, M.J., & Craig, T.J. (1982). Computers and quality of care. In B.I. Blum (Ed.), *Proceedings of the Sixth Annual Symposium on Computer Applications in Medical Care* (pp. 125–129). New York: Institute of Electrical & Electronics Engineers.

Naditch, M.P. (1994). Shifting to a new paradigm to measure outcomes. *Behavioral Healthcare Tomorrow*, *3*, 273–294.

Newman, F.L., Hunter, R.H., & Irving, D. (1987). Simple measures of progress and outcome in the evaluation of mental health services. *Evaluation & Program Planning*, *10*, 209–218.

Rodriquez, A.R. (1992). Management of quality, utilization, and risk. In J.L. Feldman & R.J. Fitzpatrick (Eds.), *Managed mental health care: Administration and clinical issue* (pp. 83–97). Washington, DC: American Psychiatric Press.

Romanczyk, R.G. (1991). Monitoring and evaluating service delivery: Issues and effectiveness of computer database management. In A. Ager & S. Bendall (Eds.), *Microcomputers and clinical psychology: Issues, applications and future developments* (pp. 155–173). Chichester, UK: Wiley.

Thompson, K.S., & Cheng, E.H. (1976). A computer package to facilitate compliance with utilization review requirements. *Hospital & Community Psychiatry*, *27*, 653–656.

Wehr, R.J. (1987). A microcomputer database for mental health program evaluation. *Canada's Mental Health*, *35*, 5–10.

Wolfe, P.C., & Haveliwala, Y. (1976). A model for program evaluation in a unitized setting. *Hospital & Community Psychiatry*, *27*, 647–649.

Computer Assisted Instruction Including Self-Help Applications

Abernathy, W.B. (1979). The microcomputer as a community mental health public information tool. *Community Mental Health Journal*, *15*, 192–202.

Alpert, D. (1986). A preliminary investigation of computer-enhanced counselor training. *Computers in Human Behavior*, *2*, 63–70.

Antonoff, M.B. (1985). New software for self-help. *Personal Computing*, *9*, 95–101.

Berven, N.L. (1985). Reliability and validity of standardized case management simulations. *Journal of Counseling Psychology*, *32*, 397–409.

Bourque, M. (1981). S.I.C. for health education. In H.G. Heffernan (Ed.), *Proceedings of the Fifth Annual Symposium on Computer Applications in Medical Care* (pp. 696–701). New York: Institute of Electrical & Electronics Engineers.

Bradt, S., Crilly, J., & Timvik, U. (1993). Computer training for the young adult patient with chronic mental illness. *Journal of Rehabilitation*, *59*, 51–54.

Brieff, R. (1994). Personal computers in psychiatric rehabilitation: A new approach to skills training. *Hospital & Community Psychiatry*, *45*, 257–260.

Budoff, M., & Hutten, L.R. (1982). Microcomputers in special education: Promises and pitfalls. *Exceptional Children*, *49*, 123–128.

Butler, D.L. (1986). Interests in and barriers to using computers in instruction. *Teaching of Psychology*, *13*, 20–23.

Chan, F., Parker, H.J., Mecaskey, C., & Malphurs, L. (1987). Computer case management simulations: Applications in rehabilitation education. *Rehabilitation Counseling Bulletin*, *30*, 210–217.

Chubon, R.A. (1986). Genesis II: A computer-based case management simulation. *Rehabilitation Counseling Bulletin*, *30*, 25–32.

Cox, G.B., Erickson, D., Armstrong, H.E., & Harrison, P. (1986). Computer simulation of community mental health centers. *Computers in Human Services*, *1*, 105–107.

Doelker, R.E., & Lynette, P.A. (1988). The impact of learner attitude on computer-based training in the human services. *Journal of Continuing Social Work Education*, *69*, 214–223.

Ferguson, D. (1986). Computer assisted training for activity professionals in long term care facilities. In F.A. McGuire (Ed.), *Computer technology & the aged* (pp. 109–119). New York: Haworth Press.

Fine, M., & McIntosh, D.K. (1986). The use of interactive video to demonstrate differential approaches to marital and family therapy. *Journal of Marital & Family Therapy*, *12*, 85–89.

Finnegan, D.J., & Ivanoff, A. (1991). Effects of brief computer training on attitudes toward computer use in practice: An educational experiment. *Journal of Social Work Education*, *27*, 73–82.

First, M.B., Williams, J.B.W., & Spitzer, R.L. (1988). DTREE: Microcomputer-assisted teaching of psychiatric diagnosis using a decision tree model. In R.A. Greenes (Ed.), *Proceedings of the Twelfth Annual Symposium on Computer Applications in Medical Care* (pp. 377–381). Washington, DC: Institute of Electrical & Electronics Engineers.

Foulds, R.A. (1982). Applications of microcomputers in the education of the physically disabled child. *Exceptional Children*, *49*, 155–162.

Genty, D.B. (1992). Using computer aided interactive video technology to provide experiential learning for mediation trainees. *Journal of Divorce & Remarriage*, *17*, 57–74.

Haydel, DC (1990). A DSM-III-R computer tutorial for abnormal psychology. *Teaching of Psychology*, *17*, 203–206.

Henningson, K.A., Gold, R.S., & Duncan, D.F. (1986). A computerized marijuana decision maze: Expert opinion regarding its use in health education. *Journal of Drug Education*, *16*, 243–261.

Hodgin, J.D. (1986). Microcomputers, interactive videodisks, and psychodynamic simulations. *Southern Medical Journal*, *79*, 451–454.

Hornby, P.A., & Anderson, M.D. (1994). Computer use in psychology instruction: A survey of individual and institutional characteristics. *Behavior Research Methods, Instruments, & Computers*, *26*, 57–59.

Hyler, S.E., & Bujold, A.E. (1994). Computers and psychiatric education: The "Taxi Driver" mental status examination. *Psychiatric Annals*, *24*, 13–19.

Isaacs, M., Costenbader, V., Reading–Brown, M., & Goodman, G. (1992). Using a computer simulation in the research, training, and evaluation of school psychologists. *Behavior Research Methods, Instruments, & Computers*, *24*, 165–168.

Kennedy, R.S., & David, J. (1994). Using computers to review case-based materials and formulate a psychiatric write-up. In S. Safran (Ed.), *Proceedings of the Seventeenth Annual Symposium on Computer Applications in Medical Care* (p. 949). New York: McGraw–Hill.

Kieley, J.M. (1993). Integrating remotely accessible information services into psychology instruction and research. *Behavior Research Methods, Instruments, & Computers*, *25*, 287–294.

Lambert, M.E. (1987). A computer simulation for behavior therapy training. *Journal of Behavior Therapy & Experimental Psychiatry*, *18*, 245–248.

Lambert, M.E. (1987). Mr. Howard: A behavior therapy simulation. *The Behavior Therapist*, *10*, 139–140.

Lambert, M.E., Hedlund, J.L., & Vieweg, B.W. (1990). Computer simulations in mental health education: Current status. *Computers in Human Services*, *7*, 211–229.

Lambert, M.E., Intrieri, R.C., & Hollandsworth, J.G., Jr. (1986). Development of a computerized reference retrieval system: A behavior training tool. *Journal of Behavior Therapy & Experimental Psychiatry*, *17*, 167–169.

Lambert, M.E., & Lenthall, G. (1988). Using computerized case simulation in undergraduate psychology courses. *Teaching of Psychology*, *15*, 132–135.

Lambert, M.E., & Lenthall, G. (1989). Effects of psychology courseware use on computer anxiety in students. *Computers in Human Behavior*, *5*, 207–214.

Lepper, M.R. (1985). Microcomputers in education: Motivational and social issues. *American Psychologist*, *40*, 1–18.

Lichtenberg, J.W., Hummel, T.J., & Shaffer, W.F. (1984). CLIENT 1: A computer simulation for use in counselor education and research. *Counselor Education & Supervision*, *24*, 155–167.

Lowman, J. (1990). Failure of laboratory evaluation of CAI to generalize to classroom settings: The SuperShrink interview simulation. *Behavior Research Methods, Instruments & Computers*, *22*, 429–432.

Mahler, C.R., & Meier, S.T. (1993). The microcomputer as a psychotherapeutic aid. *Computers in Human Services*, *10*, 35–40.

Maypole, D.E. (1991). Interactive videodiscs in social work education. *Social Work*, *36*, 239–41.

McMinn, M.R. (1988). Ethics case-study simulation: A generic tool for psychology teachers. *Teaching of Psychology*, *15*, 100–101.

Meier, S.T. (1988). An exploratory study of a computer-assisted alcohol education program. *Computers in Human Services*, *3*, 111–121.

Meier, S.T., & Sampson, J.P. (1989). Use of computer assisted instruction in the prevention of alcohol abuse. *Journal of Drug Education*, *19*, 245–256.

Moncher, M.S., Parms, C.A., Orlandi, M.A., Schinke, S.P., Miller, S.O., Palleja, J., & Schinke, M.B. (1989). Microcomputer-based approaches for preventing drug and alcohol abuse among adolescents from ethnic-racial minority backgrounds. *Computers in Human Behavior*, *5*, 77–93.

Muehlenhard, C. L., & McFall, R. M. (1988). Automated assertion training: A feasibility study. *Journal of Social & Clinical Psychology*, *1*, 246–258.

Munson, C.E. (1988). Microcomputers in social work education. *Computers in Human Services*, *3*, 143–157.

Nurius, P.S., & Hudson, W.W. (1993). *Human services practice, evaluation, and computers: A practical guide for today and beyond.* Pacific Groves, CA: Brooks/Cole Publishing Co.

Oakley–Browne, M.A., & Toole, S. (1994) Computerised self-care programs for depression and anxiety disorders. In G. Andrews, H. Dilling, T.B. Ustun, & M. Briscoe (Eds.), *Computers in mental health: 1994* (pp. 96–102). Geneva, Switzerland: World Health Organization.

Ober, B.R., Trainor, T.N., & Semb, G.B. (1985). Courseware and behavioral instruction: The design and dissemination of effective teaching systems. *The Behavior Analyst*, *8*, 273–274.

Olevitch, B.A., & Hagan, B.J. (1991). An interactive videodisc as a tool in the rehabilitation of the chronically mentally ill. *Computers in Human Behavior*, *7*, 57–73.

Park, O., & Seidel, R.J. (1987). Instructional design principles and AI techniques for development of ICAI. *Computers in Human Behavior*, *3*, 273–287.

Patterson, D.A., & Yaffe, J. (1993). Using computer-assisted instruction to teach Axis-II of DSM-III-R to social work students. *Research on Social Work Practice*, *3*, 343–357.

Patterson, D.A., & Yaffe, J. (1994). Hypermedia computer-based education in social work education. *Journal of Social Work Education*, *30*, 267–277.

Phillips, S.D. (1983). Trends & implications for training: Counselor training via computer. *Counselor Education & Supervision*, *23*, 20–28.

Phillips, S.D. (1984). Contributions and limitations in the use of computers in counselor training. *Counselor Education & Supervision*, *24*, 186–192.

Politser, P.E., Gastfriend, D.R., Bakin, D., & Nguyen, L. (1987). An intelligent display system for psychiatric education in primary care. *Medical Care*, *25*, 123–137.

Resnick, H. (1986). Electronic technology and rehabilitation. A computerized simulation game for youthful offenders. *Simulation & Games*, *17*, 460–466.

Resnick, H. (1988). "Busted": A computerized therapeutic game: Description, development and preliminary evaluation. In B. Glastonbury, W. LaMendola,

& S. Toole (Eds.), *Information technology and the human services* (pp. 103–113). Chichester, UK: Wiley.

Rosen, E.F., & Petty, L. C. (1992). Computer aided instruction in physiological psychology course. *Behavior Research Methods, Instruments, & Computers, 24,* 169–171.

Sampson, J.P. (1986). The use of computer-assisted instruction in support of psychotherapeutic processes. *Computers in Human Behavior, 2,* 1–19.

Sampson, J.P., & Krumboltz, J.D. (1992). Computer-assisted instruction: The missing link in counseling. *Journal of Counseling & Development, 39,* 395–397.

Schwartz, M.D. (1988). Computers in psychiatric education. *Psychiatric Annals, 18,* 228–235.

Seabury, B.A., & Maple, F.F. (1993). Using computers to teach practice skills. *Social Work, 38,* 430–439.

Semmel, M.I., Varnhagen, S., & McCann, S. (1981). MICROGAMES: An application of microcomputers for training personnel who work with handicapped children. *Teacher Education & Special Education, 4,* 27–33.

Smith, J.J. (1987). The effectiveness of a computerized self-help coping program with adult males. *Computers in Human Services, 2,* 37–49.

Smith, N.J., Parmar, G., & Paget, N. (1980). Computer simulation and social work education: A suitable case. *British Journal of Social Work, 10,* 491–499.

Speight, I., Laufer, M.E., & Mattes, K. (1993). CIV (Computer aided video): A novel application in neuropsychological rehabilitation. *Computers in Human Behavior, 9,* 95–104.

Summerfield, A., & Lipsedge, M. (1993). Training in microcomputing for chronic psychiatric patients. In R. West, M. Christie, & J. Weinman (Eds.), *Microcomputers, psychology, and medicine* (pp. 267–276). Chichester, UK: Wiley.

Tanner, B.A. (1990). The MMPI Assistant: A microcomputer program to assist in teaching interpretation of the MMPI. *Computers in Human Behavior, 6,* 207–210.

Van Dongen, C.J. (1984). CAI applications in mental health nursing. *Computers in Psychiatry/Psychology, 6,* 25–26.

Wallace, D.H. (1984). Microcomputer applications in self-help software. In G.S. Cohen (Ed.), *Proceedings of the Eighth Annual Symposium on Computer Applications in Medical Care* (pp. 901–907). Silver Spring, MD: Institute of Electrical & Electronics Engineers.

Wolfman, C. (1980). Microcomputer simulated psychiatric interviews used as a teaching aid. *Journal of Psychiatric Education, 4,* 190–201.

Counseling

Card, C.A.L., Jacobsberg, L.B., Moffatt, M., Fishman, B., & Perry, S. (1993). Using interactive video to supplement HIV counseling. *Hospital & Community Psychiatry, 44,* 383–385.

Erdman, H.P., & Foster, S.W. (1986). Computer-assisted assessment with couples and families. *Family Therapy, 13,* 23–40.

Ekstrom, R., & Johnson, C. (1984). Computers in counseling and development [Special issue]. *Journal of Counseling and Development, 63,* 131–196.

Fernandez, E., Brechtel, M., & Mercer, A. (1986). Personal and simulated computer-aided counseling: Perceived versus measured counseling outcomes for college students. *Journal of College Student Personnel, 27*, 224–228.

Hayden, DC (1985). Microcomputer survey of counseling centers. *Journal of College Student Personnel, 26*, 560–561.

Illovsky, M.E. (1994). Counseling, artificial intelligence and expert systems. *Simulation & Gaming, 25*, 88–98.

Katz, Y.J. (1991). Computer assisted counseling—Model for the elementary school. *International Journal for the Advancement of Counseling, 14*, 51–57.

Lambert, M.E. (1988). Computers in counselor education: Four years after a special issue. *Counselor Education & Supervision, 28*, 100–109.

Meier, S.T. (1986). Stories about counselors and computers: Their use in workshops. *Journal of Counseling & Development, 65*, 100–103.

Myers, R.A., & Cairo, P.C. (Eds.) (1983). Computer assisted counseling [Special issue]. *The Counseling Psychologist, 11*, 9–75.

Parente, F.J., Anderson, J.K., Ottenstein, R. J., & Hass–Woods, M. (1981). A computer-assisted method of counseling. *American Mental Health Counselors Association Journal, 3*, 62–71.

Sampson, J.P. (1986). Computer technology and counseling psychology: Regression toward the machine? *The Counseling Psychologist, 14*, 567–586.

Sampson, J.P., & Krumboltz, J.D. (1992). Computer-assisted instruction: The missing link in counseling. *Journal of Counseling & Development, 39*, 395–397.

Slack, W.V. (1978). Patient counseling by computer. In F.H. Orthner (Ed.), *Proceedings of the Second Annual Symposium on Computer Applications in Medical Care* (pp. 58–62). Washington, DC: Institute of Electrical & Electronics Engineers.

Smith, G.W., & Debenham, J.D. (1979). Computer automated marriage analysis. *American Journal of Family Therapy, 7*, 16–32.

Wagman, M. (1984). Using computers in personal counseling. *Journal of Counseling & Development, 63*, 172–176.

Wark, D., Kalkman, J., Grace, D., & Wales, E. (1991). An evaluation of the Therapeutic Learning Program: Presentation with and without a computer. *Computers in Human Services, 8*, 119–132.

Legal and Ethical Issues Including Confidentiality, Ethics, Privacy, and Standards

American Psychological Association. (1987). Appendix B: American Psychological Association guidelines for computer-based tests and interpretations. In J.N. Butcher (Ed.), *Computerized psychological assessment: A practitioners guide* (pp. 413–431). New York: Basic Books.

Banes, J.S. (1987). Issus in patient tracking: A former patient's perspective. In L.J. Kline & C. Cappello (Eds.), *Issues in Patient Tracking: Proceedings of the Tenth MSIS National User's Group Conference* (pp. 30–37). Orangeburg, NY: Nathan S. Kline Institute for Psychiatric Research.

Bennett, C.J. (1991). Computers, personal data, and theories of technology: Comparative approaches to privacy protection in the 1990s. *Science, Technology, & Human Values, 16*, 51–69.

Bersoff, D.N., & Hofer, P.J. (1991). Legal issues in computerized psychological testing. In T.E. Gutkin & S.L. Wise (Eds.), *The computer and the clinical decision-making process*. Hillsdale, NJ: Erlbaum.

Bongar, B. (1988). Clinicians, microcomputers, and confidentiality. *Professional Psychology: Research & Practice, 19*, 286–289.

Colby, K.M. (1986). Ethics of computer assisted psychotherapy. *Psychiatric Annals, 16*, 414–415.

Erdman, H.P., & Foster, S.W. (1988). Ethical issues in the use of computer-based assessment. *Computers in Human Services, 3*, 71–87.

Eyde, L.D., & Kowal, D.M. (1987). Computerized test interpretation services: Ethical and professional concerns regarding U.S. producers and users. *Applied Psychology: An International Review, 36*, 401–417.

Farrell, A.D. (1989). Impact of standards for computer-based tests on practice: Consequences of the information gap. *Computers in Human Behavior, 5*, 1–12.

Ford, B.D. (1993). Ethical and professional issues in computer-assisted therapy. *Computers in Human Behavior, 9*, 387–400.

Gutman, J.S. (1987). Tracking and civil liberties. In L. J. Kline & C. Cappello (Eds.), *Issues in Patient Tracking: Proceedings of the Tenth MSIS National Users' Group Conference* (pp. 23–29). Orangeburg, NY: Nathan S. Kline Psychiatric Research Center.

Hartman, D.E. (1986). On the use of clinical psychology software: Practical, legal, and ethical concerns. *Professional Psychology: Research & Practice, 17*, 462–465.

Jacob, S., & Brantley, J.C. (1987). Ethical-legal problems with computer use and suggestions for best practices: A national survey. *School Psychology Review, 16*, 69–77.

Jacob, S., & Brantley, J.C. (1989). Ethics and computer-assisted assessment: Three case studies. *Psychology in the Schools, 26*, 163–167.

Kramer, J.J. (1986). Epilogue: Why no standards for computer-based testing and test interpretation. *Computers in Human Behavior, 1*, 317–320.

Mason, R.O. (1986). Four ethical issues of the information age. *MIS Quarterly, 10*, 5–14.

Murphy, J.W., & Pardeck, J.T. (1988). Dehumanization, computers and clinical practice. *Journal of Social Behavior & Personality, 3*, 107–116.

Nycum, S.N. (1986). Legal liability for expert systems. In R. Salamon, B. Blum, & M. Jorgensen (Eds.), *Proceedings of Medinfo 86* (pp. 1069–1071). Amsterdam: North Holland.

Pardeck, J.T., Murphy, J.W., & Callaghan, K. (1993). Computerization of social services: A critical appraisal. *Scandinavian Journal of Social Service, 3*, 2–6.

Sampson, J.P., & Pyle, K.R. (1983). Ethical issues involved with the use of computer assisted counseling, testing, and guidance systems. *Personnel & Guidance Journal, 61*, 283–286.

Watson, D. (1989). Computers, confidentiality and privation. *Computers in Human Services, 5*, 153–167.

Weizenbaum, J. (1976). *Computer power and human reason: From judgment to calculation*. San Francisco: W. H. Freeman.

Wolkon, G.H., & Lyon, M. (1986). Ethical issues in computerized mental health data systems. *Hospital & Community Psychiatry, 37*, 11–14.

Zachary, R.A., & Pope, K.W. (1984). Legal and ethical issues in the clinical use of computerized testing. In M.D. Schwartz (Ed.), *Using computers in clinical practice: Psychotherapy and mental health applications* (pp. 151–164). New York: Haworth Press.

Miscellaneous

Caputo, R.K. (1988). *Management and information systems in human services: Implications for the distribution of authority and decision making.* New York: Haworth Press.

Craig, T.J. (1984). Overcoming clinicians' resistance to computers. *Hospital & Community Psychiatry, 35,* 121–122.

Cummings, N.A. (1985). Assessing the computer's impact: Professional concerns. *Computers in Human Behavior, 1,* 293–300.

Designing quality into information systems [Special issue]. (1994). *Journal on Quality Improvement, 20,* 591–656.

Farrell, A.D. (1989). Impact of computers on professional practice: A survey of current practices and attitudes. *Professional Psychology: Research & Practice, 20,* 172–178.

Figley, C.R. (1985). *Computers and family therapy.* New York: Haworth Press.

Greist, J.H. (1984). Conservative radicalism: An approach to computers in mental health. In M.D. Schwartz (Ed.), *Using computers in clinical practice: Psychotherapy and mental health applications* (pp. 191–194). New York: Haworth Press.

Fuhriman, A., & Burlingame, G.M. (1994). Measuring small group process—A methodological application of chaos theory. *Small Group Research, 25,* 502–519.

Guess, D. (1993). Chaos theory and the study of human behavior: Implications for special education and developmental disabilities. *The Journal of Special Education, 27,* 16–34.

Hammer, A.L., & Hile, M.G. (1985). Factors in clinicians' resistance to automation in mental health. *Computers in Human Services, 1,* 1–25.

Johnson, J.H., Williams, T.A., Klingler, D.E., & Giannetti, R.A. (1977). Interventional relevance and retrofit programming: Concepts for the improvement of clinician acceptance of computer-generated assessment reports. *Behavior Research Methods & Instrumentation, 9,* 123–132.

Klein, D.F. (1994). The utility of guidelines and algorithms for practice. *Psychiatric Annals, 24,* 362–367.

Kropla, W.C., Yu, D., Ross, L.L., & Ward, R. (1994). Stereotyped human behavior—A nonlinear dynamical analysis. *Journal of Behavior Therapy and Experimental Psychiatry, 25,* 1–14.

McGuire, F.A. (1986). *Computer technology and the aged.* New York: Haworth Press.

Meier, S.T., & Lambert, M.E. (1991). Psychometric properties and correlates of three computer aversion scales. *Behavior Research Methods, Instruments & Computers, 23,* 9–15.

Nickell, G.S., & Pinto, J.N. (1986). The computer attitude scale. *Computers in Human Behavior, 2,* 301–306.

O'Leary, S., Mann, C., & Perkash, I. (1991). Access to computers for older adults: Problems and solutions. *American Journal of Occupational Therapy, 45,* 636–642.

Peterson, L.L., Dana, K.O., Reisch, J.S., Hiberd, T., Korman, M., Munves, P.I., North, A.J., Van Hoose, T.A., & Trimboli, F. (1981). An information processing system for the psychiatric emergency room. *Behavior Research Methods & Instrumentation, 13*, 485–498.

Pettifor, J.L. (1982). Expectations of mental health information systems. *Canadian Psychology, 23*, 105–108.

Reynolds, R.V.C., McNamara, J.R., Marion, R.J., & Tobin, D.L. (1985). Computerized service delivery in clinical psychology. *Professional Psychology: Research & Practice, 16*, 339–353.

Romanczyk, R.G. (1985). *Clinical utilization of microcomputer technology.* New York: Pergamon Press.

Rosen, L.D., Sears, D.C., & Weil, M.M. (1993). Treating technophobia: A longitudinal evaluation of the computerphobia reduction program. *Computers in Human Behavior, 9*, 27–50.

Schmid, G.B. (1991). Chaos theory and schizophrenia: Elementary aspects. *Psychopathology, 24*, 185–198.

Shortliffe, E.H. (1994). Dehumanization of patient care: Are computers the problem or the solution. *Journal of the American Medical Informatics Association, 1*, 78.

Stoloff, M.L., Brewster, J., & Couch, J.V. (1991). *Hardware, software, and the mental health profession: The complete guide to office automation.* Washington, DC: American Psychological Association.

Weil, M.M., Rosen, L.D., & Wugalter, S.E. (1990). The etiology of computerphobia. *Computers in Human Behavior, 6*, 361–379.

Index